CLINICAL LESSONS ON LIFE AND MADNESS

The author of *Clinical Lessons on Life and Madness: Dostoevsky's Characters* draws on Dostoevsky's universe to illuminate psychoanalytic theory and practice. Using Dostoevsky's characters as case studies, the author discusses the various psychoanalytic concepts they embody, and shows how these insights can be applied to therapeutic understanding.

By considering the people who populate Dostoevsky's world as personifying a whole spectrum of human possibilities and modes of relation, Heitor O'Dwyer de Macedo's discussion of the characters – including those from *Notes from Underground, Crime and Punishment* and *The Brothers Karamazov* – allows him to explore fundamental issues constitutive of clinical practice, such as trauma, fantasy, perversion and madness.

Clinical Lessons on Life and Madness will provide an important resource for psychoanalysts with an interest in literature, as well as students of literature seeking a psychoanalytic interpretation.

Heitor O'Dwyer de Macedo is a French psychoanalyst and former theatre director of Brazilian origin, based in Paris. He has worked both in an institutional context, with psychotic patients, and in private practice.

"Located in the space between the raw reality of treating psychosis and Dostoevsky's powerful work, this book takes us to the intersection of unnamable anguish where the characters encounter the unconscious. Determined to delve into the spheres that Freud, focused on neurosis, left unexplored – trauma and madness – Heitor O'Dwyer de Macedo, with his love of literature and the acute perception of an exceptional clinician, takes us across zones filled with the cumbersome hatred of the dead, to show us that these zones can open unto love and desire. This book is essential for clinical practice, and will delight all those who find the unconscious endlessly fascinating."

– **Anna Angelopoulos**, psychoanalyst, anthropologist, President of the Fédération des Ateliers de Psychanalyse (Federation of Psychoanalytic Workshops), Paris; renowned researcher in the oral tradition of storytelling

"In this book, psychoanalyst Heitor O'Dwyer de Macedo shows us that Dostoevsky, the brilliant clinician, describes psychic processes that Freud would only formulate decades later. In simple language, de Macedo also points out that Dostoevsky's novels deal essentially with the desire to establish vibrant relationships with others, without letting ideology replace lost religion."

– **Michel Eltchaninoff,** philosopher, editor in chief of *Philosophie Magazine*

"With his considerable clinical experience and vast knowledge of literature, the author ponders the mysteries of the human soul as they are revealed by Dostoevsky. Psychoanalysis and literature are both enriched as a result. We have here what Sartre would call the work of a master."

– **Ronaldo Lima Lins**, writer, professor emeritus of literature at the Federal University of Rio de Janeiro

CLINICAL LESSONS ON LIFE AND MADNESS

Dostoevsky's Characters

Heitor O'Dwyer de Macedo

TRANSLATED BY AGNÈS JACOB

Routledge
Taylor & Francis Group
LONDON AND NEW YORK

First published 2019
by Routledge
2 Park Square, Milton Park, Abingdon, Oxon OX14 4RN

and by Routledge
711 Third Avenue, New York, NY 10017

Routledge is an imprint of the Taylor & Francis Group, an informa business

This book is a translation of a work previously published in French as *La Clinique de Dostoïevski ou Les Enseignements de la folie* by Cécile Defaut, Paris (2015).

Translation into English by Agnès Jacob.

British Library Cataloguing in Publication Data
A catalogue record for this book is available from the British Library

Library of Congress Cataloging in Publication Data
Names: Macedo, Heitor O'Dwyer de, author.
Title: Clinical lessons on life and madness : Dostoevsky's characters / Heitor O'Dwyer de Macedo.
Description: Milton Park, Abingdon, Oxon ; New York, NY : Routledge, 2018. | Includes bibliographical references.
Identifiers: LCCN 2018022491| ISBN 9781138499553 (hardback) | ISBN 9781138499560 (pbk.) | ISBN 9781351014533 (epub) | ISBN 9781351014526 (mobipocket)
Subjects: LCSH: Dostoyevsky, Fyodor, 1821-1881--Characters. | Dostoyevsky, Fyodor, 1821-1881--Psychology. | Psychoanalysis in literature. | Psychology and literature.
Classification: LCC PG3328.Z7 P7956 2018 | DDC 891.73/3--dc23
LC record available at https://lccn.loc.gov/2018022491

ISBN: 978-1-138-49955-3 (hbk)
ISBN: 978-1-138-49956-0 (pbk)
ISBN: 978-1-351-01455-7 (ebk)

Typeset in Bembo
by Taylor & Francis Books

CONTENTS

PREAMBLE

This book brings together the research underlying the bi-monthly seminar I conducted for six years, between 2009 and 2014. This means that the text you are reading was intended for oral delivery. Although I removed the repetitions that allowed the audience to take up the thread of previous sessions, I did not change the original form of the talks. I would not be able to modify the initial content without completely reorganising its structure; rewriting a text means writing a different text. Another reason for not changing the form is that psychoanalysis is a practice of the spoken word, which names the "real" that it uncovers, while presenting a point of view which makes it possible to reinterpret a conception previously regarded as definitive.

I wanted the work of the seminar to take place in a context that would make it possible to share clinical psychoanalytic experience. In France, such places, essential for the training of analysts, are disappearing. Consequently, the seminar included regular clinical presentations, made by experienced clinicians or by young practitioners, followed by extensive discussion of the cases presented, involving all of the participants.

Participants included nurses – the psychiatric nursing diploma was abolished a few years ago – psychologists, educators, social workers, psychiatric interns – whose training does not include the psychoanalytic approach, considered unnecessary by health authorities – and psychoanalysts.

Open to anyone interested in reflecting on the world around us, the seminar was attended by people in fields vastly different than mine – film, theatre, law and the arts. They exerted a marked influence on the formulation of my discourse, widened our perspective and contributed to the ease of the discussion after each presentation.[1]

Discussing analytic practice based on Dostoevsky's texts is a reminder of the close relation Freud saw between literature and psychoanalysis. In addition, I felt that this approach would facilitate transmission and the clinical training of young nurses, psychologists, psychiatrists and psychoanalysts who were lacking a structure in which to learn their profession.

As we know, Freud showed a certain resistance to philosophy – as opposed to French psychoanalysts who, after Lacan, formed closer ties with philosophy than with literature. Yet Freud always acknowledged his debt to Spinoza. This is how he phrased his refusal when he was asked to contribute an article to a book commemorating the tricentennial of Spinoza's birth (1932): "Throughout my long life, I (timidly) sustained an extraordinarily high respect for the results of the thought of the great philosopher Spinoza". In a letter to Lothar Bickel, a Spinozist interested in psychoanalysis, who asked him to specify his debt to Spinoza and explain why he so rarely cited him, Freud wrote, on June 28, 1931: "I readily admit my dependence on Spinoza's doctrine.... There was no reason why I should expressly mention his name, since I conceived my hypotheses from an atmosphere created by him, rather than from a study of his work". And, to make his position clear, he added: "Moreover, I did not seek a philosophical legitimation".[2]

As for me, I am very interested in philosophical thought – it would be difficult not to be, in France – but I agree with Setembrini, the character in Thomas Mann's *The Magic Mountain* (1996), whose advice to the young Hans Castorp was that one should explore philosophy after literature. This echoes Dante's famous maxim: *prima vivere, poi filosofare*, or Camus' comment that one must live before speaking of life. I believe that encountering very early in life an all-encompassing philosophy creates the risk of destroying sensitivity, more specifically the risk of avoiding or rejecting the psychic work of identifying affects and emotions. Such a philosophy can, in my opinion, be dangerous for those on the brink of life – the young —; therefore, it is preferable to struggle to find one's own words to describe one's feelings, taking one's inspiration from the words of great poets, than to become locked in a comprehensive system of elucidation. Of course, such a framework can provide the illusion of understanding everything and knowing everything – condemning one to impoverished experiences and the inability to learn from one's own life. Let us remember that Lacan used to warn psychoanalysts: "Take care not to understand too quickly".

In other words, encountering a philosophical system too early can constitute an obstacle to loving. This would be a handicap for anyone, but for a psychoanalyst it is an aberration – and for patients, a catastrophe. Because a psychoanalyst's work is all about love. What else does he do but prepare those he meets for this life-sustaining catastrophe, or repair the wounds, devastation and scars left by the absence of love, or caused by failed loves?[3]

Thus, one goes to see a psychoanalyst to speak of love, and, when the psychoanalyst speaks, in principle he speaks about love. Indeed, as Samuel Beckett said of his own writing, it is "only good for that"; and when a psychoanalyst speaks or writes, one can expect him to speak of exactly this: of how one loves, of how people love each other. And if we are going to speak of love, Dostoevsky is excellent company, since he is the writer who best explores this encounter.

The psychoanalytic practice I have just described is based on a political presumption: the existence of a regime which allows reflection. The military dictatorships in Latin America in the 1960s and 70s revealed that the psychoanalytic establishment judges the quality of a political power by the extent to which it serves the class interests of its members.

No Latin American association of psychoanalysts opposed military dictatorships. On the contrary. In Brazil, when the late Helio Pellegrino revealed that an analyst in training belonging to his Society, Amilcar Lobo, was working as an assistant physician at a military torture centre, he was expelled by the President of the Society, Leao Cabernite – the training analyst of the torturer denounced by Helio. Helio was excluded by his colleagues on the pretext that his public denunciation was harming the image of the Society. (Burlesque outcome of the story: Helio's status in his professional association was restored by a decision of the Superior Military Tribunal, an institution of the political regime, given that he had not committed any errors in his analytic practice!)

I believe that this kind of complicity between some psychoanalysts and terrorist regimes is based on a certain metapsychological conception of analysis, in which no psychic event escapes processing at the level of fantasy; in other words, from this perspective, the real does not exist. This way of seeing things reduces psychoanalytic transference to mere repetition of the affective and libidinal experiences of childhood. Thus, Freud's discovery is transformed into a knowledge-based practice, better suited to the philosopher's search for rational ideas.

But in fact, what is scandalous about the unconscious is that its effects lie beyond repetition, in the transference as a novel experience in the subject's life. This experience serves to perceive the other as akin to oneself and willing to help. Defined in this way, the transferential device can serve as a tool to separate the subject from his trauma.

If the shock of the unprecedented is eliminated, psychoanalysis becomes a technique, the analysis of a patient becomes a lesson involving established knowledge about a self-sufficient psyche, closed in on itself – the Freudian monad: Oedipus, castration, repression. Analysts who adopt this point of view validate Nabokov's definition of psychoanalysis: a method consisting of the daily application of Greek myths to one's genitals.

In other words, psychoanalysts become mere government-employed interpreters, and psychic health is reduced to adapting to reality – a reality defined by the ideology of the regime in power.

In Latin America in those years, the regime was totalitarian and murderous. This terrible period revealed a surprising reality: in the case of certain psychoanalysts, working with the unconscious had no effect on their relation to thinking, to culture, to morality or to truth. Having reduced psychoanalysis to an interpretative technique, they did not concern themselves with the recognition of the particular, or with openness to the unknown, the foreign, the out-of-the-ordinary.

As I said, the unsettling aspect of the unconscious, which lies in infantile sexuality and beyond repetition, emerges in transference as an unprecedented experience in the subject's life. It is possible to protect oneself from this disturbing encounter by transforming a theory into a fortification – a fetish – to justify one's psychic impotence, or phobia, or imposture, inflicting on patients the silence born of one's inhibitions, and one's dread of the "aliveness" of life.

In 1986, I organised the Latin American Psychoanalysis Meeting, whose content was published in 1988 in a book entitled *Le Psychanalyste sous la terreur* (The Psychoanalyst under Terror).[4] The Argentinian psychoanalyst Gilou Garcia Reinoso, who attended the Meeting, and who, with her husband Diego Garcia Reinoso, had been among those who had set up a support structure for the Mothers of the Plaza de Mayo, known as "the madwomen", introduced a reflection on the possibility of identifying theories that could have some compatibility with a totalitarian context. She raised the question of the relation between a closed theory and complicity with dictatorial regimes. And she pointed out the proliferation of self-referential psychoanalytic theories in Argentina, during the terrorist regime. At the Latin American Psychoanalysis Meeting, Diego Garcia Reinoso explained that, in a context of terror, there is always a *silence* that erases the trauma, rendering it mute, intimate, embedded in the psychic fibre.

In these circumstances, defending the hypothesis of the unconscious is a political act *par excellence*. To uphold this hypothesis means to affirm the possibility of naming that which must remain silent, excluded from language, unspoken and ordered to remain unconceived. To defend the hypothesis of the unconscious is to imagine the creation of new tools to unearth that which was intended to remain buried under silence, and to trust in the creation of new forms that can integrate these discoveries.

Gilou Garcia Reinoso has shown that the reign of terror aims at "killing death", at depriving life of its limit and its consistency, both of which depend on the recognition of death, a recognition intimately tied to our humanity, a recognition which makes us human.

To demonstrate, Gilou Garcia Reinoso describes this diabolical scheme of the Argentinian military regime: the disappearance of individuals:

> In my country, power is absolute power, it oversees everything, it takes care of everything, it fills the whole space, it answers all questions, it makes sure that everyone is in his place, and that anyone who is not, or who might have something to do with something that is out of place, disappears. In short, what must be made to disappear are all real or potential possibilities of a displacement not decided upon by the authorities in power. Making people disappear was a terrible procedure, but how did it manifest itself in people's daily lives? What was happening for the citizens, for individuals in Argentina at that time? Every day someone disappeared. What does it mean, for someone to disappear? It means that at my neighbour's house, or my student's house, or my father's house, or anywhere nearby, there is suddenly an "*operativo*", an operation where the army or the police arrives in force. The whole neighbourhood witnesses this. The operations are usually carried out at night, but they are

> very spectacular: someone is taken away, the house is ransacked, loot is taken – that is, everything valuable. People are taken away, no one knows where, no one knows who. Very often, the operation is carried out not by army personnel or policemen in uniform, but by people in civilian clothes in cars without licence plates. After that, no one knows anything. So a few people start to search. This is very dangerous: when you start to look for someone, you are implicating yourself. After a while, the person who is searching gets a phone call, and a voice tells him: "You had better leave everything and go away, or else the same thing will happen to you". Impossible to know who is speaking, or know anything else. Still, lawyers submit writs of habeas corpus; it is their work to denounce disappearances, but they disappear too. Many, many lawyers disappeared in this way. The denunciations are submitted to the justice system, but there is no follow-up. [...] These borderline situations are a dilemma for everyone. [...] Here, in Europe, what was happening in concentration camps was shrouded in silence.... I don't have the impression of speaking of something specific to Latin America, although there are specific characteristics, of course.[5]

The existence of these beings, neither living nor dead, but "disappeared", contaminates the entire social fabric. The citizens, who can disappear at any moment, become zombies, between life and death. People don't die anymore, they disappear. First, people are made to disappear, then the disappearance is made to disappear: this is how silence is established.

Everything is in order, we are free to be happy. Interestingly, in France proposals for the treatment of psychosis based on a normative, positivist definition of mental health have the same objective: eliminate whatever does not conform to the officially established standard of normality. Of course, as Gilou Garcia Reinoso observes, all this brings to mind the extermination of Jews and Gypsies by the Nazis. Moreover, Pierre Dardot and Christian Laval have revealed the relation between this normative and positivist definition and the neo-liberalism of our era.[6]

And it is for all these reasons that it is impossible to reject psychoanalysis and the methods it inspires. Not because psychoanalysis might constitute a system of thought that explains such horrors, but because it is the only field of applied reflection that can provide tools making it possible to name the unnamable, and to transform the impossibility to think into a means of reflection. Psychoanalysis is the only intellectual practice which can identify in repetitions the scars of silence produced by horror, which can break the silence and, above all, search for its meaning and history – both personal and political.

The Social Clinic of Psychoanalysis founded by Helio Pellegrino in Brazil, in a favela, also opposed the assassination of death (Michel Foucault considered this experiment the most important anthropological action of the twentieth century). The Social Clinic refused to exclude a portion of the population of Rio de Janeiro, considered a negligible human segment. To create a psychoanalytic clinic in the midst of an impoverished and wretched population was to assert that suffering can be placed at the service of social change, and above all, that poverty does not exclude anguish or psychic suffering. In other words, it was an acknowledgement that the residents of favelas are human beings like everyone else.

The Mothers of the Plaza de Mayo, like the Social Clinic of Psychoanalysis in the favela, are examples of the creation, through psychoanalysis, of a new kind of political tool adapted to an unprecedented situation. I will quote Gilou Garcia Reinoso again:

> Let us go back to the initial occurrence: the phenomenon of the Mothers of Plaza de Mayo. Who were the Mothers of the Plaza de Mayo? They were called the "madwomen", the government called them madwomen, and I think there was a certain truth to this. It was madness for seven women, in 1977, just after the terrorist regime took power, to show up in front of the presidential palace and ask: "Where are our children?" It was madness because until then no one had dared to ask the question directly; they hired mediators, took legal action even though there was no system of justice, pretended to have faith in the system, but the Mothers went directly to the government and asked: "Where are our children?" They do it once – they are mad, no need to pay attention. They continue to do it. They gather before the palace again and again. Soon, other women join them, and their numbers swell. One day, someone puts a gun to their chest and says: "Ladies, disperse!" [...] So these women, these mothers, go to the presidential palace to enquire about the disappearance of their children, and they are told: "Ladies, you are crazy, please keep moving." So they start to move in circles in front of the palace, around the May Pyramid (symbol of the country's independence). From that day on, every Thursday at the same time there is a procession: first the women, then women and men. The mothers lead, and they wear a white kerchief on their heads, on which, in very small letters – illegible but inscribed just the same – someone's name and a date are embroidered. They come every Thursday at 3 o'clock in the afternoon, and walk in circles, year after year. It's strange, but this circular movement allows them to cross barriers, break through the density of the space, perforate this space. Now, there is a hole in this space that was completely "filled". This turning in circles, moving in place, causes time to advance. I do not mean to say that the Mothers overturned the regime. I am saying that, in addition to the question they asked and the words they said, the fact that they were present as a signifier of absence was crucial.
>
> Because it pointed to the possibility, and demonstrated concretely, that the power was not absolute. It was not absolute as long as they were there. Their insistence accorded the population a return to the symbolic order, made it possible to symbolise, and played the role of an interpretation for those who could hear it.
>
> [...]
>
> What happened to the population? [...] The government made it an offer – an offer which is probably always made by a totalitarian regime – to identify

> with the absolute power. It is easy for the subject to accept this offer, because doing so is in his nature. Therefore, he can be tempted to respond to offers of omnipotence. [...] To identify with this offer means imagining oneself all-powerful, and escaping the distress and awareness of what happens when we contribute to supporting this absolute, destructive and terrible power. But the Mothers created an opening and maintained it. [...] They were told that they were demanding the impossible and it was true. Their slogan was "They were taken alive, bring them back alive." It may sound absurd, but it is not. There is a whole sequence of natural processes that has been disrupted. A sequence between living and what? Nothing. A void that must be filled in the legal realm and the realm of speech, and until this is done, someone must continue to demand it.
>
> [...]
>
> Why was it the mothers, why was it women? It is very important to understand. [...] [Gilou Garcia Reinoso then goes on to ask:] If the advent of the Name-of-the-Father is part of a process, if the paternal metaphoris essential to the constitution of a living subject, what happens when the father is an assassin?[7]

Is this very different than what is happening here, in our societies? In France, a minister, Marie-Arlette Carlotti, has declared publicly that she would no longer finance psychoanalytic institutions and institutions offering psychotherapy, but only those conducting behavioural therapy. In other words, a minister of a democratic government declares that a designated State therapy shall be practiced, to the exclusion of all others. And no representative of the culture, no writer takes up the pen to object. This silence on the part of the population is disturbing. Moreover, there are psychoanalysts and clinical psychiatrists who choose to ignore the constant attacks of the government on treatment institutions and on institutional psychotherapy, most clearly illustrated in France by the inadequate "Plans for Autism" introduced by the Health Ministry. This lack of solidarity, of responsible citizenship, is disturbing.

This resignation on the part of psychoanalysts (and psychiatrists), this silence, this lack of commitment, reflect their theoretical position which claims that there can be no psychoanalytic practice in hospitals, that psychoanalysis cannot be conducted with psychotics, any more than with children. This confinement of clinical work to private offices can have terrible consequences for the population. In Latin America, in the name of theory, some psychoanalysts were against the Grandmothers of the Plaza de Mayo, who were doing everything they could to find their grandchildren, some of whom had been adopted by the executioners who had tortured their fathers and killed their mothers after they gave birth. These psychoanalysts claimed that it would be traumatic for these children, who were certainly happy in their new families, to learn that the father they loved was, let us say, the assassin of their real mother. These analysts opposed the Mothers of the Plaza de Mayo, and did not support Helio Pellegrino. In some cases, they also denounced colleagues who treated militants engaged in armed combat, saying that this amounted to supporting terrorists. And their colleagues disappeared – meaning that they were killed by the military regime. Juan Carlos Pla, Uruguayan poet and psychoanalyst living in exile in Mexico, speaks of psychoanalytic crookedness.[8] The word is violent and suitable. For us, Latin-American psychoanalysts who have lived in dictatorships, this word is not an insult. It names a situation that is a fact. And facts deserve respect.

All this inspires disgust, indignation and revolt.

The essence of the psychoanalytic experience is the encounter with the unprecedented. This is a theoretical and clinical position. This position takes literally Freud's assertion in "The Dynamics of the Transference" (1912b): that the analyst is, in the patient's life, a new person and a new libidinal hope. Thus, the most important element in the transferential experience is not that which is repeated, but that which is experienced for the first time. An experience never before encountered, and never before named.

This perspective reinforces the affective productivity of transference, adding what Freud called the work of mental elaboration. It transforms psychoanalysis into a "metaphoriser". It creates metaphors allowing the passage from the particular to the universal, from trauma to taboo, from confusion of languages and times to the separation of psychic spaces.

When dealing with traumatised patients and psychotics, the psychoanalyst always offers a myth about the origins – and it is not true that this myth never varies. In psychosis, we are dealing with intergenerational short circuits. These short circuits, in and of themselves, constitute an autonomous "culture", closed in on itself, with its own values, codes and prohibitions – specific to it – which function for the entire family group as universal certainties. This is what defines madness.

To treat a psychotic subject means to enable him to rid himself of the hatred of the dead who oppress him, to bury the bodies that prevent him from having his own skin, his own body – without which there is no distinction between the space of life and the space of death; and it is the absence of this distinction that defines madness. The relationship established in psychoanalysis will be the experience providing a way out of entrapment in these intergenerational short circuits, in a manner that saves the subject from feeling guilty for being alive.

What we have learned from the experience of psychoanalysis in murderous, totalitarian regimes in Latin America is that clinical work with trauma and psychosis is an act of responsible citizenship which encourages political involvement. Indeed, a clinical practice based on separating what is life-giving from what is deadly, and the dead from the living, forces us to be aware of, or to invent, passages allowing the dead to enter – or go back to – the world of the dead, to be aware of or to invent laws allowing the dead to organise and remain among themselves, and allowing the living not to envy the peace of the dead, and not to submit to their devastating rule. Separating the deadly from the life-giving in order to give, or give back, to death its rightful place – immense but circumscribed – makes every psychoanalyst an ethnographer of the ancestors, and an archaeologist in the republic of these particular dead whose traces, not to say mummies, clutter the psyche of the despairing subject who turns to us for help. Refusing to consider these aspects of the practice denotes ignorance about psychoanalysis (let us reread Freud!). The thought process inherent to psychoanalysis makes life in its aliveness familiar and is therefore an antidote to the spiteful indifference springing from hatred of everything young, emerging, unhoped-for, contrary to the norm and to the comfort of established, idiotic knowledge.

Neither Reinoso nor Pellegrino was promoting the idea of political psychoanalysis, which would be foolishness. They are, of course, citizens taking a political stand. As Jean-Luc Godard would put it, it is not a matter of advocating political psychoanalysis, but of conducting psychoanalysis politically; and, at the same time, elaborating, as Freud never stopped doing, the politics of psychoanalysis.

Today, this question is now more timely than ever, everywhere in the world. It is urgent to conduct psychoanalysis politically and define the politics of psychoanalysis. Why?

Because there is a war going on and, at the moment, psychoanalysis is losing. It has been vanquished by the grotesque alliance between the *business* of psychoanalysis, biologically oriented psychiatry, behaviourism, systemic analysis, neuroscience and short therapies. The aim of this war is to exclude the unconscious from the field of reflection, to ward off the efficiency and productivity of its unsettling nature.

There is a war and psychoanalysis is losing for the time being. Of course, psychoanalysts themselves are the ones mainly responsible for this. In France, empty analyst chairs have left young psychiatric interns and young psychologists in a state of distress. Faced with psychosis, they are helpless, unable to invent a relational approach to madness, because they have established no relation with their analysts, who have had no clinical experience in psychoanalysis, and even less with psychosis.

In the meantime, psychoanalytic associations have focused mainly on acquiring a large number of members, in France and in the world, in order to disseminate the theory, elevated to the status of a religion, and its oracles – primarily the oracles, in fact. The *business* of analysis continues to thrive, although it is less lucrative today than in the 1980s. Other associations, which are truly concerned with the training of psychoanalysts, have done nothing to combat this state of affairs. For one thing, they considered this way of doing things a "trend" which would taper off on its own, like all momentary trends – after all, aristocrats do not mix in the common affairs of the world. For another thing, aristocrats don't mix in politics, as everyone knows; Freud's work is an inheritance not needing to be supported or reinvented, being eternal like the monarchy or the Himalayas. This erroneous assessment is not new, but in these circumstances it is proving disastrous.

There is a war and psychoanalysis is losing for the time being. My generation will not be here to see a reversal in this trend. We can only offer resistance and maintain our position, while we wait for back-up – that is, the young. Until then, we will refuse to compromise, we will make no alliances with the enemies of reflection. They must be taken for what they are: dangerous enemies of psychoanalysis and civic responsibility. And we will transmit, and never stop transmitting, the theory of analysis as we learned it from the most daring clinicians of our community.

There is a war and psychoanalysis is losing for the time being. But there have been battles, sometimes ferocious, in which psychoanalysis and humanity have gained important victories. We must acknowledge and pass on these victories to those who, with passion and courage, are ready to defend the obligation of reflection and honesty, as the minimal requirements for the practice of our profession.

For those who are interested in new art forms, it is worth noting that the fact that today's cultural institutions no longer take the unconscious into account – or very little – has resulted in the mediocrity that celebrates the setting aside of any aesthetic and ethical standard as a victory of the human mind. The corollary to this is that any demand for rigorous reflection is now considered a sure sign of being out of date.

This book was written with all these things in mind. One of its intentions springs from my constant concern with showing that psychoanalysis is not made up of a body of knowledge closed in on itself, but rather of a body of reflection, theoretical and clinical, in the service of life and the human community. The starting point was the idea that Freud found it intolerable that Dostoevsky focused his attention on something which he himself had set aside – trauma and psychosis – in favour of developing his theory of neuroses.

In Dostoevsky's work, the greatness or abjection of the main characters is associated with their discovery of the unconscious. The fact that the construction of the characters originates in the trauma of the encounter with the unconscious is certainly one of the main reasons for their timelessness. I make use of these characters to discuss essential themes involved in clinical work: trauma, fantasy, perversion and madness.

Notes

1 Special thanks go to Nurit Aviv, Lise Beaulieu, Guy Gérard (filmmakers), Joseph Scdillow (theatre critic), Claire Hocquet, Hélène Meynaud (attorney and jurist respectively), and Max Itzikovitz (leading authority on African art), for their regular attendance of the seminar.
2 Yovel, Y. (1992), *Spinoza and Other Heretics*, Princeton, NJ: Princeton University Press, p. 139.
3 See "True Love", in De Macedo, H.O. (2016), *Letters to a Young Psychoanalyst*, Routledge, p. 167.
4 De Macedo, H.O. (ed.) (1988), *Le Psychanalyste sous la terreur*, Paris: Matrice-Rocinante.
5 Reinoso, G.G., in *Le Psychanalyste sous la terreur*.
6 Dardot, P. and Laval, C. (2014), *The New Way of the World*, Elliott, G. (trans.), Verso.
7 Reinoso, G.G., in *Le Psychanalyste sous la terreur*. Here she is referring to the work of Martha Rosenberg, "Ce que les mères savent" (What the Mothers Know), in *L'Enfant dans la psychanalyse*. *Patio Psychanalyse*, No. 6, Paris: Éditions de l'éclat, 1986.
8 Pla, J.C., in *Le Psychanalyste sous la terreur*.

1

NOTES FROM UNDERGROUND

I encountered Dostoevsky several decades ago. I was 14. The first book was *Crime and Punishment.* All the others followed. Being Brazilian, I read these books in my native tongue. The books were very big, published in large print. Each volume was impressive because of its size and weight. It was a kind of big box that always filled me with emotion and respect. And pride. I was proud to feel this emotion, to be able to contain it and treasure it. Even now, the intact memory of this completely new, inaugural experience moves me and reassures me. I felt the reassurance even then. I do not believe it came first. I think it came after this discovery that changed my life. Forgive me for hesitating: we all know that it is impossible to speak with precision about such critical moments in our lives.

The size and weight of the books no doubt contributed to the feeling of reassurance. This physical aspect of the reading provided a setting for the hand-to-hand combat with the work, at once exhilarating and humanising. The physical presence of the volumes was also reassuring. It made concrete this presence I joyfully interiorised. The presence of another. Surrounded by these books – I had soon spread the volumes of the complete works of Dostoevsky all through my room – I felt very proud to have this intimate relation with someone's thinking, a relation which allowed me to recognise my own intimate being, which separated me from everything that had weighed on me, and still did. This intimacy shaped my space of solitude, where it was good to be. Looking at these books, touched and grateful for the gift life was making me, I was absolutely certain that they had been written for me and first of all for me. They were not a secret, but they were my secret.

These books were not *a* secret, since my parents knew I was reading them – they even admired my perseverance in reading them (they were, in fact, my first passion, but my parents did not know that). But they were *my* secret because, displayed in plain view, these books concealed a treasure I alone knew about: they were the aliveness of life! And for my parents – especially my mother – to accept without question my deep connection to someone other than them was, in itself, a real novelty. As well as a liberation: for the first time, I could admit without guilt to having an experience all my own. This experience changed my life: I was learning from Dostoevsky that feelings could be named, that one could feel something other than anguish, and that anguish had a name. The first thing I learned from Dostoevsky was to identify feelings.

Psychoanalysts know this: when a child of 14 develops such a passion for an author, two things can explain it: either he is doing very, very well, or he is in very bad shape. And if the author is Dostoevsky, it may be that the child will become a criminal. Or a psychoanalyst.

When Freud was a child, he no doubt heard a phrase similar to this, which could certainly have been written by Dostoevsky. Surely, the narrator in *Notes from Underground* could have used the same thought to complete the first line in his journal: *I am a sick man* [...] *I am a spiteful man* [...] perhaps a criminal.

The Underground Man

Notes from Underground is the third novel Dostoevsky wrote after his return from Siberia, where he spent four years in exile, in a labour camp, after being accused of plotting against the tsarist regime. His arrest was followed by a mock execution, a horrifying experience which affected him profoundly.

The book tells a tale of secret delight, of voluptuous pleasure. But where exactly does pleasure lie, the narrator asks himself. Still, he tells us that he writes in order to explain this pleasure.[1]

On a superficial level, we might say that he is talking about the pleasure of hating. Hating oneself, hating the other. A *spiteful man, a sick man*. An insect, a mouse, enjoying his degradation, his debasement, his despair, his nastiness. This is the impression produced by the sarcastic, mocking tone used by the author. The tone is in keeping with the contempt the narrator feels for himself, a contempt to be seen as the most spectacular effect of his abysmal solitude. All he has left is to take pleasure in his suffering.

Admittedly, the unpleasant tone is maintained throughout the novel, and solitude creates monstrous effects, but the reader must keep in mind that both – the tone and the solitude – should be seen as the symptoms of a subject who feels excluded from the world. Very quickly, it becomes clear that the narrator wants to focus on the reasons that explain his acceptance of this solitude. For instance, he is unable to resign himself to the reasonable laws of science that say "twice two makes four". Better to take pleasure in a toothache or a crime than to accept such a limiting argument. This can be seen, not without reason, as a refusal of laws and an argument in favour of perversion. But only at a superficial level.

The reading remains at this level when we look at the diffuse guilt of the Underground Man, as well as his boredom, or what he calls the weight of inertia, and his inability to love or make decisions.

On the surface, the Underground Man is an excellent example of the successful outcome of a Lacanian-Millerian analysis: he has acquired the consciousness that fundamentally a human being is worthless trash, that any impression of well-being is only an illusion, and that the only accessible truth lies in the acceptance of one's helplessness. The Underground Man takes pleasure in his non-being. I am not being sarcastic when I say this. I think a conclusion of this kind is dreadful. It is dreadful that psychoanalysts can say such idiotic things. In fact, this cynical vision of life was fashionable in a certain intellectual milieu in Dostoevsky's Russia; he was revolted by it and denounced it.

From another perspective, *Notes from Underground* speaks of the conditions required for thinking to be possible: reflection always begins beyond self-love. It is impossible to think and to protect oneself from the consequences of thinking at the same time. The absence of self-esteem makes it possible to examine with finesse the subtlest attitudes of the other.

This is why self-hatred can sometimes generate powerful thinking – but limited by the subject's inability to make use of it.

Hatred of others and of the world also generates reflection. Its destructive, murderous nature focuses on the most obscene, vile and frightening aspects of the real. Rooted in paranoid certainties, this reflection is just as sterile and deprived of usefulness for the subject.

What, then, does the Underground Man teach us? I am speaking of those of us whom Freud has taught to learn from psychopathology. He teaches that detachment from oneself, and the setting aside of self-love require a strong existential foundation – what psychoanalysts call well-structured primary narcissism. This is the prerequisite that will allow the subject to make use of his thinking and to take pleasure in his accomplishment. This existential foundation also renders reflection practical, enabling the subject to construct a new interpretation of his life story, and acquire a new place in the world. Freed of *amour propre*, thinking draws strength from its savage daring, from the ferocity of its combat with the density of the world, from the joy of reflecting the unknown.

Before accepting the pleasure, he could take in his vileness and vice, the Underground Man suffered greatly:

> But at first, in the beginning, what agonies I endured in that struggle! I did not believe it was the same with other people, and all my life I hid this fact about myself as a secret. I was ashamed (even now, perhaps, I am ashamed).[2]

This means that now, when he is writing these lines, the Underground Man knows that others have had this experience as well. But let us examine the reasons for his torment. You will see that we will not be wasting our time.

The cause of suffering

Remember that before concluding that he is a nasty, vicious creature, the Underground Man asks himself: "*whether other people feel such enjoyment*". He feels guilty, even the guiltiest of men, but *a guilty man without blame*. He is guilty of an excess of consciousness, of heightened consciousness. Indeed, he asks himself: "Can a man of [consciousness] respect himself at all?"[3] And we ask: conscious of what?

The answer is obvious and applies to all the major characters of the book. Dostoevsky presents his characters engaged in a struggle with an unsettling discovery they are unable to name, but whose effects they admit courageously. Since Dostoevsky shares with them this experience of the unnamable, the reader is invited to join in this search rooted in speech – Dostoevsky's characters speak all the time – a dizzying search for a parcel of unknown which, as we now know, is called the unconscious.

In the novel, the Underground Man, his brothers and some of his sisters accept, with courage and generosity, the effects of their relation with this component of the unknown. (It is generosity that renders the major Dostoevskian characters excessive.) This component of the unknown fascinates them and increases their self-worth: they are proud of their absolute singularity. At the same time, this element originating in the unknown appals and oppresses them: thrown into abysmal solitude, they are afflicted by an impression of exclusion from the world of their contemporaries. This contradictory position, this back-and-forth between passion and distress, accompanies the inability of a *heightened consciousness* to name the unknown it recognises. The *heightened consciousness* has an unalterable conviction: the personality (which we now call the "subject"), goes beyond the conscious (which we now call the "ego"). And when this awareness of the subject calls "unconscious" that which comes from the realm of the unknown – examples abound, as we shall see – this realm is considered a *source* rather than a *place*.

Designating the unconscious as a place was going to be Freud's work. But, through his characters, Dostoevsky gives us a glimpse of what Freud might have experienced in his self-analysis, and more specifically of the hellish universe in which he was immersed before discovering fantasy.

Before this discovery, Freud felt as miserable as the Underground Man because he could not consider all his thoughts, and all the desires he recognised in himself, as illustrating simply the field of possibilities of a human subject. *Outside of this perspective*, each thought and each recognised desire becomes the *essential truth of the being*. Within this perspective, if the subject has a perverse thought, he is a pervert; if he imagines a crime, he is a criminal, and so on. This being so, there is immense anguish to be contained, and its effects are devastating. Freud's complete, uncensured correspondence with Fliess[4], regarded as the springboard of psychoanalysis, testifies amply to this torment – which overwhelms Dostoevsky's characters.

In today's Western world, the unconscious is recognised as a self-evident fact by many people, like running water and electricity. Now that it has become commonplace, this notion no longer produces the shocking effect related to its origins in infantile sexuality. But for the man who was the first to recognise his sexual desire for his mother and his desire to kill his father, the emotional pain and the shame of this discovery must have been hard to bear.

Dostoevsky's characters are familiar with this pain and with this shame, but contrary to Freud, they will never be able to recognise the links between the scenarios constructed by their desire and fantasy life. As a result, they have only three options: they are immediately stunned by the field of possibilities they discover; or they rush into the reality of an action that will force them to live with a horrible image of themselves; or else they become saints, mystics showing infinite tolerance for the inhuman hiding in everyone. Dostoevsky's characters are spinning in circles, as Freud did during his self-analysis, because they mistake that which is only *fantasy* for *essential being*. And because they are generous and courageous in their encounters with fantasies they don't recognise as such, they admit that they are *plural beings*, but can no longer tell *who* they are. And who are they, really? They are reservoirs of dreams and reality, capable of suffering and of being serene, of feeling passion and shame, love and hate, rising to the sublime and sinking to crime; in short, they are like other people. In fact, the Underground Man, the paradigm of the dilemmas encountered by Dostoevsky's characters, sometimes admits that he is not the only one of his kind.

Encounter with the unconscious

Psychoanalysts are familiar with all the means of avoiding the pain and the shame associated with recognising unconscious fantasies. While they underwent their own analysis, they felt the strength of the resistance set up to avoid recognising as part of their internal world that which they identified as external reality. They are also familiar with the difficulty of containing the anguish of their emotional conflict instead of projecting its content onto the external world. They also know how much time it takes to stop using pain, as the Underground Man does, as a narcissistic symbol, and consider it instead simply a component of what constitutes our humanity.

Thus, psychoanalysts can understand the torment of Dostoevsky's characters. They know from personal or clinical experience, or both, how much energy is expended to *prevent* freeing the afflicted child from the shame of having had murderers for parents. To divest oneself of this shame means to leave behind once and for all the reality of a scene of destruction by transforming it into an object of reflection. To choose memory instead of the real scene of an affect is to accept a psychic wound and (perhaps) a scar, a scar marking the passage, the transporting of the real experience to a place in the unconscious. To have a perspective on the world – *a point of view*, requires abandoning infantile megalomania – which haunts and inhabits the Underground Man, the same megalomania to which he had recourse as a child to survive disaster.

If we take a look at Dostoevsky's other works and consider two major characters – Prince Myshkin in *The Idiot* and Alyosha in *The Brothers Karamazov* – we can see that psychoanalysts are familiar with them as well. It has long been the case that in the psychoanalytic community many have elevated analysis to the status of a religion. At best, they have compassion for their patients; but their compassion is of no use. Since, like Myshkin and Alyosha, they have given up on their own life and their own desire, they are not equipped to orient the analysis towards a perspective in the realm of aliveness. Then there are those who transform psychoanalysis into a secular sect serving as a steppingstone to madness. Dostoevsky speaks of them as well; we will discuss this at length in the context of the fascination exerted by assassins of the soul.

In *Notes from Underground*, Dostoevsky describes the unimaginable anguish related to the encounter with the unconscious. (All his characters experience the same anguish.) He shows how, in the case of the Underground Man, this anguish prevents spontaneity, paralyses action and inhibits the ability to decide.

> Well, such a direct person I regard as the real, normal man. [...] I envy such a man till I am green in the face. He is stupid. I am not disputing that. [...] [I]f you take, for instance, the antithesis of the normal man, that is, the man of acute consciousness [...] this retort-made man is sometimes so nonplussed in the presence of his antithesis that with all his exaggerated consciousness he genuinely thinks of himself as a mouse and not a man. [...] Apart from the one fundamental nastiness the luckless mouse succeeds in creating around it so many other nastinesses in the form of doubts and questions, adds to the one question so many *unsettled questions*, that [*his agitation*] inevitably works up around it a sort of fatal brew, a stinking mess, made up of its doubts, emotions, and of the contempt spat upon it.[5]

We would be wrong to interpret this torment as a defence mechanism constructed by an obsessive personality, as psychoanalytic practice teaches us. The Underground Man's attempt to construct such defences fails. Not that he doesn't ruminate, but his ruminations take place in a devastated psychic arena. He does not accept the Platonic idea of a normal man, he does not agree that conscious rationality is the best criterion for recognising the essence of being, but the only alternative he has to offer is his painful, wounded, confused humanity. Why? Because the encounter of the Underground Man with the unconscious takes place in a context of hate. It reminds us of the teaching passed on by Sandor Ferenczi (1949) in his essay *Confusion of Tongues*: crushed by a perverse adult, the child takes on the guilt that the other does not feel.

> And, indeed, I could never endure saying, "Forgive me, Papa, I won't do it again," not because I was incapable of saying that – but, on the contrary, perhaps just because I have been too capable of it, and in what a way, too! As though of design I used to get into trouble in cases *when I was not to blame in any way*. That was the nastiest part of it. [In the sentence above, about the "luckless mouse", this same nastiness was already internalised.] At the same time I was genuinely touched and *penitent*, I used to shed tears and, of course, *deceived myself, though I was not acting in the least and there was a sick feeling in my heart at the time.*[6]

> It is loathsome to remember it all, but it was loathsome even then. Of course, a minute or so later I would realize wrathfully that it was all a lie, a revolting lie, an affected lie, that is, all this penitence, this emotion, these vows of reform.[7]

This guilt that the subject takes on in order to protect his father will constitute the central theme of *The Brothers Karamazov*. In *Notes from Underground*, the parents have left the scene; only the tormented psychic body is left.

For the Underground Man, the question of the father is a central theme as well. In fact, the text finishes with a reflection about the father, more specifically about his absence:

> We [...] have long ceased to be born of living fathers, and we like this more and more. We're acquiring a taste for it. Soon we'll contrive to be born somehow from an idea.[8]

Facets of the character

The Underground Man resides on the border between the recognition of his unconscious and introspection. His tale is never without interest because he describes a dizzying search for a means of containing his unfathomable anguish within the limits of a representation. But none of the representations he comes up with is good enough: before having time to become an object of reflection, each one is immediately replaced by the next. All the representations are swept away by a wave of emotion that submerges the subject. He turns to hatred in an attempt to organise the chaos. But since the hatred he uses is not his own, but that of his father who keeps returning, he creates and keeps encountering a landscape of destruction.

The Underground Man encompasses three characters: the one in the first part, the one who is acquainted with Simonov, and Liza's lover. And since the interlude with Liza sheds a new light on everything and prompts a different reading of the first part, we can say that by the end there are at least four characters in the novel.

The despair of the character in the first part solicits our sympathy. He is a tragic character whose clowning does not mislead anyone. On the contrary, it underscores the dark, shadowy part of this solitary man.

The character who was Simonov's schoolmate surprises, worries and disgusts us. We imagined the man we met in the first part to be uncompromising, unconventional, despising high society manners. But the slimy, ridiculous, sentimental and pitiful character interacting with Simonov, and among the guests at Simonov's apartment the following evening, forces us to admit that what we took to be clowning in the first part was, in fact, the expression of an unbearable truth that we did not want to recognise for what it was.

This often happens in analysis; we can attribute it to our naiveness or idealisation, in short, to countertransference. Someone comes to see us and the first sessions encourage us to continue the work. Very quickly, once he is on the couch, the patient shows himself to be despicable. We attribute this to regression and we wait for developments. And some months, or years, later we discover certain things that confirm our initial impression. And we are horrified.

Some people will tell you that they never fall for such a trick, that they can't be fooled. These people are not analysts. It is not possible to be cynical and be a psychoanalyst. To be an analyst presupposes that one can be fooled. The only question is: what should be done when this happens? How can we keep in mind that if the subject accepts to appear so despicable, it is because he is in analysis and he trusts us completely?

This is one important attribute of Dostoevsky's writing: the words always mean to say what they say. Like in analysis. What happens at Simonov's apartment and at the restaurant has already been revealed in the first part. But we did not want to believe what we were reading.

And then there is Liza, and all that cruelty and hate. All that weakness. We had not wanted to believe it. Yet that too had been disclosed in the first part, all the wallowing in the mud, the taking pleasure in horror.

So, we read the first part again, and we realise that our difficulty consisted in being unable to imagine such self-hatred. The fact is that it would be unimaginable without the story about Liza, which is its clinical illustration.

Rereading the first part

A closer reading of the first part of Dostoevsky's novel reveals a number of surprises. The fact that we find it difficult to recognise the depth of the character's hatred is not unintended. He describes himself as being sick, wicked, an insect, even less than an insect, guilty. But Dostoevsky's genius presents these self-attributed traits as the result of the character's examination of his unconscious: "I did not believe it was the same with other people, and all my life I hid this fact about myself as a secret".[9] Hate is not presented as a distinct, independent element; instead, it is part of "many, very many elements [in myself] absolutely opposite to that".[10] One of these elements is the emphatic reality of desire, which the Underground Man accepts without reserve. In other words, who has not ever felt he was the most pathetic of men? It is, indeed, the universal nature of what is unfolding in the psychic reality of the Underground Man which allows us to identify – just as the reader identifies with each of the clinical cases in Freud's *Case Histories*.

All this serves to explain what I said earlier about our "reading" of the despicable portrait the Underground Man presents of himself. Perhaps it is not naiveness that makes us view this portrait with indulgence, but our conviction that the range of fantasy is infinite. One can fantasize about anything, think about anything, desire anything. But one cannot do "anything".

At first reading, the beginning of *Notes from Underground* can be taken to be a collection of fantasies which underlies the self-representation of a subject who places devastating demands on himself. We attribute the incident with the officer, and the ensuing obsessions, to these devastating demands – which Freud called the cruel superego. But the encounter with Liza changes the whole perspective, it requires reinterpreting everything from the beginning. An action does not eliminate fantasy, but such great interpenetration of the two changes our perception of the role of fantasy in psychic functioning: a crime is a crime.

Leslie Kaplan's insightful essay on this novel proposes, with good reason, that the whole monologue be interpreted in light of the events involving Liza, which she calls an "experience of murder". We shall come back to this, but first let us examine the tale from the beginning.

From the start, the reader is confronted with vastly contradictory considerations. After introducing himself as a sick man, wicked, spiteful and tyrannical with his colleagues, the character speaks of his intelligence, his abhorrence of mediocrity. This is then followed at once by the assessment that he is a fool who has the indecency of living beyond forty.[11]

Now, the reader is presented with an incredible argument intended to prove that whatever a man does, it's all completely the same, that contradictory positions have equal weight. Surprisingly, this was to be confirmed by Freud several decades later, when he spoke of an identity of opposites in the unconscious, asserting that the unconscious does not recognise negation. In other words, the psychic functioning of Dostoevsky's character is governed by the processes that Freud was to identify and describe as inherent to the unconscious: the primary process. Let us quote an example of this identity of opposites: "when I am most capable of feeling every refinements of all that is 'good and beautiful' […] it would happen to me to do such ugly things".[12] He then describes in detail the pleasure he derived from this, a pleasure which renders all action futile, and which is mixed with despair.

The inability to act results from a very particular economy of aggressivity, which stops it from manifesting itself, from turning outward. Turned inward, aggressivity reinforces the hatred that overwhelms the Underground Man. The inability to turn one's aggressivity outward prevents (or seriously inhibits) the ability to exert any effect on the reality of the world. *This knot of unexpressed unsatisfied desires* ends up distancing one from the world, which is perceived as unreal and persecutory. This distancing from the world accentuates the focus on one's own psychic functioning and creates a sensitivity that makes one feel *responsible* for everything that happens. This same sensitivity will always portray the encounter with the other as tinged with persecution.

"Can a man of [consciousness] respect himself at all?" Dostoevsky asks in the first part of the book. This question reminds us of Freud, who saw the recognition of the unconscious as a narcissistic wound. The Underground Man describes remarkably well how the encounter with the unconscious makes him *unable to control himself*, plunges him in constant doubt, doubt which in turn leads to inertia and to daydreaming, which replaces engaging with the world. After examining his crushing feelings of guilt, the Underground Man looks at his inability to express his rage, or be aggressive in any way. He observes that, in order to act, one must *be at ease with his feelings*, specifically of aggressivity – something he just cannot do. And he concludes by saying that, as a result, "throughout my entire life I've never been able to start or finish anything". Dostoevsky's astuteness is remarkable when he points out that letting oneself be carried away by one's feelings requires aggressivity. Indeed, saying "I am sad" involves choosing between a great number of possible feelings and affirming this choice – therefore affirming our difference – on the stage of the world.

In praise of the symptom and of desire

Dostoevsky praises the symptom and underscores its importance in brilliant fashion:

> Oh, if I had done nothing simply from laziness! Heavens, how I should have respect myself then. I should have respected myself because I should at least have been capable of being lazy; there would at least have been one quality, as it were, positive in me, in which I could have believed myself. Question: What is he? Answer: a sluggard; how very pleasant it would have been to hear that of oneself! It would mean that I was positively defined, it would mean that there was something to say about me. "Sluggard" – why, it is a calling and vocation, it is a career.[13]

Undoubtedly, psychopathology is helpful. Identifying oneself as a hysteric, an obsessive-compulsive or any other thing fitting into a category is reassuring. For some people, learning that they have a deadly disease can be a relief, an officially acknowledged identity.

This praise of the symptom is associated with the Underground Man's admission of his vulnerability, and even a total lack of defences. This exasperating defencelessness will help us understand what takes place when he meets his old schoolmates, and then Liza.

"And what if it so happens that a man's advantage, *sometimes,* not only may, but even must, consist in his desiring in certain cases what is harmful to himself, and not advantageous?" This is how Dostoevsky introduces his demonstration of the primacy of the unconscious over any rationality, of the existence of psychic conflict and the irrepressible nature of desire. In this segment of the monologue, the discourse becomes universal. The Underground Man describes psychic functioning in general, insisting on the fact that the truth of a particular subject is located outside the systems serving to explain the world. Speaking of this, he comments: "But man has such a predilection for systems and abstract deductions that he is ready to distort the truth intentionally".[14] He then goes even further, pointing out the links between boredom and rationality, boredom and hate, boredom and cruelty.

The next segment of the monologue begins with an ironic assault on the scientific delusion which claims that free will can be reduced to pure logic. Frightfully timely, Dostoevsky's description brings to mind the current perspective of behaviourists and neuroscientists who try to convince us that sensitivity, and even dreams, can be explained by formulas that govern them. This "scientistic" delusion is reminiscent of the effects that structuralism had on thinking in the 1970s, and particularly on psychoanalytic thinking. Jean-Paul Sartre's famous remark to Michel Foucault is worth remembering: "The important thing is not what was done to man, but what man has made of what was done to him". Dostoevsky predicts:

> But when all that is explained and worked out on paper [...] then certainly so-called desires will no longer exist. [...] And as all choice and reasonings can be really calculated [...] there may one day be something like a table constructed of them [*a Lacanian chart*? – HM], so that we really shall choose in accordance with it. [...] You see, gentlemen, reason is an excellent thing, there's no disputing that, but reason is nothing but reason and satisfies only the rational side of man's nature, while will is a manifestation of the whole life, that is, of the whole human life including reason and all the impulses. [...] Reason only knows what it has succeeded in learning (some things, perhaps, it will never learn...); and human nature acts as a whole, with everything that is in it, *consciously* or *unconsciously*, and, even if it goes wrong, it lives. [...] But I repeat for the hundredth time, there is one case, only one, when man may consciously, purposely, desire what is injurious to himself, what is stupid, very stupid – simply in order *to have the right* to desire for himself even what is very stupid and not be bound by an obligation to desire only what is sensible. Of course, this very stupid thing, this caprice of ours, may be in reality, gentlemen, more advantageous for us than anything else on earth. [...] But very often, and even most often, choice is utterly and stubbornly opposed to reason.[15]

After this definition of desire as necessarily transgressive, the discourse becomes universal again and focuses on a description of emotional conflict as a confrontation between conscious and unconscious. Here, the need for dreams is introduced, for the most *fantastic dreams*, and an explanation is given for man's need to step out of the confines of reason, even if it means having recourse to the death drive: "And if he does not find means he will contrive destruction and chaos, will contrive sufferings of all sorts, only to gain his point [...] then man would purposely go mad in order to be rid of reason and gain his point!"[16] A remarkable perspective, in which madness is the subject's final recourse for preserving his humanity. Let us remember that Dostoevsky wrote this novel in 1864!

Abysmal solitude

After pointing out that the laws of reason do not apply to the whole of human life, the monologue goes on to demonstrate the existence of a passion for chaos and destruction (what Freud called the death instinct). Dostoevsky contrasts this passion for chaos to something that is deadly: designating well-being as the goal of human life. Understanding the nature of the human is not a question of choosing between well-being and suffering, between love and hate, between life and death – these things must be taken all together.[17] The Underground Man then goes on to praise fantasy: "But what does it matter to me that [my invention] is inconsistent? That makes no difference since it exists in my desires, or rather exists as long as my desires exist?" Convinced of the universal nature of the phenomenon he is describing, Dostoevsky uses the plural: "I'm convinced that we underground folk ought to be kept on a curb".[18]

The end of the monologue, in Chapter XI, abounds with contradictions. First, the character declares that he prefers the Underground Man to the normal man. This seems coherent, in view of everything we were told previously. Yet the narrator admits that: "there is not one thing, not one word of what I have written, that I really believe". Indeed, he is unable to consider his thoughts a reality. He takes up his ruminations from the beginning, describes himself as incapable of any initiative, and in the end concludes that he is a coward. This about-face, after all his well-supported arguments, seems incomprehensible. It must be that a "memory of a distant past" insists: Liza's murder.

Although this *reminiscence* from *a distant past* might serve as a "psychological" explanation, at the end of the first part of the book, the return to the initial self-blame seems unavoidable. The discourse of the Underground Man is closed in on itself, is not addressed to another. It simply finds support in a reflection attributed to another, in order to unfold. Of course, this discourse is a desperate call for help, but since the subject never expects anyone to hear him, his discourse produces no impression. Although the reader may be surprised by the astuteness of the narrator's arguments, for the latter they fail to constitute a point of view, and his thinking retains an unreal quality.

In fact, the Underground Man speaks like someone in analysis. In this respect, he demonstrates clearly that the psychoanalytic process goes beyond free association. Although free association is an essential tool, its use presupposes the real presence of another subject – the therapist. It is he who must see to it that the patient uses this method appropriately, and not merely for sterile introspection. In order to avoid this, the patient must feel accompanied, supported and recognised in the course of the demanding and sometimes disorienting experience of discovering the unconscious.

The Underground Man's extreme solitude is the fundamental attribute of all Dostoevskian characters. Nevertheless, Dostoevsky's topic *par excellence* is the encounter.

Of course, his focus is the failed encounter, but this failure points directly to its opposite: the psychic event that would have taken place if the character could have transformed his desperate appeal into a desire to be met by another, if he accepted the risk of separating from his solitude in order to experience the feeling of accomplishment associated with the recognition of his debt, and his dependence on another subject.

The greatest sin

According to Kafka, the greatest sin is impatience. But according to Dostoevsky, it is lying.[19] *Notes from Underground* develops this idea through an assertion maintained throughout the tale: that it is better to be mad than to be an imposter.

The Crystal Palace is a modern architectural monument built for the Great London Exposition of 1862. When Dostoevsky visited London, he saw this huge iron and glass structure as the symbol of Baal, the demon from Hell, a debauched, godless creature, rationalist and greedy, embodying the secular utopia of European culture.[20] I refer to these remarks made by Dostoevsky because, in my opinion, they illustrate two haunting themes present in all his work. Here, they are associated and condensed in the figure of Baal. One is the dissociation between feelings and the mind, and the other is sexuality.

Dostoevsky confronts the threat of an ideal not rooted in sensuality directly and relentlessly. It is his way of combating European capitalist rationalism, and the effect of this ideology on the psychic functioning of a subject: rationalisation and the use of reason to justify everything. Let us recall how the Underground Man concludes his *Notes*: "We [...] have long ceased to be born of living fathers, and we like this more and more. We're acquiring a taste for it. Soon we'll contrive to be born somehow from an idea".

The threat of sexuality is only alluded to by inference, but it is a theme present in all the novels. In my opinion, the subject of women holds a major place in Dostoevsky's reflection. This may seem to contradict the assertion that he perceived sexuality as a threat. But a psychoanalyst is very familiar with such apparent contradictions.

Dostoevsky's views on thinking cut off from affect, or on sexuality, are not at all unintended or circumstantial. The theme of ideas disconnected from affect is a key element in his fight against rationalism and materialism, which he considers the two greatest catastrophes threatening what is most valuable in Russian culture and tradition. European materialist rationality is a lie; and for Dostoevsky, lying is the greatest sin.

The Dream of a Ridiculous Man, a fantastic tale published in a *Writer's Diary* in April 1877, sheds the clearest possible light on these questions. This text was written thirteen years after *Notes from Underground* and four years before Dostoevsky's death. The narrator in the 1877 tale has certain points in common with the Underground Man, who also considers himself ridiculous.

A cynical man, to whom nothing has mattered for years, decides to kill himself after a boring evening spent with acquaintances. On his way home, after making this decision, he meets a little girl in distress who asks him for help. He pays no attention to her, but later notices that her pain has not left him indifferent. Still, he tells himself that it makes no sense to care about a little girl's despair when one has decided to end one's life. (In Dostoevsky's work there are other important encounters between adult men and little girls. These encounters are associated with death: Svidrigailov in *Crime and Punishment* and Stavrogin in *Demons*. In *Notes from Underground*, Liza is also portrayed as a child in relation to the narrator.)

Back in his miserable lodgings, the ridiculous man sits at his table and places his revolver on it. He thinks about his decision and, to his annoyance, also about the little girl he met on the street. He then falls asleep and has a dream that will change his life.

In his dream, he is in paradise, before the Fall. All the people there love each other, they know neither fear nor violence. They live in harmony with nature and the animals. He, the ridiculous man, feels ashamed, and is filled with wonder at what he sees. But, after a while, he corrupts the people around him: he teaches them to lie – the greatest sin – and introduces them to sensuality. Finally, hate, envy and rivalry will fill their whole world. When he awakens, the ridiculous man decides to stay alive in order to let humanity know that it is possible to live in a world of love and peace. Indeed, the reader will remember that the inhabitants of paradise chose to keep their humanity, despite its dark side.

On second thought

I said earlier that what takes place between the narrator and his schoolmates seems unbelievable after everything the Underground Man related in the first part of the book. But we must remember that the events involving his classmates and Liza took place first. The reflections in the first part of the book are the outcome of the experiences recounted in the second part.

At the end of the first part, the Underground Man says: "Every man has reminiscences [...] which [he] is afraid to tell even to himself. [...] Anyway, I have only lately determined to remember some of my early adventures. Till now I have always avoided them, even with a certain uneasiness". In short, we have been forewarned: the second part presents the material that was repressed in the first part, that which existed before hate succeeded in filling the whole space and ruling over all aspects of life.

The second part of the book is entitled *Apropos of the Wet Snow*. It starts with a passage from a poem by N.A. Nekrasov, that I quote here in full. This quote makes it clear that after the encounter with Liza nothing can ever be the same, that she would always haunt the Underground Man, like a relentless ghost, that she would eat away at him like a cancer. Here is the extract from the poem:

> When from out of error's darkness
> With a word both sure and ardent
> I had drawn the fallen soul,
> And you, filled with deepest torment,
> Cursed the vice that had ensnared you
> And so doing wrung your hands;
> When, punishing with recollection
> Forgetful conscience, you then told
> The tale of all that went before me,
> And suddenly you hid your face
> In trembling hands and, filled with horror,
> Filled with shame, dissolved in tears,
> Indignant as you were, and shaken ...
> Etc., etc., etc.[21]

The events recounted in the first chapter of the second part took place twenty years before what was narrated in the first part. The character is only 24 years old. He is ill-at-ease, tries to put on a good face, feels alone, is only a child.

His solitude becomes his hallmark, the thing which distinguishes him from those he considers "romantics", sentimental Russians, about whom he speaks with contempt. When his solitude becomes unbearable, he takes refuge in debauchery – that is, sexuality, bordellos, prostitutes. As I said earlier, Dostoevsky's characters perceive sexuality as a threat. The Underground Man confesses that his sexual encounters leave him with a feeling of "shame which never deserted me, even at the most loathsome moments, and which at such moments nearly made me curse". I found the end of the sentence so incredible that I looked it up in all available translations. Indeed, the shame associated with his sexuality, a "filthy vice" undertaken "in solitude", "furtively", never abandoned him. It was even the sign – most interestingly – that, as he says: "I had my underground world in my soul".

It was after such a night of debauchery that he met the lieutenant with whom he would be obsessed for two years. Passing by a little tavern, he witnessed some men fighting with their billiard cues; one of them was thrown out the window. He envies this man so much that he wishes he too could be beaten and thrown out the window. He enters the tavern and stands beside the billiard table.

> [An officer] wanted to pass; he took me by the shoulders and without a word – without a warning or an explanation – moved me from where I was standing to another spot and passed by as though he had not noticed me. [...] I had been treated like a fly. This officer was over six foot, while I was a spindley little fellow.

In my understanding, the narrator was looking to this officer for the punishment that would assuage his guilt about his "dissipation", his guilt for having a sexual nature. But he considers himself so ridiculous that he feels unworthy of this well-deserved punishment. He has only one desire: to become worthy of a confrontation with this admirable man, a duel, or at least a collision of their bodies on the street – an event for which he is preparing unwittingly, like a bridegroom. With this duel in mind, he wrote a letter. He imagined that if the officer read it, he would come running to him and

> flung himself on my neck and [...] offered me his friendship. And how fine that would have been! How we should have got on together! He could have shielded me with his higher rank, while I could have improved his mind with my culture, and, well [...] my ideas, and all sorts of things might have happened.

In the end, he does not send the letter, but starts to prepare for a collision, for literally bumping into his idol. But first, he has to see to his attire. He buys a hat and black gloves; he prepares "a good shirt with white bone studs". Thanks to an advance on his salary, he changes the raccoon collar of his coat to one made of beaver. He imagines the scene:

> "Of course, I shall not really push him", I thought, already more good-natured in my joy. "I will simply not turn aside, will run up against him, not very violently, but just shouldering each other – just as much as decency permits.

And the long-awaited moment finally arrived:

> Suddenly I closed my eyes, and we ran full tilt, shoulder to shoulder, against one another! I did not budge an inch and passed him on a perfectly equal footing! He did not even look round and pretended not to notice it; but he was only pretending, I am convinced of that. [...] Of course, I got the worst of it – he was stronger, but that was not the point. [...] I was delighted. I was triumphant and sang Italian arias.

Mood changes

As a reader, I am surprised by the narrator's sudden changes of mood. He hates his colleagues yet goes to play cards with them; he stifles his rage and says pleasant things to people, and so on. We recognise his contradictions, his inconsistent ego, made vulnerable by extreme proximity to primary processes. But what I find most interesting is the particular tension in the narrator, which makes him bored, irritated, changeable, agitated, in danger of "losing his mind". This type of tension characterises almost all male characters in Dostoevsky's work. Since we are repeatedly told that the Underground Man sleeps little, or poorly, and sometimes not at all for several nights in a row, I conclude that the nature of this tension resembles that produced by insomnia. The tension of insomnia: tiredness and, at the same time, the inability to relax and the exasperation created by this situation; inability to sleep combined with the need to act: one rearranges the books on a shelf, cleans the kitchen, does housework, hallucinates, kills an old woman or kills one's mother, develops theories on suicide or kills oneself.

We have already noted how the Underground Man acts out his sexuality. Another way for him to escape from solitude is to daydream. He says:

> There were moments of such positive intoxication, of such happiness, that there was not the faintest trace of irony within me, on my honour. I had faith, hope, love [...] though it was fantastic love, though it was never applied to anything human in reality, yet there was so much of this love that one did not feel afterwards even the impulse to apply it in reality; that would have been superfluous.

In short, like an adolescent, the Underground Man refuses to spoil the perfection of the fantastical scenario by trying to fit it into reality. Indeed, like an adolescent, he sees himself as a hero, saviour of the world and, in this role, loved by everyone. But after a while, he tires of dreaming; he then decides to go out and see his department chief, who could be visited every Tuesday. At the end of the evening he returns home, after having remained silent for hours, paralysed with boredom. He is then glad that he has a means of escaping from such a mediocre reality.[22]

On one occasion, when this need "to plunge into society" manifested itself on a Thursday, not the day his chief received guests, he went instead to visit Simonov, a former classmate he had not seen for a year.

At Simonov's, he meets two former classmates he hates. He also hates the man for whom a dinner is organised for the following day. Yet, most surprisingly, he offers to join in. Why? He tells himself that it's a generous gesture. His old schoolmates point out the incongruity of it, but he won't budge, defending his proposition against all logic. Thus, he places himself in an absurd situation, and is forced to spend money he does not have.

The scene is charged with embarrassment, the narrator is clearly becoming trapped in a painful scenario of his own making, unrelated to his reality as he described it to the reader. Back in his flat, he remembers his school years:

> I hated them [his schoolfellows] from the first, and shut myself away from everyone in timid, wounded and disproportionate pride. [...] I was struck by the pettiness of their thoughts, the stupidity of their pursuits, their games, their conversations. [...] Everything that was just, but oppressed and looked down upon, they laughed at heartlessly and shamefully. They took rank for intelligence; even at sixteen they were already talking about a snug berth.

As for the schoolmate in whose honour the dinner to which he so absurdly agreed to participate was given, the narrator portrays him as a young man "vulgar in the extreme", who suddenly declared that

> he would not leave a single village girl on his estate unnoticed, that that was his *droit de seigneur*, and that if the peasants dared to protest he would have them all flogged and double the tax on them, the bearded rascals.[23]

Why, then, did he agree to spend an evening with people he hates and who are hateful?

To show his generosity, he thinks. In his own words: "It seemed to me that to invite myself so suddenly and unexpectedly would be positively graceful, and that they would all be conquered at once and would look at me with respect". In short, he wants to be loved by all, *conquer them, triumph over them, charm them.*

Ridicule

The events taking place in the second part of the tale relate to a period when the narrator, who was to become the Underground Man, was 24 years old. He was isolated, didn't know how to behave in society, and was unable to feel anger. His anger quickly changed to hate, and since hate was not yet integrated into the ego, its emergence had to be masked by obvious artifice, by absurd and inadequate reaction formation. What rendered him ridiculous was precisely the fact that this mechanism was inadequate. The ridiculous is always related to the failure of the camouflage. This failure reveals precisely what it wants to hide. This disharmony also contributes to the feeling of painfulness associated with the impression of being ridiculous: the disharmony reveals the subject's inability to handle conflict, which always burdens, submerges or paralyses him.

In the third chapter of the second part, the reader learns certain facts about the narrator's history which help to explain the latter's attitude towards Liza. The narrator speaks of a friend he had during his school days:

> But I was already a tyrant at heart; I wanted to exercise unbounded sway over him. [...] I frightened him with my passionate affection; I reduced him to tears, to hysterics. He was a simple and devoted soul; but when he devoted himself to me entirely I began to hate him immediately and repulsed him.

The narration goes on to describe the catastrophe, the narcissistic slaughter, the self-massacre of the psychic body. We left the narrator in the exaltation of the dreams where he was triumphant, able to charm people, and loved. Now, still exalted, he is in the throes of the tension of a sleepless night. Exalted, tense, agitated, overwhelmed by megalomaniacal images, unable to develop a symptom that would provide a satisfactory solution to his despair, the young man who would later become the Underground Man is now in the grip of the utmost suffering. Badly dressed, fearful and persecuted, rendered ridiculous by his vulgar arrogance, he is a sentimental figure of human misery. The exaggerated poses he strikes to appear self-confident, and his appreciation of his own extravagance, that he sees as a sensible reaction to the absurd situations he invents, render him similar to Don Quixote.[24]

Here, we have the proof of Dostoevsky's remarkable sense of observation of the development of a pathology. His precise, meticulous description of the collapse of what is left of the disturbed young man's self-esteem explains the ensuing scenario: the emergence of the Underground Man, who has transformed a narcissistic catastrophe into hate, and uses perversion as a defence against psychotic breakdown.

Dostoevsky teaches us that when the work of imagination is insufficient for constructing a life, what dominates is the encroachment of images upon the internal world. Using imagination to construct a world is what Freud identified as the ego ideal. If, as in the case of the Underground Man, this agency does not emerge, what takes its place is an unproductive proliferation of images produced by the ideal ego. In practice, what is the difference between the ego ideal and the ideal ego? When a child says that he wants to grow up to be Superman, he speaks with the voice of the ideal ego. If he says that he will be a physical education teacher, it means he has already constructed an ego ideal. The ego ideal refers to shared reality, it relies on the symbolic. The ideal ego can exist at the level of dreaming, which is connected with the level of the ego ideal. But the ideal ego can also be limited to freewheeling dreaming, a narcissistic drunkenness with no reference to the other. Like Cervantes, Dostoevsky describes the characteristics of the ideal ego. But in Don Quixote's case, contrary to the Underground Man, the ideal ego is always referred to an ideal: Dulcinea. Don Quixote's battles are fought to defend truth, while the Underground Man fights to survive. Don Quixote cares about his place in the world; the Underground Man seeks support in his own psychic world. What is ridiculous about Don Quixote reassures and humanises us, while what is ridiculous about the Underground Man afflicts, worries and frightens us. The disasters caused by Quixotic extravagance reveal the reality of the world and reaffirm the hero's fight to survive; the Underground Man's failures lead him into inescapable spheres of infernal destruction. Don Quixote lives in a state of manic exuberance which invites others, Sancho and Dulcinea, to witness his battles. The Underground Man is engaged in a fruitless war against a persecutory superego, in an uninhabited sphere. Drawn into catastrophic scenarios of his own making, he cannot resist them for fear of taunting himself afterwards, and accusing himself of turning coward: "So you funked it, you funked it, you funked the *real thing*!"[25]

What Don Quixote tries to achieve is narcissistic repair to avert traumatic catastrophe; the young narrator who became the Underground Man is engaged in the erotisation of trauma to avoid drowning in apathy.

In these two chapters (2 and 3), Dostoevsky gives a clinical description of how the disturbed young man creates a masochistic orgy. Because this scenario is unbearable for his ego, he must direct his hate in another direction, must assign it a different destiny; this is how the Underground Man is born. Can we then say that the Underground Man, instead of eroticising hate by practicing moral masochism, as the young man does, will direct his hate towards others? Can we assert that from now on he will find pleasure in murder? Yes and no. Masochism is a very complex clinical question. If we go back to the first part of the book, we can see that twenty years later the tendency to turn hate against himself persists. François Perrier has written about the "subjectivation of hate", in the context of the work allowing a subject to own his feelings of hate. This expression can also apply to the uselessness of a subject's rumination. As for me, I can only speak of the impossible subjectivation of hate, because subjectivation presupposes the existence of a subject, and where there is hate the existence of a subject becomes very problematic, if not impossible.

The experience of murder

When he arrives at the bordello, the Underground Man enters a murder scene. Kill or be killed, his clothes wet with snow, in a state of extreme agitation, his features distorted. This is how the narrator meets Liza, who works as a prostitute, in the very room where, in keeping with his resolve, he was going to avenge himself for the offences inflicted by his old schoolfellows.

Two hours later, during which time he has not spoken a word to the woman in bed beside him, Liza, he recovers from his stupor. He realises clearly "the hideous idea – revolting as a spider – of vice, which, without love, grossly and shamelessly begins with that in which true love finds its consummation". He has the unpleasant sensation of having entered "a damp and mouldy cellar".

The disgust with which Dostoevsky regards sexuality, and particularly the female genitals, is very clear. Through this disgust, he associates himself with the narrator of *Notes from Underground*. (Let us point out that Stavrogin, in *Demons*, sees a spider when the little girl is about to hang herself.)

When the narrator starts a conversation with Liza, the candle lighting the room goes out altogether, leaving them in the dark. As if they were underground? More precisely, as if they were in a dark tomb, in which the Underground Man speaks of a corpse with which he wants Liza to identify – the dead body of a prostitute. For maximum effect, he starts by saying that he and Liza are alike; "I am, perhaps, worse than you are", he adds to draw her in. He tries to be gentle, to find out her secret. To this end, he tells her the truth. Here, the truth is not a bridge favouring an encounter. Instead, it is a tool in a process of seduction intended to enslave her, "to turn a young soul like that".

But why go to all this trouble, why make all this effort? Because, at the age of 24, the one who would later become the Underground Man is not yet completely submerged by hate. He still suffers from boredom and anguish, which encroach upon him, and of which he must rid himself by transferring them to someone else – in this case, Liza.

This is the distinguishing feature of perversion: the need to make the other carry one's anguish. The attempt to drive the other insane is manifest in the pervert's insistence to drown the other in the despair that he denies and rejects. The psychotic is one who has become the reservoir of this unavowed dejection.

Liza's defences are not very solid. When the Underground Man speaks of a "girl like her", she asks in a whisper: "A girl like me?" Now, he knows he has scored a point – we must keep in mind that the game consists of drawing the other into a trap in order to gain power over him. To reinforce his advantage, the Underground Man uses identification: he tells Liza about his childhood, when he was abandoned by his family. It is a clever strategy: he offers to replace the earlier identification to a corpse with identification to an abandoned child. The device he uses to this end is brilliant, worthy of a very astute clinician: what we have come to know, since Freud, as the feminine Oedipus. When he describes a loving father, he is obviously offering to play that role. Touched, Liza confesses her secret: she was sold by her father.

The pervert and his discourse

Let us make some clinical observations, starting at the end of the story. I was saying that the Underground Man offers to take the place of a loving father. But it is not something he ever says explicitly. This means that the pervert is extremely skilled at manipulating the effects of discourse. Nothing is stated openly – so that he cannot be held responsible for any commitment he may have made – but a message is conveyed and expected to produce certain effects.

It is also interesting for the reader to learn that the narrator was abandoned as a child. This can be seen as the breeding ground for the hatred he carries. Abandonment is what he reenacts in his relations with his old schoolmates, as well as in the way he excludes himself from the world, the way he sequesters himself in the underground, the way he actively inflicts on himself, again and again, the trauma of his childhood. Psychoanalysts see this repetition as a need to cultivate the death instinct, recognisable by the fact that the subject has a way of placing himself regularly in a painful, traumatic situation similar to one he has already experienced. Why this repetition of something undesirable? Because it is a manifestation of the unconscious: as long as suffering has not been recognised and named, it keeps calling out to the subject, reminding him that it is there. Lacan described this phenomenon by saying that when the signifier is foreclosed, it will return in the real. Of course, the difficulty is to help the subject caught in this bind to recognise that he himself creates the repetition.

When we see the outcome of the narrator's encounter with Liza, we understand that he did to her what was done to him. Sometimes, in the relation between a patient and his analyst the same thing happens: the patient causes the analyst to feel the emotions he went through in his childhood, without being able to identify them or name them. To this end, the patient inflicts upon the therapist the psychic violence he himself endured. By doing so, he forces the battered therapist to put words on an experience previously unnamed and unnamable. This process is clearly unconscious and is usually experienced as very painful by both protagonists. I will give a remarkable example of this unconscious, mysterious exchange: in a psychodrama group for adolescents organised in a psychiatric hospital, the caregivers participating in the sessions as therapeutic actors were not permitted to meet the parents of the adolescents. After several sessions, the group leader, who knew the parents, started to notice that the therapists were adopting gestures and intonations identical to those of the parents they had never seen. Psychoanalysts call this experience *projective identification*.

Let us return to Dostoevsky's text. Now that Liza has confessed her secret, the Underground Man takes it upon himself to acquaint her with the world of love, whose messenger he becomes. He announces the possibility of a world of love, into which he invites the loved and joyful child. She is deeply moved, she feels understood, but he misinterprets her reaction and thinks she is making fun of him. To punish her, he takes on another approach. He goes back to the corpse, or rather to what came before the corpse – all that is vile – the abjection of sexuality. Sexuality which hinders love, which turns her into a bitch obeying any master – in short, a slave.

After the time of all that is vile, just before the time of the corpse, there is the time of madness – let us remember that the scene takes place in total darkness.

The narrator tells Liza that she will not always be young and beautiful but will become trash; he depicts a figure straight out of Dante's *Inferno*, repulsive and fascinating at once, a figure for Liza to identify with.

Here again, we can admire Dostoevsky's talent in describing the perverse manipulation carried out by his character. The latter sets aside the tragic facts he has just learned – that Liza was sold to the madam by her father – and assigns the entire blame of her condition to her alone. She is responsible for the life she leads, for being cast out of society, for the foreseeable fate awaiting her; she is responsible for being trash, for the insanity, and for being destroyed. Finally, she is guilty of eventually becoming the corpse that will be buried in a grave where there is "sleet, filth, wet snow – no need to put themselves out for [her]".

The goal has been reached, the young woman is heart-broken, she has fallen to pieces:

> But now, having attained my effect, I was suddenly panic-stricken. Never before had I witnessed such despair! [...] Suddenly I felt a box of matches and a candlestick with a whole candle in it. As soon as the room was lighted up, Liza sprang up, sat up in bed, and with a contorted face, with a half-insane smile, looked at me almost senselessly.

She makes a quick move as if to embrace him, but doesn't dare. He gives her his address, tells her to come to see him. She says she will:

> Her eyes now were imploring, soft, and at the same time trustful, caressing, timid. The expression with which children look at people they are very fond of, of whom they are asking a favour. Her eyes were a light hazel, they were lovely eyes, full of life, and capable of expressing love as well as sullen hatred.

Now, the worst can happen.

The worst

This is where Leslie Kaplan's essay on this novel acquires its full relevance. Familiar with psychoanalysis, this French writer demonstrates clearly the universal nature of Dostoevsky's character, makes an accurate sketch of his defensive traits, and defines the experience of murder as being the betrayal of a promise made to a child. This definition can be applied to trauma in general, since trauma is always rooted in betrayal by those we love, those to whom we give our trust with the openheartedness of children.

Leslie Kaplan shows that murder is the overstepping of a limit, a threshold beyond which everything is overturned, where one becomes "like Macbeth, 'a walking shadow'. Murder aims at destroying the other, but the other is the support of language which, when not addressed to another, becomes lost, is diluted, unravels". The text goes on to assert the need for

> exploring language to the end, for recognising that words have always already been addressed and are crossed by other words, and for maintaining this; otherwise, there are only new "formulas", the same old strategies for enslaving the other, killing him.[26]

To conclude, I would like to come back to the more imaginary aspects of Dostoevsky's work. First, Dostoevsky gives his character all the chances he can possibly have. When Liza meets him, she is aware of the full extent of his weakness. It is certainly thanks to this awareness that she can guess that his hatred is a defence that protects him from infinite distress, the distress of the abandoned child he once was. Liza's attitude, when she takes the Underground Man in her arms as one would hold a child, after he has attacked her sadistically, is an impressive illustration of Dostoevsky's clinical astuteness. In other words, we are forced to recognise not only that all the conditions favouring a true encounter are in place, but that *an encounter actually takes place*. In that case, why doesn't the encounter change anything for the Underground Man, why does it not open a new field of possibilities?

The last chapter of the novel provides some answers to this question. The first concerns hatred: "She realized that my outburst of passion [he had just made love to her] had been simply revenge, a fresh humiliation, and that to my earlier, almost causeless hatred, was added now a *personal hatred*, born of envy".[27] This answer has to do with the dynamics of the relationship, and specifically with its psychopathological aspect. Let us note, in passing, that here, once again, sexuality is presented as something bad in itself, the greatest humiliation that can be inflicted.

The second answer is even more interesting. It concerns the self-image of a character who is not able to love. For him, to love is to tyrannise the other.[28] And as is often the case with Dostoevsky's characters, the Underground Man's knowledge of the unconscious is impressive. Speaking of Liza, he observes "that it was strange I should not to love her, or at any rate, appreciate her love". And he concludes:

> *I was out of touch with "real life"*. [...] I was [...] insufferably oppressed by her being there. [...] I wanted peace, to be left alone in my underground world. Real life oppressed me with its novelty so much that I could hardly breathe.[29]

These brutally honest self-reflective observations shed a different light on the narrator. The reader understands that the Underground Man does not embody an extreme figure generated through the cultivation of the death drive. Indeed, in most "underground men" we see, hate is not what organises their relation to the world. Although it determines the sensibility of the subject, its influence is less overt, more subdued. Silencing the hate has an immediate consequence: the great difficulty to recognise the perverse aspect of a relation – an aspect the subject himself is often unaware of.

In a social context, these subjects can behave admirably. Their tyrannical tendencies contribute to turning them into fervent ideologues, rigorous scientists, conscientious functionaries. Their need to exercise close control, and even to achieve perfection – without which they are in danger of imploding – makes them natural leaders in any situation involving team work. Their detachment makes them appear pleasant, calm and objective; their sarcastic irony is mistaken for humour.

It is only in the intimacy of daily life that they will show themselves to be psychically impotent, envious of any living life, insensitive and indifferent. Incapable of any generosity, self-centred, they are unwilling to make any effort that will not profit them. In everyday life, their apathy, inability to take initiatives and chronic lack of imagination become apparent. All their energy is needed to maintain a very fragile narcissistic economy. Consequently, anything asked of them is seen as a threat, any desire for another or sign of desire on the part of the other is experienced as violence. This narcissistic economy necessary for survival generates a practice of destruction in which psychic murder is a defensive device, a strategy for avoiding the encounter – since any encounter reopens an old narcissistic wound. This practice of destruction also transforms any suffering into moral pain – a means of definitely excluding the other as the source of any feeling, and of entrapping in advance any occurrence, any novelty, in the predictable spinning wheel of rumination. This rumination reduces temporality to the reflections of a monstrous subjectivity which wants to remain insensitive to circumstances, impermeable to change, always invariably itself.

The emergence of this monstrosity in the reality of a love relationship, or in the reality of transference, leaves the witness stunned, as if he sees a hallucination. This paralysing shock is the effect of the burst onto the relational scene of the combination of two unprocessed states that had always been insisting to be heard: madness and perversion, the latter being the case in which the former is enclosed.

Notes

1 Dostoevsky, F. (1960), *Notes from Underground*, Garnett, C. (trans.), Dell Publishing, p. 28.
2 Ibid., p. 29.
3 Ibid., p. 37.
4 Masson, J.M. (Ed.) (1985), *The Complete Letters of Sigmund Freud to Wilhelm Fliess*, 1887–1904. Cambridge: Harvard University Press.
5 Ibid., p. 32. My emphasis.
6 Ibid., p. 37. My emphasis.
7 Ibid.
8 Dostoevsky, F. (1993), *Notes from Underground*, Pevear, R. and Volokhonsky, L. (trans.), Vintage Classics, p. 130. In the French POL edition, *Notes du sous-sol*, 1993, Dostoevsky's novel is introduced by Leslie Kaplan's essay "L'Expérience du meurte" (The Experience of Murder), re-edited in her book *Les Outils* (The Toolbox), Paris: POL, 2003.
9 Dostoevsky, F. (1960), *Notes from Underground*, op. cit., p. 29.
10 Ibid., p. 26.
11 Ibid., p. 27.
12 Ibid., p. 29.
13 Ibid., pp. 39–40.
14 Ibid., p. 43.

15 Ibid., pp. 47–49. My emphasis.
16 Ibid., p. 50. My emphasis.
17 Ibid., Chapter IX. Those who know my views on psychoanalytic treatment will recall that I insist on the fact that what applies to compulsion and repetition also applies to life. See my book *Letters to a Young Psychoanalyst*, Letter 11, on the insistence of Eros.
18 Ibid., p. 55.
19 Dostoyevsky, F. (2016), *The Dream of a Ridiculous Man*, Garnett, C. (trans.), CreateSpace Independent Publishing Platform.
20 Dostoevsky, F. (1997), *Winter Notes on Summer Impressions*, Patterson, D. (trans.), Northern University Press.
21 Dostoevsky, F. (1993), *Notes from Underground*, op. cit., p. 42.
22 Let us remember that in *The Dream of a Ridiculous Man*, the narrator decides to kill himself after a boring evening at the home of his superior.
23 Dostoevsky, F. (1960), *Notes from Underground*, op. cit., pp. 77–78.
24 There is also a similarity to Goliadkin, the protagonist of *The Double*, a work we will examine later.
25 Dostoevsky, F. (1960), *Notes from Underground*, op. cit., p. 85. Dostoevsky's emphasis.
26 Kaplan, L., "L'Expérience du meurtre" in *Les Outils*.
27 Dostoevsky, F. (1960), *Notes from Underground*, op. cit., p. 136. Dostoevsky's emphasis.
28 This is what he says about a friend he had in school, in Chapter III of Part II: "But I was already a tyrant at heart; I wanted to exercise unbounded sway over him. [...] I frightened him with my passionate affection; I reduced him to tears, to hysterics. He was a simple and devoted soul; but when he devoted himself to me entirely I began to hate him immediately and repulsed him".
29 Dostoevsky, F. (1960), *Notes from Underground*, op. cit., pp. 136–137. My emphasis.

2

CRIME AND PUNISHMENT

I. Raskolnikov

Woody Allen once wrote: "If God exists, I hope he has a good excuse". This statement results from a century and a half of reflection elaborated within the institution of culture. It is the prism through which I will undertake to examine *Crime and Punishment.*

The Underground Man, huddled in the depths of his solitude, confronts the other with a mad act of defiance. Incapable of loving, and mean and sick as a result, he wants to prove – to himself above all – that he needs no one, that his hate is enough to keep him alive. The other is placed in the role of a non-interlocutor, who has simply to be there in the Underground Man's existence, and to point to his crime, the murder of Lisa. The Underground Man's words are not addressed to anyone. But in order for his thoughts to unfold, he needs the presence of another, of a powerless spectator. He needs the tension created by this presence; from it, he draws the energy for his frantic insistence on the uselessness of this presence. This is what gives his speech its sterile, repetitive, dizzying, interminable and tragic character. What makes the Underground Man a tragic figure is, as Leslie Kaplan says, the fact that he wants to be free of the other to think, although "the other is the support of speech, since speech addresses to no one is lost, diluted, frayed".[1]

Raskolnikov introduces a different set of tragic figures. He is the first in a series of tragic characters Dostoevsky was to develop until the end of his life. Here, the intention is not to appeal to another only to deny his existence, but rather to answer the question: if there is no God, how can man live? And the questions that follow from this: If there is no God, what referent can attest to the reality of life and of thought? If there is no God, what becomes of the Law?

Despite the fact that Dostoevsky formulated this question a century and a half ago, it has not become a universal theme for reflection. The return of religion, and the dominant position gained by fundamentalisms, testify to the immediate relevance of this question in today's world.

What is certain, is that in a world without God the other has an unquestionable place. But this place has to be defined, its connection with the world and with oneself has to be established – particularly since God is no longer there to proclaim it, making it totally dependent on the encounter. If there is no God, the community of men is left with the task of granting precarious and shifting meaning to human existence. This state of uncertainty generates anguish. A godless community is one necessarily composed of a plurality of particular individuals, where each member recognizes the difference of others as a factor stimulating reflection and providing support for desire.

Raskolnikov has preceded us all on this adventurous journey pursued without God, in anguish, with only desire to guide us. Completely alone when we first encounter him, he wants to be accountable to no one but himself. Of course, this requires a "change in the frame for thought" (Loup Verlet's concept; 1993). To understand what this could mean, imagine how difficult it is to think outside the framework of established knowledge, be it in the academic, philosophical, medical … or psychoanalytic field. Then imagine a world where religion is a compulsory referent, unavoidable, a world where religion is the framework for all thought, the only ideological frame of reference, which, for this very reason, cannot be recognised – just as the gaze which examines, searches, judges or contemplates does not see the exploring eye. In The *Disenchantment of the World*, Marcel Gauchet notes that "to understand the novelty of our present, we must delve into religion, the key to our entire past".[2] All "primitive" societies are governed by religion. This universal primacy of the religious is very probably due to living conditions and survival requirements in stateless societies. "In these societies, cohesion must be established and maintained through mechanisms needing no active intervention by society members." Indeed, in Tsarist Russia, where Dostoesvky and Raskolnikov lived, religion still played a crucial role. The dawn of capitalism – the end of serfdom – and a slight lightening of censure were causing social upheaval. In such circumstances, it is easy to understand that those in power count on the religious referent to provide coherence at a time when new institutions are being introduced. This is also understandable given that, while the usual order tumbles, the social body strongly needs religion as a glue, to maintain the cohesion of its members.

In his book, Loup Verlet points out that changing the frame of thought is an enormously difficult enterprise. When the old conceptual framework becomes shaky and the new frame is not yet in place, the "founder" – and Raskolnikov is a founder – finds himself in a very uncomfortable intermediary space, where it is extremely difficult to think.

Creating a new frame of thought is a frightening experience for the subject. To understand this frightening transition, I will use the concept of an "interim". This "interim" designates the time necessary between the moment when the subject starts to abandon a certain frame for thought, and the moment when a new set of references is set in place. Loup Verlet describes this interim by invoking the concepts of "crossing over" and "paradox". When a subject takes the psychic risk of overstepping the boundaries of a certain conceptual framework in order to venture towards the inconceived, he enters a paradox. Indeed, this overstepping involves "the more or less radical suspension of the epistemological premises on which the frame for thought is built" and obliges the subject to "seek grounding in that which [does] not yet [exist]".[3] Of course, this set of circumstances, characteristic of all creative thinking, constitutes a borderline psychic situation in which the subject draws his energy from the excessive nature of his desire. Indeed, he needs an abundance of energy for everything he is creating: a new conceptual framework for a new subject. But throughout this intermediary period of creating, there is a constant danger that he might go mad for good.[4]

Through Raskolnikov, Dostoevsky introduces the tragedy that was to be the foundation of modernity: the frightening phenomenon that consists of rejecting the conceptual framework in which God is the universal referent, and finding in oneself, despite persistent anguish, that which authorises desire and the aliveness of life.

In Ancient Greece, tragedy was the act of rebelling against a fate written by the gods. From this perspective, the outcome could only be catastrophic; therefore, what was singular and worthy of interest was the particular manner in which the hero undertook this impossible confrontation, through which he asserted his humanity.

After Dostoevsky, rebellion was replaced by anguish and by the unknown. Singularity unfolded against a blank background, morality receded before a demand for truth, ethical concerns replaced the consolation provided by group cohesion. Thus, Dostoevsky's major characters, ushered in by Raskolnikov in *Crime and Punishment*, are archetypes of possible answers to this borderline situation in which the subject, at the risk of madness, must invent everything in a life where nothing can be expected from heaven, a life whose only limit is death.

A Greek tragedy starts when the citizen uses the myth to judge the hero's excesses and transgressions. The chorus represents the citizens, ambivalent and wavering between the hero's reasons and those of the gods. In the end, the scales always tip in favour of the gods; the time of men, where chance predominates, carries little weight compared to the time of the gods. Pierre Vidal-Naquet comments:

> Of course myths contain all the transgressions found in tragedies: incest, patricide, matricide, the devouring of one's children. But they do not include any agency that judges these acts, such as the one created by the city, the one whose voice is embodied by the choir. [...] Reacting to the excesses of the hero, the choir voices the collective truth, the truth of the average citizen, the truth of the city.[5]

Dostoevsky's hero does not have the choir for an interlocutor, to act as a "regulator" of his actions. He alone is responsible for his fate, before his own conscience and, more specifically, before his superego, which invariably represents the conceptual framework the hero opposes and wants to leave behind. As Aristotle says in *The Politics*: "he who is unable to live in society … must be either a beast or a god: he is no part of a state".[6]

Dostovsky's hero is a god transformed into pure beast, since he is absolutely human, and human only. Like a god, Dostoesvky's hero is not tied to time constraints: when he changes, his transformations are always and above all internal changes resulting from his dialogue with himself. In this dialogue, as I said earlier, the other holds an essential place. Most often a double, sometimes a radically different being, the other provokes contradictions, intensifies the sense of solitude and lack of any recourse – unless it be the assertion of his desire in the absence of any certainty.

The character and time

Reality as such has no hold on the tragic Dostoevskian hero. What counts, every time, is the interpretation of this reality, the meaning conferred to it by the hero – a meaning and interpretation often highly influenced by the hero's emotional state at the time. Even the character's biography, although sometimes crucial (as in *The Brothers Karamazov*), never refers to the temporal and never provides the reasons for the drama which is unfolding. These reasons always constitute a struggle to assert an idea unrelated to any divine safeguard. From this point of view, the struggle in which the character engages contrasts sharply with everything that existed before and, since this struggle is unprecedented, the outcome cannot be foreseen. The tragic Dostoevskian hero does not live in linear time; he does not refer to a "before", and pays no attention to "development". He is invariably insomniac, stuck in the present moment, constantly in crisis and in conflict. This is no doubt why we always read Dostoevsky as we would read a crime novel, in which a crisis calls for and leads to a resolution. But in this case the crisis is the peculiar entity of the battle fought by every man in order to survive in a world abandoned by God. An idiosyncratic representation of this unavoidable battle, each tragic Dostoevskian hero, disconnected from time and stuck in his own struggle to change the existing frame for thought, becomes a mythical figure among the modern Gods of Olympus. This is, in fact, the definition of a *Dostoevskian character.*

Between the time when Dostoevsky submitted the idea for *Crime and Punishment* to his editor and the time when he had a definite plan for the novel, two versions of the manuscript were completed. His initial letter of proposal, written after two months of work, presents a plot which is, essentially, the one in the final version. The main character is described as a young man who has "come under the influence of some of those strange, 'incomplete' ideas which go floating about in the air". The crime is committed for altruistic reasons: "to bring happiness to his mother" and to rescue his sister, and is presented as legitimate – "if one can actually call a crime his act against a deaf, stupid, wicked and sick old crone, who doesn't know herself what she lives for, and who may die anyway in a month or so".[7]

Dostoevsky found the character's name easily. It derives from that of Old Believers, members of a movement aimed against the official church in the seventeenth century. In Russian, the word for Old Believers is *raskolniki*, meaning "schismatics".

Thus, the name Raskolnikov condenses several concepts. First, that of separation. Then, that of a separation from the Church – which is important for a character who will try to think outside the religious frame of reference, without alluding to God. Finally, the name suggests a split, a division – an idea consistent with the situation in which the character finds himself, since he is caught between two conceptual frameworks.

According to Joseph Frank, Dostoevsky's biographer, the final version of *Crime and Punishment* came into being "when, in November 1865, Dostoevsky shifted from a first-person to a third-person narrator". Frank points out that this shift (from the first person) "was the culmination of a long struggle, present through all the early stages of the composition".[8] I believe that this choice was not merely a matter of form: a narrator speaking in the first person is forced to relate events after the fact, so that the possibility that he will surprise himself is greatly reduced. In fact, it seems unlikely that one can describe a subjectivation process of the unprecedented at the very moment when it takes place. Moreover, narration in the first person must present a coherent construct; but what most interests Dostoevsky is being able to present simultaneously several levels of consciousness and several affective states experienced by the character, which are often contradictory and even antithetical.

The coexistence of such a plurality of affective states and levels of understanding is essential for the transmission of the difficulties, impasses and solutions encountered by the character, causing him to shift from one frame of thought to another (or not).

Raskolnikov is the first of a series of Dostoevskian heroes who are solely responsible for their fate before their conscience, synonymous for them with their superego – a superego which invariably represents the frame for thought the hero wishes to leave behind. Their superego impels these heroes to oppose a frame of thought they no longer accept. In this sense, Raskolnikov is very different from the Underground Man, who has great contempt for himself, and who fights a useless war against a persecutory superego in a deserted world: "'You are a scoundrel,' a thought flashed through my mind, 'if you laugh at that now.' 'No matter!" I cried, answering myself. "Now everything is lost!'"[9]

Crime and Punishment starts with Raskolnikov leaving his lodgings to visit an old moneylender. Here, the superego manifests itself through an injunction: he *must* do this. Specifically, this injunction springs from the comparison with an Ideal, not revealed to the reader until much later: "'I want to attempt a thing *like that* and am frightened by these trifles,' he thought with an odd smile. 'Hm […] yes, *all is in a man's hands* and he lets it all slip from cowardice.'"[10] My emphasis is intended to point out that right from the start, in addition to the sordid situation described, sordid and frightening indeed, there is the challenge Raskolnikov sets himself to be a man who can achieve anything. What is remarkable here is Dostoevsky's mastery in telling the story, his intimate knowledge of the character: the article written by Raskolnikov, not revealed to the reader until much later in the novel, is the main impetus for all his actions, the ideal which animates him.[11]

In *Notes from Underground*, Dostoevsky has his narrator say: "We … have long ceased to be born of living fathers, and we like this more and more. We're acquiring a taste for it. Soon we'll contrive to be born somehow from an idea". Raskolnikov wants to be born – or rather, be reborn – from an idea, the idea that a man can accomplish anything, if he is an extraordinary man. This is the idea, and the Ideal, by which his superego impels him to measure himself, up to the moment he commits the murder and beyond.

This idea can take two forms, depending on the circumstances. At times, it can be inflated by the Imaginary, in which case the confrontation with the superego is catastrophic. But the idea of being an *extraordinary man* can also be rooted in the Symbolic, in which case the superego tolerates more easily its presence in consciousness.

In psychoanalytic theory, all this concerns the relations between the ego, the ideal self, the ego ideal and the superego. When the idea is inflated by the Imaginary, the ideal self is produced: I want to be Marlon Brando. When the idea is rooted in the symbolic, it constitutes the ego ideal: I want to be a good actor. The ego ideal can serve as a passageway through which the superego comes to tolerate that an idea (for instance: I want to be a good actor) becomes permanently incorporated in the ego.

Let us come back to Raskolnikov. We will discuss the question of the absence of a *living father* a little further. For the moment, I would like to insist on the conditions required to carry out the idea: in effect, the absence of any emotion or affect. The scene in which Raskolnikov intervenes to prevent a young woman from falling into the hands of an old pervert on the prowl clearly shows that he confuses sentimentality with sensitivity and, by extension, that the ideal he sets for himself demands the abolition of all empathy for others and for the world.

After his vigorous intervention, and after entrusting the young woman to a policeman, Raskolnikov shouts after him, because

> something seemed to sting [him]; in an instant a complete revulsion of feeling came over him: "Let him amuse himself," he pointed at the dandy. "What is it to do with you?" The policeman was bewildered. […] "And why did I want to interfere? Is it for me to help? Have I any right to help? Let them devour each other alive – what is it to me?"

But, unlike in the case of the Underground Man, here the superego does not fill the entire space: "In spite of those strange words, he felt very wretched. […] 'Poor girl!' he said, looking at the empty corner where she had sat – 'She will come to herself and weep, and then her mother will find out'".[12]

And he went on to imagine a cruel sequence of events, such as life is able to inflict, thereby showing himself to be more of a realist than an embittered man.

Marmeladov

Before the murder, three other situations escape the hold of the superego. The first is the meeting with Marmeladov, this fallen Shakespearean king, lost in a tavern in some seedy corner of Saint Petersburg. This encounter is critical for the novel as a whole and plays a secondary role in the murder; it also provides valuable insight into Raskolnikov's personality before the crime.

Raskolnikov is the one who sees Marmeladov first. Dostoevsky introduces the scene by observing: "There are chance meetings with strangers that interest us from the first moment, before a word is spoken. Such was the impression made on Raskolnikov by [Marmeladov]. [...] He looked repeatedly at [him], partly no doubt because the latter was staring persistently at him".[13] Thus, we know that before the murder Raskolnikov can take a great interest in another person. In my view, this trait of generosity in the character is crucial for the unfolding of the events that follow. I shall return to this. For now, let us ascribe this generosity to the passion that fills Raskolnikov. I also want to point out that the nature of the encounter with Marmeladov, a sudden and enigmatic encounter – enigmatic because it is grounded in the real – is recurrent in Dostoevsky's writing.

While Raskolnikov is intently focused on distancing himself from his feelings, Marmeladov is, on the contrary, immersed in the depths of suffering. "And the more I drink, the more I feel it. That's why I drink too. I try to find sympathy and feeling in drink. [...] I drink so that I may suffer twice as much!"[14] And he had detected on Raskolnikov's face "some trouble of mind. When you came in I read it, and that was why I addressed you at once".[15] Indeed, Raskolnikov had entered the tavern after visiting the moneylender, and the reader is vaguely aware that something terrible is being repeated here. The sorrow on his face reflects the great struggle he wages against his feelings. There are many similarities between Marmeladov and the Underground Man: his clear knowledge of himself, his indignity, his sordid condition, his self-hatred. Like the Underground Man, Marmeladov forces a child into prostitution, and this child is his own daughter. Yet we find this character, this murderous father, moving. Why? Because, contrary to the Underground Man, who embodies a perverse position, in Marmeladov's eyes there is "a gleam of madness": "there was something very strange in him; there was a light in his eyes as though of intense feeling – perhaps there were even thought and intelligence".[16] Unlike the Underground Man, Marmeladov is constantly appealing to the other, always supposing him to be able to hear his plea, his infinite distress. And if this other does not exist on earth, on the Day of Judgment God will welcome him into His kingdom, even if he is a swine, a beast. And the wise and reasonable will not understand,[17] no doubt because reason is not enough to sustain absolute acceptance.

This belief in unconditional divine kindness confers a pathetic and grotesque dimension to Marmeladov's character. At the same time, this belief is central to the frame of thought Raskolnikov wants to leave behind, in order that he may be solely responsible for his actions, and be the only one to whom he has to account for the meaning of his life, the only one responsible for throwing away or redeeming his life. But Marmeladov's faith reveals the extent of the task undertaken by the man who tries to establish a new way of perceiving the world. Marmeladov's faith presupposes the existence of elements without which no reliable link to the real is possible, and which, for this reason, must be included in the new frame for thought: a referent (in Marmeladov's case, God) making it possible for different singularities to coexist. This referent also allows excess, and even madness, to be included in our humanity. From this point of view, Marmeladov reflects Dostoevsky's position, a position to which he confronts Raskolnikov, without forcing him to take it. Indeed, one of the characteristics of Dostoevsky's genius is the respect and affection he shows his characters, whom he leads into spheres where he himself feels unable to venture.

For the construction of the novel, the encounter with Marmeladov is essential. It is through him that Raskolnikov will meet Sonya who, identifying with her father's desire, develops a personality allowing complete acceptance of the other. (Incidentally, when constructing his characters, Dostoevsky shows astonishing insight into unconscious identification processes).

Regarding the murder: Sonya's relation to her father is identical to Dunya's relation to her brother Raskolnikov; on their mother's insistence, Dunya is ready to "sell herself" to enable her brother to study and have access to a good career. There is also a similarity in the sordid aspect of the situation: Marmeladov and his lifestyle present the protagonist with a picture of what might be his own miserable future. This could mislead the reader momentarily, making him believe that the crime is committed purely for financial reasons.

The other two situations which escape the hold of the superego before the murder are:

- the letter from the mother – which acquaints us with a horrible, perverse, dominating mother who pimps her child;
- the dream about the killing of the horse – which acquaints us with a weak, fearful, spineless father: "We [...] have long ceased to be born of living fathers".

These two facts about Raskolnikov's family background are doubly important. First, they indicate that the solitude in which he was immersed just before the murder is not an unusual state for him, that he was alone before he became a student, just as he had been in his childhood – in other words, always. The son of a perverse mother and an absent father, Raskolnikov had to build very solid defences to protect himself from the pain produced by such deep solitude, and to be able to go on. Freud has taught us that these defences built by a child abandoned early by his parents are megalomanic defences, thanks to which the child tries to convince himself that he does not need others to live, and that he can only count on his fantasies of omnipotence. All this is understandable: to rely on the dependability of the other's presence means to risk being disappointed again, and be exposed again to the initial pain against which the subject defends himself to keep from falling apart. Treating trauma always involves respecting this manic defence constructed to alleviate immeasurable psychic pain. Dostoevsky had things to teach us about this constellation of symptoms serving as a defence in these circumstances.

Learning about Raskolnikov's family also allows us to grasp the nature of his superego – an essential bit of information for understanding the events that follow.

Once again, we cannot help being amazed by Dostoevsky's acute awareness of these psychic processes that Freud was to conceptualise decades later.

The construction of the superego depends entirely on the real relations the child establishes in very early childhood. If the parents are unable to recognise the enormous psychic needs of the baby, a cruel superego will be constructed, combining idealisation with persecution. A megalomanic defence is an attempt to escape this cruelty. It is always a failed attempt, because such a defence does not take into account the needs of the ego but, on the contrary, subjects it to a cruel demand for omnipotence.

As another consequence of the early construction of a cruel superego, the subject will project, starting in childhood, the original idealisation and persecution on every new person he meets. Idealisation will turn this person into a perfect being, who can fulfil all expectations. But deep narcissistic wounds render the least difference between the other and oneself intolerable and, as a result, the newcomer will quickly become the new persecutor. The slightest lapse, the least difference between an expectation and the response it produces, will be seen as indubitable proof of abandonment, and will assign the other the role of lifelong persecutor. Of course, this whole process is unconscious. Consciously, the subject is convinced that, once again, his confidence has been betrayed, and that his new acquaintance is incapable of love. On the conscious level, what makes the newcomer a persecutor is not the slight difference between expectation and response; consciously, this impossible coincidence is experienced as a refusal of love on the part of the other. Refusal is an act of desire: the other who refuses to give the love he could have given becomes a deliberate and destructive persecutor. Betrayed and abandoned, the subject apparently – that is, on the conscious level – returns to his familiar state of abandonment; in fact, he inflicts it on himself, repeating the original abandonment of his early childhood.

An unconscious factor reinforces the effects of the superego's cruelty: unconsciously, the subject knows that he is the one who sets up the events in which he is involved; he knows that his attacks are what turned the other into a persecutor. Feeling guilty, he punishes himself for these attacks.

All these considerations enable us to understand the enormous difficulties Raskolnikov has in being able to love Sonya and in recognizing the genuineness of her love for him. Only the daughter of Marmeladov could have borne for so long Raskolnikov's sadistic attacks. Sonya represents the figure of the therapist who treats trauma.

Razumikhin, the friend

Still, the superego is not solely the product of our earliest relationships. It is also related to communal law, to cultural references that sustain the desire and life of community members – a law and references that parents transmit to their children. Therefore, we can imagine the extent of the difficulties facing Raskolnikov. He wants to change the frame of reference in effect in his society. The legitimacy of such a project is to be found in his biography: since his initial other cannot serve as a referent, he is justified in acknowledging his desire to search for new modes of encounter in order to establish new links with the other and with the world. But he will be hindered in this search by the attributes of his superego, which will prevent him from recognizing the never-before-seen character of the other and the unprecedented nature of the encounter.

Psychoanalytic practice teaches us that diminishing the cruelty of the superego requires caring for the body, both psychic and physical, as well as inventing and sustaining the encounter with fellow human beings. A fellow man is the "small other", embodied in a casual acquaintance, be it a stranger on a train or a friend. Psychoanalytic theory holds that interest in the body and in one's fellow men designates interest in the ego, and in reinforcing the ego. To simplify, the ego is the place, the dwelling, where internal entities – memories – and external entities – the skin, the other, the world – can come together. Dostoevsky, the brilliant clinician, pays close attention to the ego. As far as the body is concerned, he keeps pointing out that Raskolnikov neglects his. As for a fellow man, there is Razumikhin.

Just before and just after the murder, he is the one Raskolnikov goes to see. Razumikhin is a generous, faithful friend, of his own generation, close and yet different – in short, his alter ego. Raskolnikov had not seen him in a long time. And given that it has only been two months since he has conceived of the murder, it might be supposed that if this friendship had been maintained uninterrupted during this period, things might have taken a different turn. But let us not speculate. One thing is certain: in Dostoevsky's work, Razumikhin is the figure of the friend and, as such, represents the importance of this "small other" in a person's life. I shall discuss Razumikhin at length further on. For the moment, I would like to make two observations.

The first concerns the plot of *Crime and Punishment*. In this novel, the crucial encounter with Sonya flounders and goes awry because Raskolnikov has no friends. Finally, the encounter can take place because he has internalized his friendship with Razumikhin, the friend, this "small other" who mitigates the cruelty of the superego and, as a result, prepares the encounter with the real of love, where the other represents Everything. The encounter with the real of love is a profoundly intense upheaval, a founding event. But when the ego is fragile, this great, unprecedented intensity is experienced as persecutory and murderous.[18]

The second observation is intended for clinicians. When dealing with trauma, it is essential for the therapist to understand and take into account the importance of this "small other" in transference. I discussed this subject some years ago, drawing attention to the importance of the transferential handling of elements of reality; when I discussed this topic again, I described friendship as the foundation of what is worked out in transference.[19]

To convey the importance of the "small other", I will conclude with a clinical scene, a conversation overhead in a restaurant. An adult says to a child who has just done something she shouldn't have: "Why did you do that?" And the little girl replies: "Don't you think it would save time if you started smacking me right away?"

There are two possibilities. The first: the adult is someone new in the child's life. In that case, the child refers back to the usual violent behaviour of the familiar adult; by doing so, she projects on the unprecedented the shadow of repetition. In this way, she avoids discovering a new mode of relating to an adult, based on a spoken exchange. This avoidance has an advantage: it enables the subject to avoid making the hugely demanding psychic effort of establishing a new manner of relating. Based on this hypothesis, the little girl's question – "Don't you think it would save time if you started smacking me right away?" – concerns her, first and foremost. Indeed, it is more economical for her to experience the usual trauma than to undertake the psychic work of recognising that all adults are not the same. Of course, all this takes place at the unconscious level. She is not aware that she herself is reestablishing her usual mode of relating to adults. On the contrary, like all those who have recourse to the same unconscious process, she is certain that the repetition comes from the real, which only produces violent adults.

The other possibility is that the adult in the restaurant is the one normally in charge of her. In that case, the little girl's statement shows her understanding of a situation that occurs regularly, in which words are of no use and which always ends in violence. In either case, the child has no "small other" and remains captive in a totalitarian relation to the adult in charge of her.

II. Razumikhin

As soon as he wakes up the day after the murder, Raskolnikov goes to see Razumikhin. He has just left the police station, where he was summoned concerning his debt to his landlady. He is surprised to find himself in front of Razumikhin's residence.

> He stopped suddenly [...] near the bridge. [...] "Why, he lives here, in that house," he thought; "why, I have not come to Razumikhin of my own accord! Here it's the same thing over again. [...] Very interesting to know, though; have I come on purpose or have I simply walked here by chance. Never mind, I said the day before yesterday that I would go and see him the day *after*, well, so I will![20]

Two days ago was the day before the murder. That day, Raskolnikov had already been surprised:

> And what put the idea of going to Razumikhin into my head just now? That's curious. [...] The question why he was now going to Razumikhin agitated him even more than he was himself even aware. [...] "*Could I have expected to set it all straight and to find a way out by means of Razumikhin alone?" he asked himself in perplexity.* [My emphasis] He pondered and rubbed his forehead, and, strange to say [...] a fantastic thought came into his head. "I shall go to [him] [...] on the next day after It, when It will be over and everything will begin

> afresh." And suddenly he realized what he was thinking. "After It," he shouted, jumping up from the seat, "but is It really going to happen? Is it possible It really will happen?"[21]

This doubt expressed at the end of his reflection indicates, in fact, that a visit to Razumikhin could have changed the course of events, *resolved everything, bring solutions to all his weighty questions.*

It was after standing in front of Razumikhin's lodgings that Raskolnikov has the dream about the horse, after which he can clearly picture committing the murder. Indeed, in the dream, the horse also represents the moneylender.

> "Good God!" he cried, "can it be, can it be that I shall really take an axe, that I shall strike her on the head, split her skull open [...] that I shall tread in the sticky warm blood, break the lock, steal and tremble; hide, all spattered in the blood [...] with the axe. [...] Good God, can it be?"[22]

Right after imagining the murder in full detail, he admits that he would *not be able to bear it.* Then: "In spite of his weakness he was not conscious of fatigue in himself. It was as though an abscess that had been forming for a month past in his heart had suddenly broken. Freedom, freedom!"[23]

It is clear that these reflections, which sprung to the character's mind after he found himself in front of Razumikhin's home, are not fortuitous (Dostoevsky leaves nothing to chance). Obviously, for Raskolnikov, Razumikhin is an ego-support resource – and Raskolnikov's reflections do in fact concern the ego.

Razumikhin is the friend. In fact, among all of Dostoevsky's major characters, he is the only figure of a friend. Between him and Raskolnikov, there is neither the permeability nor the interpenetration present between Prince Myshkin and Rogozhin in *The Idiot*, between the characters in *Demons*, or between the brothers Karamazov. Indeed, Razumikhin is not Raskolnikov's double, but is, on the contrary, radically other. In fact, Razumikhin often does not understand what his friend is feeling and thinking – which does not diminish his affection for him, or his loyalty. Razumikhin likes and admires Raskolnikov, but is not fascinated by him. He is impressed by his friend, but does not envy him. Clearly, Razumikhin loves life, loves women, has a simple, direct relation with the real. He finds, of course, that Raskolnikov complicates his life needlessly, something he points out to him patiently and affectionately. This patient tenderness is an essential characteristic which makes Razumikhin an exceptional figure in the whole of Dostoevsky's work. He is the likeable fellow who does not bother with questions he considers too complicated for him. He does not envy those who take these questions seriously, nor does he regard them with condescension or irony. These things are simply not his concern. His interest in people is founded on other characteristics: sincerity, strength of character, moral fortitude, generosity, a talent for living.[24]

The threat of madness

Thus, Razumikhin is the friend, the "small other" *par excellence*, the one whose presence is vital for recovering from trauma, because he reinforces the ego. This "small other" is also needed for undertaking any important project. And if the one whose support we expect is not there, we feel betrayed and abandoned, with good reason.

In Dostoevsky's other novels, men try to escape the spheres of trauma with the help of women. But these attempts are always unsuccessful, partly because of the women they choose, of course. But, above all, they do not succeed because these men don't have someone like Razumikhin in their lives, a male friend whom they trust and whose support they can count on. For a man, recognising and being able to accept the homosexual undertones implicit in such a relationship is an essential precondition for being able to meet a woman. When, after a long time, Raskolnikov was able to draw psychic nourishment from Sonya's love, it was because Razumikhin had begun to exist in his internal world.

Dostoevsky portrays Razumikhin as an exceptional man, whose mood never varies:

> He was an exceptionally good-humoured and candid youth, good-natured to the point of simplicity, though both depth and dignity lay concealed under that simplicity. [...] Another thing striking about Razumikhin: no failure distressed him and it seemed as though no unfavourable circumstances could crush him.[25]

And indeed, when Raskolnikov came back to his senses after the murder, Razumikhin was there, by his side. And he took care of everything. A man of action with a practical sense, he found his friend's address – a fact which, considering the circumstances of their last meeting, shows the extent of his loyalty. He succeeded in befriending the landlady – and even in obtaining the promissory note signed by Raskolnikov, which had been the reason for the summons to the police station. Above all, Razumikhin takes care of Raskolnikov's body – that is, of his ego: Raskolnikov has nourishing food, good pillows to sleep comfortably, covers and new clothes.

When Razumikhin goes to Raskolnikov's lodgings, he finds his friend weak, feverish and delusional, and far removed from the concerns of the world. After the murder, little by little, Raskolnikov becomes oblivious to everything. Before killing the old woman, during the incident with the young girl, he had forced himself to become unfeeling, to act like a clown.[26] Now this insensitivity surprises and horrifies him. There can be no better description of the depersonalisation associated with disinvesting the body – a disinvestment that signals the onset of psychosis. Raskolnikov had noticed the first signs at the police station:

> he suddenly felt completely indifferent to anyone's opinion, and this revulsion took place in a flash, in one instant. [...] Now if the whole room had been filled, not with police officers but with those nearest and dearest to him, he

> would not have found one human word for them, so empty was his heart. A gloomy sensation of agonising, everlasting solitude and remoteness took conscious form in his soul. [...] Something was happening to him entirely new, sudden and unknown. [...] He had never experienced such a strange and awful sensation. And what was most agonising – it was more a sensation than a conception or idea, a direct sensation, the most agonising of all the sensations he had known in his life.[27]

This *agonising sensation* is the result of an ego which disintegrates and disappears – a disappearance which follows upon the disinvestment of the body – which, as a result, becomes empty, disincarnated.

His condition worsens and he is aware of it. Like the Underground Man, he tells himself: "'It is because I am very ill,'" he decided grimly at last. 'I have been worrying and fretting myself, and I don't know what I am doing [...] all this time I have been worrying myself.'"

But contrary to the Underground Man, he is still able to be frightened by this state, and able to wish not to remain locked in it: "I shall get well and I shall not worry. [...] But what if I don't get well at all? Good God, how tired I am of it all!"[28]

The feeling of exhaustion comes from his inability to find "some distraction": "He longed terribly for [it], but he did not know what to do or what to undertake". This feeling of powerlessness is mixed with a pervasive hatred that overpowers everything, and signals the onset of psychosis:

> A new, overwhelming sensation was gaining more and more mastery over him every moment: this was an immeasurable, almost physical repulsion for everything surrounding him, an obstinate, malignant feeling of hatred. All who met him were loathsome to him – he loathed their faces, their movements, their gestures. If anyone had addressed him, he felt that he might have spat at them or bitten them.[29]

He was in this state when *his legs automatically carried him to Razumikhin's lodgings*. Unconsciously, just when his own body no longer offers support, he turns to the friend, a "small other", another ego, another body. This attempt to find some support proves that he is not entirely destroyed, that a living space inside him has remained intact. This attempt testifies to the existence of the psychic conditions necessary for the subsequent encounter with Sonya. But this attempt cannot succeed immediately; for the time being, Raskolnikov cannot transform it into an encounter.

"He almost choked with rage at himself as soon as he crossed Razumikhin's threshold." It was no use telling himself that his friend was *the best*, that he was *intelligent and able to judge*, the anger he felt with himself prevailed. Indeed, like the Underground Man, he chose a megalomaniacal position. (The Underground Man is the paradigm of the relation to psychosis seen in all of Dostoevsky's major tragic characters): "now I see that I want nothing. Do you hear? Nothing at all [...] no one's services [...] no one's sympathy. I am by myself [...] alone. Come, that's enough. Leave me alone".[30] In other words, during this conversation with Razumikhin, Raskolnikov, like the Underground Man, calls upon the other only to assert his disinterest in his existence, to place him in the position of a powerless spectator.

But in this case, unlike in the case of the Underground Man, the other is not virtual. And Razumikhin, like a true friend, shouts at Raskolnikov: "'Are you raving, or what?' Razumikhin shouted, roused to fury at last. 'What farce is this? You'll drive me crazy too [...] what did you come to see me for, damn you?'" But as soon as he understands that Raskolnikov can't hear reason and that he will leave, his anger disappears and is replaced by concern for his friend: "Hey, there! Where are you living?"[31]

Two things about this visit are worth noting. First, it makes it clear to Razumikhin that his friend is *very ill*, that he is *delusional*, that he is *a kind of madman*. This is why he looks for Raskolnikov's address and takes care of him – with the beneficial effects that ensue. Although Raskolnikov's attempt to encounter a "small other" fails, it is not useless, since it allows his friend to recognise both his despair and his call for help.

Second, an important aspect of the visit has to do with Razumikhin's anger when he shouts: "What is this farce you're playing? You've even got me all screwed up. [...] Ah, the devil, what did you come for then?" This statement is not that of a "small other", but that of a trustworthy authority, someone who invokes the common consensus, in this case the fact that one does not treat others as if they do not exist and have no feelings. Indeed, fortunately, the friend does not play only the role of "small other"; a true friend often serves as a spokesman for reality. In fact, what other type of relation, other than true friendship, creates a space in which the encounter is founded and maintained through recognition of the singularity of each partner? – a difficult, demanding and joyful practice of reciprocity requiring the creation of an ethical code.

Indeed, it is from the perspective which places the friend in the role of a trusted authority that I postulated a common matrix for friendship and transference. Of course, I was aware that this proposition raised a serious epistemological problem: how can we suggest that friendship could be the origin and support of transference, when the analytic process is based on an essential *asymmetry*, while friendship presupposes *reciprocity*?

Before answering this question, we must specify that when we claim that transference is founded on friendship, we are keeping in mind that the former has a more restricted scope; it is a powerful tool, but limited by its function, which allows the subject to acquire a new perception of his relation to himself and to the world. In fact, our experience has taught us that certain transferential relations are characterised by the fact that the friendship we feel for the patient is what allows us to conduct the analytic process. When the analysis is over, we hope that he will be able to meet us in the sphere in which our support of him and of the transference originated.[32]

This leads us to conclude that while asymmetry establishes the psychoanalytic dialogue, it is the desire to think together which provides a setting for the process. Psychoanalytic treatment requires a *circularity* and *reversibility* of the subjective places held by the two protagonists. Without this *circularity* and *reversibility*, it would not be possible to assert, as every Freudian does, that analysis is the central element of training – since today's analysand could be tomorrow's analyst. This possible reversibility of places is also the foundation of the mobility and transmission of the unconscious as an object of thought. In addition, recognising this circularity and reversibility defines a certain clear conception of ethics in psychoanalysis, which are based on friendship.

I was surprised that when I outlined these ideas in *Letters to a Young Psychoanalyst*, they did not give rise to strong opposition from the analytic community. I now I believe that this implicit agreement was due to the fact that in my discussion I placed the friend in the role of a trusted authority – which is undoubtedly the essential role of a true friend. This conception is compatible with the theory of transference, which considers the psychoanalyst, rightly, the authority figure Lacan designated as "Big Other".

Of course, the authority granted to the analyst constitutes the key factor in analytic treatment. But while this role is at the centre of transferential events from the start in a context of neurosis, in the treatment of trauma both protagonists struggle to establish it. This is so because the traumatised patient and the psychotic are all too willing to place the other in the role of an ideal "authority". Having done so, they will quickly be able to transform him into the persecutor they have always known. These patients need time to be able to use the analyst as an agent allowing passages between the plurality of internal spaces in their own psyche, or as a guarantor of the passages and exchanges between oneself and the world. In order for the psychoanalyst's function as an authority to make possible this mobility, this flexibility of the relation to oneself and to the reality of the world, the patient must first make sure that the analyst is a real person. For this to happen, the psychoanalyst must consent to be a "small other" as well, a simple Razumikhin. This is not always easy for psychoanalysts.

Who has not experienced or heard the ludicrous story of a patient who notices that the analyst is tired and expresses concern, only to be asked: *Why are you bringing this up?*

III. Porfiry

Porfiry Petrovich, an investigating judge, is first mentioned by name to the reader during the exchanges between Razumikhin and Zossimov, the young doctor who is looking after Raskolnikov, and is Razumikhin's distant relative.[33]

Porfiry is Raskolnikov's double. The good double.

The double is a fundamental element in Dostoevskian narration. It serves to structure relations between characters in a powerful manner. So much so, that it could constitute a clue to deciphering each novel, an incomplete but enlightening clue, based on the question: who is the double of whom?

The concept of the "double" appears early in Dostoevsky's work. *The Double* is the title of his second book, published after *Poor Folk*, which was highly acclaimed and enjoyed great popular success. This was not the case for *The Double*. The great literary critique Belinsky, whose enthusiastic review of *Poor Folk* had been crucial for the book's success, hated *The Double*, saying that "a character like Mr. Golyadkin, a victim of schizophrenic break-up, might be more suited for a lunatic asylum than literature".

Porfiry is also worth examining as the character who teaches us to interpret perverse defences.

Learning about this starts with Razumikhin, during his conversation with Zossimov about the crime, and about the questioning of Nikolai, the painter suspected of having killed the moneylender. Razumikhin goes over the exchange between the policeman and the accused:

> "And why did you run away?"
> "Because I was awfully frightened".
> "What were you frightened of?"
> "That I should be accused".
> "*How could you be frightened if you felt free from guilt?*"
> "Now, Zossimov, you may not believe me, *that question was put literally in those words. I know it for a fact, it was repeated to me exactly*! What do you say to that?"
> "Well, anyway, there's the evidence".
> "I am not talking of the evidence now, I am talking about the question, of their own idea of themselves."[34]

Razumikhin's indignation concerns the perverse manipulation implicit in the words used by the policemen. We note, in passing, that Dostoevsky expresses his great respect for words through Razumikhin's remarks.

The latter is also indignant in the scene where Luzhin, the newly arrived fiancé of his friend's sister, visits Raskolnikov. Luzhin speaks of the neighbourhood where he rented an apartment for his future wife. Razumikhin's reply is unambiguous:

> A disgusting place – filthy, stinking and, what's more, of doubtful character. Things have happened there, and there are all sorts of queer people living there. And I went there about a scandalous business. It's cheap, though.[35]

Following Luzhin's attempt to make a good impression by repeating commonplaces about good society in the "new" Russia of his day – which also bear witness to the beginnings of capitalism in Russia,[36] Razumikhin replies mercilessly:

> I've grown so sick during the last three years of this chattering to amuse oneself, this incessant flow of commonplaces, always the same, that, by Jove, I blush even when other people talk like that. You are in a hurry, no doubt, to

> exhibit your acquirements; and I don't blame you, that's quite pardonable. I only wanted to find out what sort of man you are, for so many unscrupulous people have got hold of the progressive cause of late, and have so distorted in their own interests everything they touched, that the whole cause has been dragged in the mire. That's enough![37]

Razumikhin is neither angry nor indignant when he asserts these truths. His calm detachment is certainly due to his indifference to what Luzhin is saying. He reminds the latter that he has heard this discourse countless times, uttered by members of the lower middle class on the verge of climbing the social ladder. But he remains *unrelenting*.

The interpretation of perverse defences relies on a calm attitude, detachment and relentlessness. Detachment results from a lack of narcissistic stakes for the one who interprets. Razumikhin is not trying to convince Luzhin of anything. He simply tells him what he thinks, and leaves it up to him to make use of what he has conveyed, or ignore it. Relentlessness has to do with concern for the truth. What Razumikhin lacks is receptivity – something Porfiry is very concerned with. But strangely, Razumikhin is very shocked by Raskolnikov's anger and by what he tells Luzhin. Anger reveals an essential aspect of the interpretation of perverse defences: the affective aspect of countertransference, that is, the introduction of the therapist's feelings in the transferential relation. Here, Raskolnikov is furious with Luzhin, with good reason. The content of Raskolnikov's discourse points to yet another aspect of the interpretation of perverse defences: in order to foresee the destructive effects, in the sphere of the real, of the pervert's manipulation of words and of his encounter with the other, these effects must be *imagined* in advance. The therapist's ability to guess the real that is to come depends on his proficiency in imagining. As we know, Razumikhin is perfectly capable of anger, and he would have no difficulty imagining how Luzhin might behave in other circumstances. But he has no interest in making this effort.

Let us remember what Raskolnikov tells Luzhin:

> "But why do you worry about it? […] It's in accordance with your theory! […] Carry out logically the theory you were advocating just now, and it follows that people may be killed. […] Economic ideas are not an incitement to murder."
>
> "And is it true," Raskolnikov interposed once more suddenly, again in a voice quivering with fury and delight in insulting him, "is it true that you told your *fiancée* […] within an hour of her acceptance, that what pleased you most […] was that she was a beggar […] because it was better to raise a wife from poverty, so that you may have complete control over her, and reproach her with your being her benefactor?"[38]

At this point, let us review the requirements for the interpretation of a perverse defence:

1. ability to be receptive;
2. detachment;
3. concern with truth;
4. relentlessness;
5. anger and the taking into account, by the therapist, of his emotional responses (use of countertransference);
6. based on this emotional reaction, to guess the real that is to come.

Porfiry is Raskolnikov's double. His good double. This becomes clear to the reader at the end of the novel, when Porfiry promises to have Raskolnikov's sentence reduced if he gives himself up. And he keeps his promise.

It is obvious that Porfiry respects Raskolnikov. He understands him well because, in some ways, Raskolnikov is what he himself was – before ageing prematurely and succumbing to a certain cynicism. In a way, Porfiry wants to protect Raskolnikov from himself, wants to prevent him from going completely mad. By saving Raskolnikov, Porfiry safeguards a part of himself, something Raskolnikov has revived in him: a combination of passion, excess and generosity. Raskolnikov represents that which is repressed in Porfiry. But in order for Raskolnikov to have a chance of reestablishing contact with the buried portion of himself the investigating judge perceives in him, Porfiry must look for it behind Raskolnikov's perverse defences.

When I speak of perverse defences, I am not referring to Raskolnikov's theatrical behaviour when he first meets Porfiry, a meeting Razumikhin arranged at his request. This playacting through which he presents a false image of himself illustrates the psychoanalytic concept of *false self*. In Raskolnikov's case, this "fake personality" is under close scrutiny by a relentless Superego which points out the character's faults, his shortcomings with respect to the ideal of a carefree man not burdened by excessive sensitivity, with a sharp mind, able to exert control over everything and – above all – have total control of the other and of his thoughts.

Of course, in Raskolnikov's case, this control over the other and over his thoughts remains an unfulfilled wish. It never becomes an active strategy of taking hold of the other in order to transfer one's anxiety and insensitivity to him – the strategy used by Svidrigailov, the most notable pervert in the novel. What we see in Raskolnikov could more accurately be called a perversity, that is, an ever-failed *attempt* at setting up perverse defences. This attempt provides glimpses of the failings, the anguish and the confusion that characterise him. This is the confusion Porfiry explores, the confusion of which he wants to free Raskolnikov – taking all the time he needs. But what exactly is this confusion?

Raskolnikov's confusion and theories

Raskolnikov's confusion is rooted in his inability to distinguish love from hate. Regarding this hate, let us recall the conversation Razumikhin and Dunya have about him:

"You've told us a great deal that is interesting about my brother's character [...] and have told it impartially. [...] I think you are right that he needs a woman's care"

"What?"

"He loves no one and perhaps he never will," Razumikhin declared decisively.[39]

This lack of distinction between love and hate is characteristic of psychosis. The pervert acts it out in his relation to the other. The most common example is the act of betrayal: the friend, the loved-one, the lover, turns out to be a monster, a murderer. The pervert enjoys the horror felt by the other in the face of his sudden transformation, his abrupt passage from love to hate. This disturbance he causes in the other – a disturbance associated with the horror of the indistinction between love and hate – manifests the expulsion from his internal world of an experience to which he is subjected constantly: his inability to distinguish love from hate. This experience which haunts him, which is his private hell, is the place from which the pervert contemplates the abyss of psychosis lying in wait and beckoning to him. And he expels that as well: the encounter with a pervert sometimes leads to madness.

It was no doubt when he read Raskolnikov's article on crime that Porfiry understood this confusion. He referred to it when they first met, right after warning Raskolnikov of his plan:

"Are you such a good dissembler?" Raskolnikov asked carelessly. "You wouldn't have supposed it, eh? *Wait a bit, I shall take you in, too. Ha, ha, ha*! No, I'll tell you the truth! All these questions about crimes, recall to my mind an article of yours which interested me at the time. 'On Crime' or something of the sort, I forget the title. I read it with pleasure two months ago in *Periodical Review*."[40]

Interestingly, what stands out in Porfiry's mind is that the article stated that

the act of carrying out a crime is always accompanied by illness. Very, very original, but [...] as a matter of fact, what interested me was not that part of the article, but a certain thought tossed in at the end. [...] The whole point is that in this article all people are somehow divided into the "ordinary" and the "extraordinary". The ordinary must live in obedience and have no right to transgress the law, because they are, after all, ordinary. While the extraordinary *have the right to commit all sorts of crimes and in various ways to transgress the law, because in point of fact they are extraordinary*. This is how you had it, unless I'm mistaken?[41]

But Raskolnikov's intentions were more complex, as he explains:

I admit that you have stated it almost correctly. [...] The only difference is that I don't contend that extraordinary people are always bound to commit

> breaches of morals. [...] I maintain that if the discoveries of Kepler and Newton could not have been made except by sacrificing the lives of one, a dozen, a hundred, or more men, Newton would have had the right, would indeed have been in duty bound [...] to *eliminate* the dozen or the hundred men for the sake of making his discoveries known to the whole of humanity. [...] Legislators and leaders of men, [starting from the most ancient] were all without exception criminals, from the very fact that, making a new law, they transgressed the ancient one, handed down from their ancestors and held sacred by people. [...] As for my division of people into ordinary and extraordinary [...] [or] into two categories: inferior [...] that serves only to reproduce its kind, and men who have the gift or the talent to utter a *new word*. [...] The second category all transgress the law; they are destroyers or disposed to destruction according to their capacities.[42]

Raskolnikov is speaking of the difficulty of changing the frame for thought,[43] which is a hugely difficult question.

Clearly, Porfiry has grasped the scope of Raskolnikov's article. His genius consists in having guessed the existential interpretation given to these essential ideas by a very young man challenging himself to put them into practice. Porfiry imagines the anguish and the desire for the insensitivity needed to transform into concrete experience what the article presents solely in the form of ideas. In fact, he discusses this with Raskolnikov – Dostoevsky makes *everything* explicit in his dialogues:

> there are various practical possibilities that make me uneasy! What if some man *or youth* imagines that he is a Lycurgus or a Mahomet – a future one, of course – and suppose he begins to remove all obstacles. [...] He has some great enterprise before him and needs money for it [...] and starts to get it [...] do you see?[44]

Porfiry knows. Now, he has to make Raskolnikov admit his crime. But how? His strategy is to uncover the anguish, the affect in the young man.

Porfiry knows. And he makes this clear to Raskolnikov right away. First, by his official demeanour when he discusses the reasons for his visit: "'You have to give information to the police,' Porfiry replied with a most businesslike air". Then by the small hints inserted into their conversation:

> "I have been expecting you here for a long time [...] I heard, indeed, that you were in great distress about *something. You look pale still.* [...] Really *delirious*? You don't say so!" Porfiry shook his head *in a womanish way*. [...] "Quite the contrary, quite the contrary! If only you knew how you interest me! It's interesting *to look on and to listen* [...] *and I am really glad you have come forward at last.*"[45]

Let us remember what is needed to interpret perverse defences: detachment, concern with truth, relentlessness, taking one's own affects into account, being able to surmise the real that is to come. And being receptive.

Porfiry *knows* how Raskolnikov feels because he can, at least minimally, identify with him. This means that he has experienced, in his own way, overwhelming anguish as a result of the indistinction between love and hate. The same anguish is experienced very early by children who later become therapists.

After Raskolnikov's long monologue about the difference between *ordinary* and *extraordinary* men, Porfiry asks him if he believes in God and in the resurrection of Lazarus. He is probably trying to assess the degree of guilt of which his interlocutor is capable. This question makes such a strong impression on Raskolnikov that when he first visits Sonya, he asks her to read the passage about Lazarus in the Bible.

Then Porfiry lays his cards on the table. Despite his warm, friendly welcome, he takes on a *peculiar, impudent* and *careless* tone.[46]

> "Excuse the natural anxiety of a practical law-abiding citizen [...] if confusion arises and a member of one category imagines that he belongs to the other, begins to "eliminate obstacles" as you so happily expressed it, then [...] are there many people who have the right to *kill others,* these extraordinary people?"

This is followed by the question quoted earlier:

> "there are various practical possibilities that make me uneasy! What if some man *or youth* imagines that he is a Lycurgus or a Mahomet – a future one, of course – and suppose he begins to remove all obstacles. [...] He has some great enterprise before him and needs money for it [...] and starts to get it [...] do you see?"

And he goes on:

> "When you were writing your article, surely you couldn't have helped – he-he! – fancying yourself [...] just a little, an 'extraordinary' man. [...] That's so, isn't it? – Allow me to observe [...] that I don't consider myself a Mahomet or a Napoleon. [...] Oh, come, don't we all think ourselves Napoleons now in Russia?" Porfiry Petrovitch said with alarming familiarity. Something peculiar betrayed itself in the very intonation of his voice.

To top it all off, Zametov blurted out from the corner: "Perhaps it was one of these future Napoleons who [killed] Alyona Ivanovna last week?"[47]

Those who are familiar with Inspector Colombo will remember that it is just when he is about to leave a suspect that Colombo comes back to ask the most pertinent question. This is just what Porfiry does at the end of his meeting with Raskolnikov, when, *suddenly happy about something* and saying that he *just remembered,* he asks the question which lays the trap, enquiring if Raskolnikov saw the painters as he was going up the stairs. In fact, the painters were there on the day of the crime, not on the day Raskolnikov says he visited the moneylender for the last time.

Porfiry knows, and Raskolnikov knows that he knows. This is how things stand when the two men meet for the second time.

Porfiry's treatment of Raskolnikov

Raskolnikov was surprised at how long he was kept standing in the waiting room at the police station before seeing Porfiry for a second interview. Although he was calm when he arrived, the thought that the stranger who had called him an assassin the previous day on the street was, after all, only a phantom, suddenly made him tremble. But in the next instant the intense hatred he felt for Porfiry stopped his trembling.

The judge met him with a cheerful and affable air. Filled with suspicion, Raskolnikov needed some time to realise that Porfiry was not at all uncomfortable, as it seemed to him at first, but on the contrary, completely at ease.

Raskolnikov becomes very nervous when he faces the judge – and everything around him contributes to his discomfort. Porfiry's body, in particular, fills him with disgust: "His plump, little round figure [...] the little wrinkles on his forehead [that] smoothed out".[48]

Indeed, Porfiry is quite agitated and makes no attempt to hide it. He has reason to be, since he has just seen the man who harassed Raskolnikov, "the phantom", who told him about going to the apartment, ringing the bell, asking about blood. Porfiry is absolutely sure: Raskolnikov is the one who killed the old moneylender. Porfiry's pacing back and forth is an attempt to calm down, to find the right tone to use with Raskolnikov.

He has just uncovered a crucial element of the problem he is responsible for solving. But the identity of the criminal, as such, is not what interests him. Porfiry is too intelligent to be satisfied with placing people in categories. What interests him is the crime, and each crime is unique, as he likes to say – just like each therapy.

What Porfiry wants is to present *mathematical* proof of the crime. But in dealing with Raskolnikov, he is determined to prove that a judge must turn each crime *into a completely particular case* – just as a psychoanalyst must do with every interpretation.

In other words, Porfiry wants to bring the young man – formerly a law student – to confess and admit that the game is over.

The scene with Nikolai, the painter, who accuses himself of the murder, testifies to the fact that Porfiry can be very direct, extremely brutal and pitiless. This contrasts sharply with the very special, even deferential manner in which he treats Raskolnikov.

Of course, Porfiry's pride would be flattered if he succeeded in making the extraordinary young man admit that he has been unmasked. But this is not what most matters to him. What Porfiry most wants is to make Raskolnikov admit that the war is over. The war between the two of them and, above all, the war Raskolnikov wages with himself. Porfiry knows that a transgression of this magnitude has transformed Raskolnikov – that he has become his act. The criminal becomes the crime and depriving him of his crime means thrusting him into a dizzying abyss.

Porfiry's greatest concern is to avoid Raskolnikov's suicide – to which he refers directly during their third meeting. Thus, Porfiry is torn between two contradictory desires: bringing the young man to confess his crime, and preventing his breakdown.

The method he chose to reconcile these two opposing objectives was one Raskolnikov knew well: "He [...] simply babbled on, uttering empty phrases, letting slip a few enigmatic words and again reverting to incoherence". And without warning, he would state a fact quite directly, for instance: "they begin by disarming him with irrelevant questions (as you so happily put it) and then deal him a knock-down blow, he-he-he!"[49]

Despite Porfiry's great kindness towards Raskolnikov, this method produces devastating effects, as Porfiry admits when they meet for the third time. Faced with Raskolnikov's resistance, the examining lawyer gets carried away and reveals the reasoning which led him to conclude that the young man is the murderer.[50]

Raskolnikov becomes completely desperate: he shouts, he bangs his fist on the table, he insults Porfiry. And the latter is really frightened by the consequences of his determined pursuit of Raskolnikov.

But why does Porfiry show so much concern? What is the nature of his ties to Raskolnikov?

As I said earlier, Raskolnikov represents everything Porfiry has repressed. Indeed, contrary to Raskolnikov, Porfiry has not taken the risk of overstepping the boundaries set by the frame for thought of his society; he is not engaged in a process of *liberation* from conventional rules. Aware of this, his greatest concern is to make sure that the young man, unlike him, should have a living life after the disaster. Because he has faced similar challenges, in a different context, Porfiry can identify with Raskolnikov. He can recognise – beyond madness, beyond pretentiousness, arrogance and the Ideal Ego – Raskolnikov's striving for truth and for the new Ego Ideal he seeks. Porfiry admires his courage – insane courage, but courage just the same – in taking up these challenges, in attempting to invent an absolutely personal manner of living. Porfiry knows from experience that the one who sets such standards of authenticity for himself is condemned to great solitude. This knowledge explains his affection and feeling of friendship for Raskolnikov. But there is more.

Porfiry's secret

Porfiry's effeminate gestures are the traces of the battle he fought with himself, and which he lost. Not having had the courage to admit his homosexuality, with the hardships it involves, turned him into a prematurely old man. He said as much to Raskolnikov: "You see, I'm a bachelor [...] I'm running to seed"[51]; "'listen to an old man [...] Rodion Romanovitch' (as he said this Porfiry Petrovitch, who was scarcely five-and-thirty, actually seemed to have grown old; even his voice changed and he seemed to shrink together)".[52] "I am a man with nothing to hope for, that's all. [...] But you are a different matter".[53]

Raskolnikov, the gloomy, presumptuous, impertinent, out of the ordinary, daring young loner fascinates Porfiry. Porfiry truly loves him, and desires him. His love is mixed with envy and rage, born of the knowledge of the hopelessness of this passion. But Porfiry has the generosity of a man in love: "I'm a candid man [...] am I a candid man or not? What do you say? I fancy I really am: I tell you these things for nothing and don't expect a reward for it, he-he!"[54] And later: "I desire now to do all I can to efface that impression and to show that I am a man of heart and conscience. I speak sincerely".[55]

At times, envy and rage turn him into a cruel, sadistic man. His cruelty and sadism are mixed with a brutal desire for penetration, for sodomy:

> "What a wily person you are!" Porfiry tittered, "there's no catching you; you're a perfect monomania. So you don't believe me? But still you do believe me, you believe a quarter; I'll soon make you believe the whole, because I have sincere liking for you and genuinely wish you good".[56]

But the man who loves gives the younger man the indications necessary for living a life beyond the immediate horror: "I regard you in any case as a man of noble character, and not without elements of magnanimity. [...] When I made your acquaintance, I felt attracted by you".[57]

> "That you were bold, head-strong, in earnest and [...] had felt a great deal, I recognized long before. *I, too, have felt the same*, so that your article seemed familiar to me. It was conceived on sleepless nights, with a throbbing heart, in ecstasy and suppressed enthusiasm. [...] Your article is absurd and fantastic, but there's a transparent sincerity, a youthful incorruptible pride and the daring of despair in it. It's a gloomy article, but that's what's fine in it".[58]
>
> "Ah, don't disdain life!" Porfiry went on. "You have a great deal of it still before you. [...] You've lost faith and you think that I am grossly flattering you; but how long has your life been? How much do you understand?[...] How do I regard you? I regard you as one of those men who would stand and smile at their torturer while he cut their entrails out, if only they had found faith or God. Find either and you will live. You have long needed a change of air. Suffering, too, is a good thing. Suffer![...] I know you don't believe in it – but don't be over-wise; fling yourself straight into life, without deliberation; don't be afraid – the flood will bear you to the bank and set you safe on your feet again. What bank? How can I tell? I only believe that you have a long life before you. [...] But keep a good heart and have less fear! Are you afraid of the great expiation before you? No, it would be shameful to be afraid of it. [...] I know that you don't believe it, but indeed, life will bring you through. You will live it down in time. What you need now is fresh air, fresh air, fresh air![...] Perhaps God is saving you for something. [...] Come, what does it

> matter that you will be passing into another class of men? *It's not comfort you regret, with your heart!* What of it that perhaps no one will see you for so long? It's not time but yourself that will decide that. The point lies in you, not in time. Be the sun and all will see you. The sun has before all to be the sun".[59]

We must not forget that everything Porfiry is saying is reinforced by a promise:

> I've come to you with a direct and open proposition – that you should surrender and confess. [...] Secondly: Don't you know how it would lessen your sentence? [...] *I swear before God* that I will so arrange it that your confession shall come as a complete surprise. We will make a complete sweep of all these psychological points, of all the suspicion against you, so that your crime will appear to have been something like an aberration, for in truth it was an aberration. I am an honest man, Rodion Romanovitch, and will keep my word.[60]

It is no exaggeration to say that Porfiry is acting like a true therapist. Once he has destroyed all the perverse defences, he accompanies Raskolnikov in the process of facing the most terrible aspects of his trauma. He strives to pull him out of the catastrophic mire in which he is voluptuously ensconced, to attempt to bring him back to life, to the community of the living.

Before discussing what connects Porfiry and Raskolnikov on the emotional-sexual level – what Freud calls the libidinal level – I would like to examine their relation from the perspective of the place Porfiry is able to gain in Raskolnikov's psychic life.

Porfiry frees Raskolnikov from absolute subjection to an ideal which has been transformed into pure image (ideal ego). Thanks to Porfiry, Raskolnikov can glimpse the possibility of a relation to himself in which the law, his own law, is no longer cruel and persecutory, where the law becomes a point of reference, a criterion on the basis of which the other and the world can meet. Porfiry transforms the cruel superego into a protective superego;[61] this transformation is achieved by creating a place for the friend. The creation of this place is the result of all the psychical work Raskolnikov was able to do in their relationship, thanks to Porfiry. The existence of this place enables Raskolnikov to admit the necessity of his friendship with Razumikhin, and later of Sonya's love.

The work Porfiry succeeds in inciting Raskolnikov to do is a powerful example of the difficulties encountered by a therapist in his efforts to establish the role of the protective superego in the internal world of a subject caught in the snare of trauma. Those who tend to believe that it is naïve on my part to propose, as Freud did, a theory of the protective superego, associated with the joy of reflection, may find reason here to reconsider.

Leaving behind the world of the morbid to admit that the encounter with the other is a necessity constitutes a passage, but one which is traumatic. It is so painful, in fact, that the psychotic who has abandoned his delusions becomes so fragile, so sensitive to the joys and pains of existence, that he may prefer to end his life. Sometimes, because he cannot contain the unbearable; sometimes because he does not yet recognise life as a collection of fleeting moments, and therefore chooses death in order not to risk losing the fullness of living he is experiencing now.

As I said earlier, a theory of the interpretation of perverse defences relies on receptivity, detachment and relentlessness. To discuss relentlessness in greater detail, I must first open a parenthesis.

I have never liked the concept of "guilt". Not having an alternative, I accepted the difference introduced by Melanie Klein between good and bad guilt, as a temporary compromise. The religious overtones of the word disturb me. Like Winnicott, I do not like turning an idea contaminated by its morbid significance into a metapsychological tool. We all know that the introduction of guilt in a relationship has ravaging effects and is completely unproductive. I encountered these difficulties when reflecting on Claude Lanzmann's film *Shoah*. In regard to an extreme situation, what there is to think about is not guilt, but our entire responsibility. If, in the face of such a situation, responsibility is absent, then hate is present: either hate felt by the other, or my own hate which takes root in the incurable wound of self-deception.

Porfiry can be relentless because he feels responsible for Raskolnikov's fate. (Just as Claude Lanzmann feels responsible for the work of memory he carries out in his film.) Porfiry seeks neither complicity nor gratitude. What he wants is to shift the position of death, bring it into the sphere of life as a shared destination, and not let it remain the trophy mounted on the ruins of Raskolnikov's narcissism.

Finally, let us look at Porfiry's libidinal functioning. Raskolnikov is his double, but he is also his contrasting other. Porfiry loves him as he would like to love life, with the intensity with which he once loved life. Raskolnikov is his sunshine, his hope, his redemption, his revenge.

In *The House of the Dead*, there is a very surprising description of a homosexual passion. It shows, once again, Dostoevsky's astute understanding of unconscious processes. But, above all, this passion provides another clue to the meaning of the relation of opposition and complementarity of the characters portrayed two-by-two in Dostoevsky's work (Raskolnikov and Porfiry, Myshkin and Rogozhin, Ivan and Smerdyakov). In *The House of the Dead*, the relation between two men is *obviously constructed on the massacre of a woman's sexuality*.

A convict tells the following story. In his village, his friend was boasting of being the lover of a young woman. He persuaded the future convict to smear tar on the door of Akulka's house (Akulka is the young woman's name). To punish their daughter for having dishonoured them, the parents beat her regularly, several times a day. Later, the future convict is offered money to marry the girl, and accepts. And then, surprise, *Akulka is still a virgin*. The future convict spreads the news in the village, telling everyone that his friend is a scoundrel. Akulka cries with joy, her parents ask for her forgiveness. But the friend persuades the future convict that he is a fool, that he was drunk on his wedding night and couldn't be sure of anything, and that he has been duped. After this, the husband starts to beat his wife morning, noon and night – it is the price to pay for his friendship with his wife's supposed lover. He keeps beating his wife and proclaiming his loyalty to his friend.

And one day this friend falls to the ground on the street before Akulka, declares his love and asks her forgiveness for all the lies he spread about her. She forgives him and tells her husband that she loves this other man *more than the whole world*. Her husband ends up slashing her throat, and leaving her to bleed to death.[62]

What is surprising here is the representation that emerges from this story: two men mistreating a woman to the point of murder, to punish her for awakening sexual desire in them. Later, we will encounter twice more in Dostoevsky's work the same cruel scenario in which passion between men leads to madness. Although the monstrous aspect of these scenarios will remain the same, in the subsequent narratives it will not be made obvious that the two men are associated in the massacre of a woman whose suffering they sustain because it constitutes a source of pleasure that strengthens their bond. Let us note that Dostoevsky points out Akulka's love for her defamer; this is a stupefying clinical observation: she was able to recognise the power of a desire so great that the man was unable to bear it, and which made his internal world burst into a million pieces.

Of course, the homosexual relation between Porfiry and Raskolnikov is not consolidated by the hatred of a woman, contrary to that between Myshkin and Rogozhin, between Stravrogin and Shatov, or between Ivan and Dmitri. A thoughtful reader could learn here what psychoanalytic practice was to teach us later: because Porfiry recognised his passion for the young man, this relation between the two men had decisive consequences for Raskolnikov's life: first, he was able to accept Razumikhin's friendship, and the tenderness associated with it; then, he was able to accept Sonya's love. In fact, for a man, accepting to be loved by a man is a way of feeling the tenderness which until then he had been unable to have for himself. One thing is certain: one cannot accept the love of another if he does not love himself.

After Raskolnikov's third meeting with the judge, he "was hurrying to Svidrigailov".[63] Dostoevsky's clinical astuteness is astonishing, as he shows us: Raskolnikov has to choose between accepting Porfiry's offer or opting for the Svidrigailov solution. Indeed, while Raskolnikov represents everything Porfiry has repressed, Svidrigailov represents what is repressed in Raskolnikov.

IV. Svidrigailov

Murder without guilt

What I just said above can be stated differently. Raskolnikov has to make a psychic choice: either he accepts Porfiry's proposition, which Sonya supports in her own way, or he must invent a way out of the impasse where he finds himself. Suicide is, of course, the least likely probability. Raskolnikov would certainly agree with Woody Allen, who said that the trouble with suicide is that it never provides a good answer to the problem it is supposed to solve.[64]

The problem Raskolnikov must solve concerns his own ideals, as they apply to the manner in which he should live his life. Although, after the murder of the moneylender and her unfortunate sister Lizaveta, he doubts that he is an extraordinary man, he has not given up the idea that he will find an *extraordinary* answer to the conflict in which he is caught. We can, of course, invoke the young man's pride or the merciless superego which torments him – as I said earlier. But these are secondary considerations compared to the highest stakes: not to forfeit a representation of himself worthy of his ideal. In light of these stakes, the idea of suicide appears as a base, cowardly act, an easy way out, an obscene betrayal.[65]

But this does not mean that for Raskolnikov the risk of suicide is eliminated. Dostoevsky states several times that it could have happened. But it would have been a frantic act, carried out in a moment of unbearable pain, not a deliberate option.

We know what Raskolnikov chose to do, with Porfiry's and Sonya's help. I shall go on to show how extraordinarily heroic his decision is – and therefore in agreement with his ideal, – and how very dangerous. You will then see that my interpretation of his choice is very far removed from the sentimental explanations often given for the novel's ending.

But first, let us look at the Svidrigailov solution. This is a possibility Raskolnikov never ceases to consider. Given his view of his own conflict, this solution seems the most obvious and is the most tempting. It is so familiar and at the same time so uncanny that Raskolnikov's meeting with Svidrigailov takes place in a hallucinatory mode:

> "Can this be still a dream?" Raskolnikov thought once more. He looked carefully and suspiciously at the unexpected visitor. "Svidrigailov! What nonsense! It can't be!" he said at last aloud in bewilderment.
>
> His visitor did not seem at all surprised at this exclamation.[66]

Dostoevsky goes on to describe the meeting. It is like the *continuation of a dream*, in other words, an expression of Raskolnikov's *desire*. The meeting is described in a strange fashion: it is as if Raskolnikov *recognises* Svidrigailov, whom he has never seen, as if he had been waiting for him.[67]

Raskolnikov remembers well the role Svidrigailov played in his sister Dunya's life, and it is precisely the amoral behaviour of the man which intrigues and fascinates him. This curiosity[68] and fascination were already there before their first meeting. It is no doubt for this reason that Raskolnikov is interested in what Svidrigailov has to say.

And he is not going to be disappointed. Svidrigailov begins with a discourse on the excessive nature of love: *reason is the slave of passion.*[69] Considering the hold of desire, man is a *victim* rather than a *monster*. Svidrigailov is asking whether an action motivated by love can still be called monstrous. Of course, this idea is not completely strange to someone who refuses to consider as *murder* an action born of a *higher ideal*.

In fact, murder is what Raskolnikov wants to discuss with Svidrigailov. The latter says that, technically speaking, he has not murdered his wife. This was formally established. He did ask himself if he had contributed morally to her death.

But this questioning clearly involved no guilt, a fact which lends strength to the very act of raising the question. Raskolnikov feels no guilt either for murdering the moneylender, but contrary to Svidrigailov, he does not wonder about any moral responsibility.

After delivering a whole discourse on feminine masochism, Svidrigailov tells Raskolnikov why he is willing to answer him, despite *the rudeness of his questions*: "You know, there's hardly anything I take interest in. [...] But I'll confess frankly, I am very much bored. [...] I am not particularly interested in anyone's opinion".[70]

Like the Underground Man, Svidrigailov is able to listen to the truth coming from anyone because a veil of indifference covers his relation to the world, and because he has no pride left. This is where he draws his strength, and it is this strength which disconcerts the student. Raskolnikov is learning: if being indifferent to everything – as he had wanted to be indifferent to the plight of the young girl harassed by the pervert in the park – makes one accept everything he is told, it means he has no pride left. But Raskolnikov is unable to imagine such a possibility – and this is at once his saving grace and his torment.

Svidrigailov then speaks of his life with his deceased wife. This relationship lasted because it was founded on that which forces a pervert into stability: something that gives the other a hold over him. Marfa Petrovna, his wife, always kept the document Svidrigailov had signed with a false name.[71]

The pervert's solution, which Raskolnikov finds tempting, can keep psychosis at bay. But indifference, an external threat or the eroticisation of hatred, do not provide an absolute guarantee against the return of horror. After his wife's death, that is, once no one had a hold over him, Svidrigailov had to struggle with hallucinations. This is something that preoccupies Raskolnikov:

> "What made me think that something of the sort must be happening to you?" Raskolnikov said suddenly. At the same moment he was surprised at having said it.
>
> "What! Did you think so?" Svidrigailov asked *in astonishment*. "Did you really? Didn't I say that there was something in common between us, eh?"[72]

The conversation continues and it is obvious that Svidrigailov is happy to be able to speak openly to someone who understands him. The reader learns that the rigid parameters of Svidrigailov's marriage did not prevent him from experiencing a hallucinatory event following the death of a serf whom he treated badly. But when Raskolnikov suggests that he consult a physician, he replies: "I know I am not well, without your telling me, though I don't know what's wrong; I believe I am five times as strong as you are".[73]

Choosing perversion to defend against madness

Svidrigailov speaks of perversion as a defence against psychosis in very clear terms:

"What do people generally say?" muttered Svidrigailov as though speaking to himself, looking aside and bowing his head. "They say, 'You are ill, so what appears to you is only unreal fantasy.' But that's not strictly logical. I agree that ghosts only appear to the sick, *but that only proves that they are unable to appear except to the sick, not that they don't exist.*"

Raskolnikov is upset at hearing this, since it is clear that this question has been on his mind.

"Nothing of the sort," Raskolnikov insisted irritably.

"No? You don't think so?" Svidrigailov went on, looking at him deliberately. "But what do you say to this argument? (Help me with it.) Ghosts are, as it were, shreds and fragments of other worlds, the beginning of them. A man in health has, of course, no reason to see them, because he is above all *a man of this earth* [Note that this takes up the reasoning of the *Underground Man*] and is bound *for the sake of completeness and order* to live only in this life. [In other words, Svidrigailov, like the Underground Man, considers normal life to be insipid, because it consents to obeying the law.] But as soon as one is ill, as soon as *the normal earthly order* of the organism is broken, one begins to realise *the possibility of another world;* and the more seriously ill one is, the closer becomes one's contact with the other world."[74]

Here, Svidrigailov mixes a romantic view of psychosis with a discourse in praise of perversion – which allows transgression of the law, giving access to a mysterious, transcendental world. This linking together of desire and transgression of the law, with no guilt casting a shadow over the pleasure it makes possible, is the fascinating legend told by the pervert. This fascination has exerted sufficient power over certain psychoanalysts to make them mistake perverse desire for desire in general. Such a mistake is the result of inadequate knowledge or of banalisation of two major aspects of perversion: the place held by hate, and specifically the eroticisation of hate; and the defensive function of perversion against psychotic breakdown – the situation we are examining here. Poor pervert: when he is taken at his word, he reinforces his exclusion from human society.

Let us return to Svidrigailov, who ends his monologue by saying: "and the more seriously ill one is, the closer becomes one's contact with the other world,"[75] "*so that as soon as the man dies he steps straight into that world. [...]* If you believe in a future life, you could believe in that, too".[76] Here again, we can admire Dostoevsky's clinical astuteness: through Svidrigailov, he presents a continuum between perversion, psychosis and death. To be in a perverse world or in a psychotic universe means to have an intimate relation to the death drive. Raskolnikov must understand what his visitor is saying quite well, since he himself is haunted by ideas of this kind. He tries to cut the conversation short.

"I don't believe in a future life," said Raskolnikov.

> Svidrigailov sat lost in thought. "And what if there are only spiders there, or something of the sort?" he said suddenly.
>
> "He is a madman," thought Raskolnikov.[77]

Indeed, one has to be mad to describe the future in terms of abandonment and vermin.

And to leave no doubt about his perception of things, Svidrigailov speaks of time in order to deny all temporality, to reduce it to trash. A future time can only be imagined as uninhabited, motionless, forever frozen as the remnants of all absences and forgettings. In Svidrigailov's words:

> "We always imagine eternity as something beyond our conception, something vast, vast! But why must it be vast? Instead of all that, what if it's one little room, like a bath-house in the country, black and grimy and spiders in every corner, and that's all eternity is. I sometimes fancy it like that".
>
> "Can it be you can imagine nothing juster and more comforting than that?" Raskolnikov cried, *with a feeling of anguish.*

We should note that in addition to anguish, there is tenderness in Raskolnikov's response. It is clear that he is experiencing the same torments as his visitor.

Svidrigailov continues, smiling vaguely: "Juster? And how can we tell, perhaps that is just, and do you know it's what I would certainly have made it?"[78] We know that he is deeply depressed and, as his subsequent remarks will indicate, that he has decided to kill himself.

At this point, Svidrigailov starts to speak of the gift of ten thousand roubles he wishes to make to Dunya. Raskolnikov is shocked by the offhand, impudent manner in which the visitor speaks of this, and scolds him as he would a child: "I beg you to finish. [...] In any case, it's unforgivably impudent". This is another example of Dostoevsky's genius: here he draws attention to the infantile irresponsibility of all perverts, a characteristic which often fascinates his interlocutors and renders him loveable in their eyes.[79]

Continuing in the same irresponsible vein, Svidrigailov explains that his love for Dunya was short-lived. The blunt manner in which he says these things is one of the particularities of the pervert which fascinates others, and which contributes to their idealisation of him for this very freedom of expression in regard to the most intimate matters. But this impression is false; it is merely the result of his indifference to everything, and of the boredom which governs his relations to the world.[80]

Finally, Svidrigailov speaks of what we will later understand as his plan to commit suicide: "On [...] determining on a certain [...] journey, I wished to make some necessary preliminary arrangements". And when Raskolnikov asks about this journey again, he adds: "'Well, that's a wide subject. [...] If only you knew what you are asking,' he added, and gave a sudden, loud, short laugh".[81]

As he was leaving, Svidrigailov ran into Razumikhin in the doorway. After explaining to his friend briefly who his visitor had been, Raskolnikov says: "I don't know why, but I'm afraid of the man". Then he asks Razumikhin if he actually saw him there, in his room. And he quickly reveals what he is really afraid of: to be as mad as his visitor, to have hallucinations like him:

> Hm! [...] that's right. [...] Do you know, I fancied [...] I keep thinking that it may have been an hallucination. I thought just now that perhaps I really am mad, and have only seen a phantom. [...] Why, who can tell? Perhaps I am really mad, and perhaps everything that has happened over the last few days may be only imagination.[82]

The two men met again shortly after a brief exchange that took place between them after the death of Katerina Ivanovna, Marmeladov's wife and Sonya's stepmother. On that occasion, Svidrigailov's allusions made Raskolnikov very uneasy, since they had to do with his confession of the murder to Sonya, a confession Svidrigailov overheard through the partition between his room and Sonya's lodgings.

This second meeting occurs in circumstances that are very particular for each of the two men. Raskolnikov has just left Porfiry, who declared him to be the murderer. This confers special importance to his meeting with Svidrigailov, in terms of the choice he has to make: accept Porfiry's proposition – supported by Sonya – to give himself up or choose the cynicism which the perverse solution promises as an antidote to any moral suffering. Even though the first time he saw Svidrigailov the reality of this promise was brought into question, he is still attracted to it, fearing it at the same time – as he tells his friend Razumikhin. As for Svidrigailov, this second meeting takes place shortly before he is to see Dunya, Raskolnikov's sister – a crucial encounter for him, a matter of life or death.

On his way to see Svidrigailov, Raskolnikov told himself that "the man had some hidden power over him [...] could it be that he expected something *new* from him – directions, a way out?" For Raskolnikov, there is a connection between Svidrigailov and Porfiry, as well as Sonya:

> He was afraid of Sonya, too. [She] stood before him as an irrevocable sentence. He must go his own way or hers. At that moment especially (*after the conversation he has just had with Porfiry*) he did not feel equal to seeing her. No, would it not be better to try Svidrigailov? And he could not help inwardly owning that he had *long felt* that he must see him for some reason. But what could they have in common? Their very evil-doing could not be of the same kind.[83]

These are the terms of his ties to Svidrigailov, clearly stated. As for the Sonya "option", the reader becomes aware that it is just as terrible; we will examine this point more closely later, guided by Dostoevsky.

The two men meet in a sordid place, a setting Dostoevsky often chooses for crucial meetings between his protagonists, as his biographer, Joseph Frank remarks. "Svidrigailov was obviously in an excited state, but only a little; he had drunk only half a glass of wine". In fact, this excitement has to do with the prospect of seeing Dunya again.

Sexuality gone mad

Svidrigailov sets the tone for the meeting by saying that he has often observed Raskolnikov walking on the street. He goes on to describe a madman; his words are insidious: "Someone may be watching you besides me, and it won't do you any good. It's nothing really to do with me and I can't cure you, but, of course, you understand me".[84]

Both of them reveal their intentions at once, since these are pressing matters that cannot wait.[85] Dostoevsky, who neglects no detail, does not forget to introduce the uncanny dimension of the double existing between the two characters. It is made evident by each man's ability to identify completely with the other, an ability giving each of them direct access to the unconscious desire of the other. This device is used in all of Dostoevsky's work, and always produces an unbearable feeling of anxiety. Svidrigailov, for instance, says:

> "I must admit that your question [about why he has been following Raskolnikov] is rather complex, and is difficult for me to answer. Here, you, for instance, have come to me not only for a definite object *but for the sake of hearing something new*. Isn't that so? Isn't that so?" persisted Svidrigailov with a sly smile.[86]

In fact, Raskolnikov had been thinking exactly these thoughts about Svidrigailov just before their meeting. And the latter insists on pointing out that he counts on him to learn something *new* about himself;[87] he even invites Raskolnikov to eat the food on his own plate. (Incredible Dostoevsky!)

Svidrigailov resembles the Underground Man in many ways. At times, he even says, like the Underground Man: "If only I'd been something, a landowner, a father, a cavalry officer, a photographer, a journalist. [...] I am nothing, I have no specialty".[88] For the Underground Man, this idea is also related to the question of identity. But contrary to the Underground Man, Svidrigailov is not afraid of sexuality:

> Vice! [...] Tell me, what should I restrain myself for? Why should I give up women, since I have a passion for them? *It's an occupation, anyway*. [...] In this vice at least there is something permanent, founded indeed upon nature and not dependent on fantasy, something present in the blood like an ever-burning ember, forever setting one on fire and, maybe, not to be quickly extinguished, even with years. You'll agree it's an occupation of a sort. [Let us note that here again the elements sustaining the argument are the ones used earlier by the Underground Man, in a different context: nature, boredom, desire.[89]] Oh, that's what you think, is it! I agree that it

> is a disease like everything else that exceeds moderation. And, of course, in this *one must exceed moderation.* [...] If I hadn't this [occupation], I might have to shoot myself.

Raskolnikov is visibly startled by this idea: "And could you shoot yourself?" Svidrigailov is deeply disturbed by his question, and answers with loathing: "'Oh, come! [...] Please don't speak of it,' he added hurriedly and with none of the bragging tone he had shown in all the previous conversation. His face had quite changed".[90]

Raskolnikov got up to leave. "He felt both oppressed and stifled and, as it were, ill at ease at having come here. He felt convinced that Svidrigailov was the most worthless scoundrel on the face of the earth".[91] Raskolnikov wanted to leave because he was embarrassed to hear talk about sexuality, since he is prudish like many of Dostoevsky's male characters. His decision would be taken after what he would hear now, because this talk was no longer about a theory that could justify perversion, but about its actual practice.

The second part of the meeting is divided into two parts: the first is the one in which Svidrigailov talks about Dunya, and the second the one in which he describes his perverse practices more explicitly. Regarding the first, I shall focus on what Svidrigailov says about women.

He starts off by commenting on jealousy in women. He speaks of his wife, Marfa Petrovna, who took his crude frankness for a guarantee of fidelity. According to him: "She thought it showed I was unwilling to deceive her if I warned her like this beforehand and for a jealous woman, you know, that's the first consideration".[92]

For a jealous woman only? Through the concept of jealousy, Dostoevsky invites reflection on feminine desire, which, in my opinion, always goes hand in hand with love. This question is central in the construction of all of Dostoevsky's major female characters – keeping in mind, nevertheless, that in Dostoevsky's work sexuality is always disconnected from love. But this separation is also taken into account in the construction of Dostoevsky's women.

Svidrigailov then goes on to speak of homosexuality in women – a factor I believe to be decisive in women's psychic development, in the constitution of their femininity.[93] Speaking of his wife, Svidrigailov asks himself:

> And however she came to risk taking such a beautiful creature into her house as a governess. [...] My explanation is that Marfa Petrovna was an ardent and impressionable woman and simply fell in love herself – literally fell in love – with your sister.[94]

If we think of Marfa Petrovna's outrage when she catches Svidrigailov and Dunya together, of her subsequent remorse and the visits she makes to all the village families to defend Dunya's honour, it becomes clear that Dostoevsky's reasoning resembles the Freudian conception of paranoia and jealousy.[95]

Next, Svidrigailov speaks of the danger for women of feeling pity for a man. He observes:

> And if once a girl's heart is moved to *pity*, it's more dangerous than anything. She is bound to want to "save him", to bring him to his senses, and lift him up and draw him to nobler aims, and restore hm to new life and usefulness.[96]

This, of course, brings to mind hysteria, both masculine and feminine. But what clinical practice has taught me is that the man a woman very often chooses as her first life partner occupies the place of the mother, or is someone she wants to "save" from himself, to redeem.

When he occupies the place of the mother, the relationship is one where he acquires a hold over her; the woman may, for instance, be delighted to have this other person tell her what to think and what to wish for. She participates willingly in this alienating relationship in which she suffocates, makes herself as unobtrusive as possible, and is willing to remain mindless.

When the man is to be saved, sacrifice is the dominant attitude. More precisely, self-sacrifice which, together with dissatisfaction and sadness, contributes to a constant tension bordering on paranoia under the guise of manic defences. It goes without saying that these two possibilities can be combined, and that hate is never far from the surface.

Regarding this hatred, the wife of the alcoholic probably gives the clearest illustration of the reaction formation masked by this "devotion". I am reminded of the late François Perrier's definitive conclusions on this subject, with which he was, unfortunately, only too familiar. He shared them in a talk on alcoholism given before a very large audience, as part of Piera Aulagnier's seminars at the Sainte-Anne Hospital. During that final period of his life, one could see in him the distressing mix of strength and despair reminiscent of Marmeladov, Sonya's father. What he said was: "You want to know what an alcoholic is, don't you? I will tell you, in the most abbreviated form: the alcoholic is a child. And he only meets fri-i-i-igid women". The man whom a woman intends to save, and the man whom she places in the position of an all-knowing authority, are also unhappy children she comforts, contrary to the wife of the alcoholic, who tortures them. But unconscious psychic functioning makes no such distinctions: self-sacrifice for the sake of saving the other may be a mere disguise of the constant torture to which the other is subjected.

The last point Svidrigailov makes about women concerns the effects flattery has on them. He speaks of "the most powerful weapon in the subjugation of the female heart, a weapon which never fails one. It's the well-known resource – flattery". And he goes on:

> Nothing in the world is harder than speaking the truth and nothing easier than flattery. If there's the hundredth part of a false note in speaking the truth, it leads to a discord and that leads to trouble. But if all, to the last note, is false in

> flattery, it is just as agreeable and is heard not without satisfaction. It may be a coarse satisfaction, but it is still a satisfaction. And however coarse the flattery, at least half will be sure to seem true.[97]

Of course, this philosophy is that of the pervert *Don Juan*, whose teachings were likely well-known to Svidrigailov. The fact is that this conception points to a complication in the constitution of feminine desire: the integration of phallic function and narcissism. This integration is always difficult, but is seriously jeopardised in a woman whose mother failed to provide an adequate container for the child's psychic needs, and later did not adequately transmit the symbols of femininity.

Desire and flattery

While Freud succeeded in formulating rather precisely the major problems of masculine sexuality, which taken together amount to his refusal to accept the feminine component of his personality, he was less successful in defining the problems of feminine sexuality. He did, however, point to the heart of the matter by speaking of penis envy (even speaking of the "impossibility" to overcome it). And then the Women's Liberation Movement arrived on the scene.

The feminist movement of the 1960s took up this concept where Freud had left it, and brought a refreshing perspective to it. Sometimes awkwardly, wildly, even laughably, women in those years nevertheless promoted the right idea by setting aside penis envy and presenting the problem of women as related to being a subject, to desire and to involvement with thought.

Their work focused on the social and political aspects of the place assigned to women in institutionalised culture. They objected to the unequal treatment of women, and demanded that this difference be acknowledged.

But although the Movement produced undeniably positive political and cultural effects, on the theoretical level it remained within the framework of ideological sociology. The Movement examined the important questions mentioned above, but did not contribute to resolving the question of the feminine version of phallicism.

During that period, Lacan was also losing interest in penis-centred theories and developing theories on the relation of the desiring subject to the phallus, whose relation to the penis is one of metonymy.

How valid is this? It's hard to say. Lacan never considered the question in terms of feminine phallicism. On the contrary, he solved the problem by employing a witticism: "The Woman does not exist". At the same time, the conditions were in place for women to reflect on the radical affirmation of desire and of thought as fundamental psychic stakes in women's lives. (Of course, this has nothing to do with the inanities invented at the time about feminine thinking, feminine writing, and so on.)

Women analysts did not solve the problem either. Those classified as "culturalist" put forth simplistic ideas such as breast or womb envy in men – a childish reversal of Freud's concept of penis envy. In France, there was even a naturalist theory of two types of unconscious, to which was added the assertion that unless a woman accepts the actual back-and-forth movement off the penis, she remains captive of her own nature – a concept that seduced many male psychoanalysts, even among the best.

All these detours bring us back to the truth of the perverse idea that flattery is a means of seduction. This idea expresses the obvious: everyone likes being admired and valued for one's qualities. People love to be loved. Men, women and children alike. What is perverse is to lie when saying the things that the other expects to hear, consciously and unconsciously, the things that can be expected of life, and which an encounter promises. The lover says these things to his beloved, who is, for him, the most marvellous being in the world. These words seduce, of course, but most importantly, they serve to root narcissism in desire. Nevertheless, our clinical practice confirms the Freudian hypothesis that narcissism is more fragile in women. This is not a question of nature but is due to the fact that the relation of a girl to her mother is much more complicated than that of a boy.

Thus, as far as love is concerned, and therefore analysis – every analysis is a love story – the awareness of another person's desire enhances narcissism and is a celebration of life. For a woman, two things are at stake, simultaneously, and they both reinforce her narcissism: one is the fact that her desire is welcomed in all its force (something many men have trouble doing), and the other is her being recognised as other, with her own way of thinking – this is what it means to have her phallicism recognised. The disappointment provoked by the pervert usually concerns the first of these elements: it is narcissistic disappointment. Although it is painful, this disappointment does not affect expectations related to the ideal of having one's phallic position acknowledged. On the contrary, if perverse deception goes so far as to promise the welcoming of desire and of the woman's singularity, disappointment causes the collapse of dreams of narcissistic fulfilment, as well as dreams of the recognition of a phallic position as legitimate. This can propel the woman into madness, as illustrated by Liza, who was destroyed by the Underground Man.

But if the promise is made by a man who is in love, or by an analyst, things will not be simple for these men. A woman whose narcissism is exalted by love, whose thinking and desire are celebrated – in short, a phallicised woman – will attempt by any means available to her to place the lover or the analyst in the role of the good primary maternal figure who accepts everything and never contradicts her, who is pure affirmation. This strategy is aimed at extinguishing desire, in order to spare oneself the huge psychic effort of maintaining a phallic position in harmony with an encounter which makes it possible for the other to be recognised as different, a position providing an opening that leads to new possibilities. This processing of the encounter is completely unconscious, and legitimate. It is up to the lover or the analyst to hold his ground.

We have now come to the end of the second stage of the meeting between Raskolnikov and Svidrigailov. The next stage is absolute horror: a married woman the latter seduces in classic Don Juan style, a young girl found drowned, a 16-year-old fiancée ("When I go now I take her on my knee at once and keep her there. [...] The present betrothed condition is perhaps better than marriage"), a 13-year-old girl and her mother whom he meets in a shady dance hall and takes under his wing by offering to provide for the girl's education. [...] In short, the erotisation of hate.[98]

Raskolnikov had thought that choosing the perverse solution could protect him from suffering through indifference, which allows distancing from pain. But listening to Svidrigailov convinces him that this solution involves endlessly repeated murder. He is frightened and is afraid for Dunya. The perverse solution is rejected, bringing about Raskolnikov's decision to give himself up.

Strongly repulsed by Svidrigailov, Raskolnikov wanted to get away from him as fast as possible. He was thinking:

> "To think that I could for one instant have looked for help from that coarse brute, that depraved sensualist and blackguard!" [...] And as far as his sister was concerned in all this, here Raskolnikov remained convinced quite assuredly that Svidrigailov would not leave her alone.[99]

The inhuman as part of the human

The meeting between Svidrigailov and Dunya provides a glimpse into the enigma of what love is for a pervert, an enigma we have already encountered in *Notes from Underground*. Dostoevsky warns us discreetly to be careful when he introduces this meeting by making what seems to be a strange comment. Just after Raskolnikov tells himself that Svidrigailov is a depraved and loathsome man, Dostoevsky comments: "Raskolnikov's judgment was uttered too lightly and hastily: there was something about Svidrigailov which gave him a certain original, even a mysterious character".[100] (Let us note, in passing, Dostoevsky's respect and affection for his characters – all of them – as well as his amoral attitude. These traits contribute to the powerful quality of his writing.)

Let us, like him, be vigilant and subtle, and speak first of affection. Svidrigailov's affection for Dunya is already visible when Raskolnikov meets him in the tavern, just before his rendezvous with Dunya. Then, when he speaks of Dunya to her brother, his mocking tone is not enough to cover up his feelings. He says:

> And however she [his wife] came to risk taking *such a beautiful creature* into her house as a governess. [...] Hang it all, why is she *so handsome*? [...] How your dear sister's eyes can flash sometimes! [...] I assure you that this glance *has haunted my dreams*; the very rustle of her dress was more than I could stand at last. I really began to think that I might have a fit or something. I could never have believed that I could *be moved to such a frenzy*. It was essential indeed, to be reconciled, but by then it was impossible.[101]

His feelings for Dunya are obvious, and not only in what he says. At times, he is overwhelmed with passion; for instance, when speaking of her marriage to Luzhin, "Svidrigailov struck the table with his fist impatiently".[102]

There is no doubt that Svidrigailov uses cynicism to distance himself from his feelings of love. But I believe this to be a secondary defence. His primary defence consists in attempting to transform his feelings of love into mere sexual excitement. As we shall see subsequently, this attempt fails. But this is how he presents things, and to a certain extent he believes what he is saying. For instance, speaking of his feelings for Dunya, he says: "it began on my side with a most irresistible [sensual] desire".[103]

Svidrigailov can be seen as a good illustration of the economy of enjoyment. This type of pleasure is related to a psychic functioning which does not admit satisfaction. In this economy, *for the subject to feel that he exists*, a high level of tension must be present at all times, and everything must constitute a source of tension. In this economy of enjoyment, even sexual excitement is merely tension which *takes the place* of psychic excitement that the subject cannot experience as such. But Svidrigailov's attempt to transform psychic excitement into purely sexual excitement – or just pure tension – fails.

It is precisely at the moment when he must admit that Dunya does not love him that Svidrigailov is stunned to discover that he loves her. This discovery causes the diminished internal world he has left to disintegrate, and reinforces his suicidal intention, because the sudden emergence of love destroys the unconscious theory governing his psychic functioning. This is the theory asserting that hate weaves relationships and fear provides the hold that makes them last. In this regard, let us remember what Svidrigailov told Raskolnikov, speaking of Dunya: "Do you know, I was *so wild about her* at that time that *if she had told me* to poison Marfa Petrovna or to cut her throat [...] it would have been done at once!"[104]

This unconscious theory takes the form of a conviction when it penetrates consciousness. This is why Svidrigailov sees no contradiction between his feelings of love and the setting of a trap and is sure that doing this will not diminish Dunya's possible tender feelings for him. This same conviction sustains him when Dunya threatens him with a revolver, and even more when she shoots at him – "She is trying to frighten me, which proves that she loves me" – might be the unconscious thought explaining Svidrigailov's relative calm when Dunya becomes frenzied like a hunted animal.[105] Psychoanalytic practice teaches us that, more often than is generally believed, the certainty that violence and hate are intimately related to love provides psychic comfort.

Svidrigailov suddenly loses this conviction:

> Suddenly she flung away the revolver. "She's dropped it!" said Svidrigailov with surprise, and he drew a deep breath. A weight seemed to have rolled from his heart, – perhaps not only the fear of death. [...] It was a deliverance from another feeling, darker and more bitter, which he could not himself have defined.[106]

This deliverance from a heavy burden, from pain, is no doubt the result of a sudden and fleeting bursting forth of the belief that the terrible solitude in which the pervert is drowning has come to an end. This fleeting moment is enough for Svidrigailov to recognise the reality of love:

> He went up Dounia and gently put his arm round her waist. She did not resist, but, trembling like a leaf, looked at him with suppliant eyes. He tried to say something, but his lips moved without being able to utter a sound.
> "Let me go!" Dounia implored.
> Svidrigailov shuddered. Her voice now was quite different.
> "Then you don't love me?" he asked softly.
> Dounia shook her head.
> "And [...] and you can't. [...] Never?" he whispered in despair.
> "Never!"
> There followed a moment of terrible, dumb struggle in the heart of Svidrigailov. He looked at her with an indescribable gaze. Suddenly he withdrew his arm. [His belief is destroyed, denial disappears. He is a dead man standing.] "Make haste! Make haste!" [he] repeated still without turning or moving. But there seemed a terrible significance in the tone of that 'make haste'." [It is clear that it took all the self-control he had not to kill her.]

Once the one he loved was gone,

> Svidrigailov stood by the window for about three minutes. [...] A strange smile twisted his face. [...] The revolver Dunya had thrown aside [...] had landed near the door. [...] It could be fired one more time. He thought for a moment, put the revolver into his pocket, took his hat, and went out.[107]

He would later kill himself with Dunya's weapon. Outside, rain is pouring down in a steady stream. Dostoevsky lets Svidrigailov get drenched to the skin – this man whose eyes never shed a tear. And he has him go from one end of the city to the other – a ghostly vision – going from house to house to distribute his money before he kills himself.

He spends his last night in a small, stuffy room under the stairs of an out-of-the-way hotel – a kind of sordid *underground*. But, unlike the Underground Man, he does not complain. Now he is no longer one of the living dead, but already a corpse with mice scurrying across his body. And this corpse dreams of dead children, of defiled children.

Indeed, there is no place for living children in a world without movement, without play, without surprises, without beginning or novelty. This is why, as he had told Raskolnikov, time and the future are old, abandoned things, already dead.

For Svidrigailov's final gesture, Dostoevsky generously – and brilliantly – gives him back the coherence of his perverse defences. Thus, Svidrigailov kills himself before a simple soldier, in whose frightened gaze he tries to see the reflection of the hatred he feels for his own unthinkable suffering.[108]

V. The Sonya solution

After leaving Svidrigailov, Raskolnikov walked several times by the Neva; he "wanted to end it there, but [...] [he] couldn't make up [his] mind",[109] he would later tell Dunya. It is after six in the evening when he finally goes to visit his mother. He has decided to denounce himself to the police and goes to say good-bye to her.[110] He finds her reading for the third time his article "Ordinary and Extraordinary Men". I believe Dostoevsky provides this detail to remind us of the ideological framework in which Raskolnikov's reflection takes place. In fact, during his visit to his sister, right after leaving his mother, he says:

> "Crime? What crime?" he cried in sudden fury. "That I killed a vile noxious insect, an old pawnbroker woman, of use to no one! [...] Killing her was atonement for forty sins. She was sucking the life out of poor people. Was that a crime? *I am not thinking of it, and I am not thinking of expiating it,* and why are you all rubbing it in on all sides? 'A crime! A crime!'"[111]

Thus, Raskolnikov is not at all thinking, as his sister imagines, of expiating or washing away anything.

> "All men shed [blood]," he put in almost frantically, "which flows and has always flown in streams, *which is spilt like champagne, and for which men are crowned in the Capitol and are called afterwards benefactors of mankind.* Look into it more carefully closer and understand it! I too wanted to do good to men and would have done hundreds, thousands of good deeds to make up for that one piece of stupidity – not stupidity even, simply clumsiness, for the idea was by no means so stupid as it seems now that it has failed... (*Everything seems stupid when it fails.*) [...] *if I had succeeded I should have been crowned with glory, but now I'm trapped.*"[112]

It is important to note that there is no difference between what he says now, a few minutes before giving himself up to the police, and what he was thinking before killing the old moneylender. He even makes a terrible comment with which we can't help agreeing: "Ah, it's not picturesque, not aesthetically attractive! *I fail to understand why bombarding people by regular siege* [...] *is a more honourable.*" And he goes on: "*The fear of appearances is the first symptom of impotence. I've never, never recognised this more clearly than now, and I am further than ever from seeing that what I did was a crime*".[113]

If he does not consider himself a criminal, if he does not believe in expiation or in God – "I didn't believe, but just now, with mother, I wept as we embraced each other" – then why is he giving himself up?

> *Only now I see clearly the imbecility of my cowardice, now that I have decided to face this superfluous* [shame]. *It's simply because I am contemptible and have*

> *nothing in me that I have decided to, perhaps too for my advantage, as that* [...] *Porfiry* [...] *suggested!*[114]

Thus, Dostoevsky excludes the possibility of purely masochistic pleasure, since he speaks of the *needless shame* of Raskolnikov's decision. Therefore, we must look elsewhere for the meaning of his decision. For now, the words to remember are "absurdity" and "giftlessness". He gives himself up because he sees himself as "not gifted" and therefore ordinary. And since he is not an extraordinary man, everything he does becomes "absurd". And if everything is absurd, he must admit that there was madness in what took place. So Raskolnikov decides to face his madness. But what is he doing exactly when he goes to the police?

By doing this, he takes the first step on a path, without knowing where it leads. He can take this path because, at his request, Sonya shows him the way. Therefore, two questions have to be answered: first, after telling Sonya his secret, why does Raskolnikov ask her, and no one else, what to do about his failure? And second, how does he imagine what awaits him if he follows Sonya's advice?

He hesitates between two options. At times he questions his innermost thoughts: "everything now is going to [...] be broken in two. [...] Everything, everything, and am I prepared for it? Do I want it myself? They say it is necessary for me to suffer!"[115] At other times, he thinks about his situation in more general terms: prison life, the years spent in captivity, being a broken man afterwards. His last meeting with Sonya before giving himself up and just after saying good-bye to his sister does not put an end to his hesitation, but gives the reader valuable insight.

On his way to see Sonya, at nightfall, his thoughts indicate clearly that he accepts this hardship – whose meaning we are trying to discern – because he knows he is loved: "But why [do they love me so] if I don't deserve it? Oh, if only I were alone and no one loved me, and I myself had never loved anyone! *Nothing of all this would have happened*".[116] Indeed, if he was "alone and no one loved me and I myself had never loved anyone!", hate would have taken over and he would have chosen the "Svidrigailov solution". Once he rejects this option, the love others have for him, especially Sonya, is what persuades him to confess the double murder to the police. But what is this love made of?

Raskolnikov's last meeting with Sonya before he gives himself up does not provide a clear answer to this question. When he asks her to give him *her crosses*, he says: "It was you who told me to go to the crossroads; why is it you are frightened now it's come to that?"[117] Sonya had, in fact, turned pale when she heard him, "but in a moment she guessed that the tone and the words were a mask".[118]

Raskolnikov took one of her crosses, and then crossed himself several times, as Sonya asked. Then he went out. When he reached the middle of the square, in the Haymarket, he fell on his knees and kissed the earth – because Sonya had told him to do this. Then he went to the police to confess his crime, so that Sonya's wish could be fulfilled. But he says that what most annoys and angers him is that "all those stupid brutish faces will be gaping at me directly, pestering me with their stupid questions, which I shall have to answer".[119] But in that case, why does he do everything Sonya advises?

Raskolnikov takes Sonya's advice as a newcomer follows the rituals that include him in the symbolic order of the community which takes him in. In the same way as in Africa a stranger first sees the elders of the tribe; and just as a Jew must observe the *mitzvot* – all the commandments in the Torah – to belong to the community.

What is essential here is that by following Sonya's instructions Raskolnikov agreed to enter a symbolic order. He knew "that Sonia was with him for ever and would follow him [...] wherever fate might take him".[120] But where is she taking him? Certainly not to Siberia. Siberia is a place of penal punishment – something Raskolnikov considers a mere detail. What, then, is this path Sonya points to, and which he takes without knowing where it leads? And why Sonya? And who is Sonya?

We know very little about Sonya. Marmeladov's description of her focused on her abnegation: she sold herself to feed her family, and she submitted to his drunken tyranny. The reader may attribute this to masochism, but this hypothesis falls away when we see her interacting with the other characters in the novel. Raskolnikov was drawn to her kindness, her artlessness and her modest, childish look. After she meets her for the first time, Dunya tells her mother: "I am sure that she is a good girl, and that [what people say about her] is all nonsense!"[121] After their second meeting, Dunya

> *looked at Sonia almost with reverence.* [...] Dounia gained one comfort at least from that interview, that her brother would not be alone. [Sonia] would go with him wherever fate might send him. Dounia did not ask, but she knew it was so [...] Sonia [...] felt herself, on the contrary, hardly worthy to look at Dounia. *Dounia's gracious image, when she had bowed to her so attentively and respectfully at their first meeting in Raskolnikov's room, had remained in her mind as one of the fairest visions of her life.* [122]

Grace, beauty, purity. Sonya recognises them in another because she possesses them herself. She says not a word, yet one knows she is reliable and loyal, and people even venerate her. Why?

Later, in the Siberian prison, another question Raskolnikov can't decide is:

> why were they all so fond Sonia? She did not try to win their favour; she rarely met them, sometimes only she came to see him at work for a moment. [...] She never gave them money, did them no particular services. [...] And when she visited Raskolnikov at work, or met a party of the prisoners on the road, they *all* took off their hats to her. "Little mother Sofya Semyonovna, you are our dear, good little mother," coarse, branded criminals said *to that frail little creature*. She would smile and bow to them and everyone was delighted when she smiled. *They even admired her gait* and turned round to watch her walking; they admired her too for *being so little*, and, in fact, did not know

> what to admire her for most. They even came to her for help in their illnesses.[123]

To be a speck of dust

Even Svidrigailov respects and admires Sonya. Raskolnikov's mother is the only one who doesn't like her and finds her strange.[124] One is reminded of the story where a mother surprises her son by guessing that he is in love with a certain woman. When he asks how she knew, she says: "Because I hate her already".

Katerina Ivanovna, speaking with the clarity of madness, vouches for the young woman's purity, selflessness and honesty. Despite appearances, she defends Sonya against Luzhin's accusations, even before hearing the two testimonies that were to destroy the slanderer's scheme.[125]

What does Sonya think about? Apparently, not very much. Dounia and Razumikhin

> at first found Sonia's letters [from Siberia] *dry and unsatisfactory*, but later on they came to the conclusion that the letters could not be better, for from these letters they received *a complete picture of their unfortunate brother's life.* [Her] letters were full of the most matter-of-fact detail, the simplest and clearest description of all Raskolnikov's surroundings as a convict. *There* was no word *of her own hopes* [...] *no descriptions of her feelings.* [...] The picture of their unhappy brother stood out at last with great clearness and precision.[126]

How are we to understand this setting aside of oneself to allow the real to emerge clearly?

Of course, women are the obvious source of suffering for men. But in the Dostoevskian universe, they are, as they should be, a source of hope. Insisting on truth, they expect men to keep their word and to respond to love. All this is well and good, and everything could unfold in the usual manner, that is, with the anxiety foreseeable when love is involved. But, for Dostoevsky sex is a sin. His women protagonists are either fascinating because they accept their sexuality – and then feel too guilty to allow themselves to be in love – or they ignore sexuality and become madwomen or maternal figures. In addition, in Dostoevsky's work women do not have an active relation to thinking. Although they exemplify truth or use it to denounce lies or cowardice in men, they usually construct only a narrative of common sense. In short, Dostoevsky portrays women who are hysterics, hysterical madwomen, or hysterically maternal. Since Dostoevsky's men are perverse, psychopathic, psychotic or are themselves hysterics, we can see that real love between them is bound to be very difficult. In fact, *true love* does not exist in the Dostoevsky work. What does exist are remarkable descriptions of the pitfalls which usually prevent its appearance.[127]

In this panoply of women, Sonya stands out. But, after all, who is this Sofya Semyonovna Marmeladova?

Sonya is a speck of dust, inconsequential, a little frail thing, a fluffy cloud. In one of her plays, Leslie Kaplan wrote:

> I want to be a speck of dust
> it's quite pleasant
> dust floats
> lightly
> in the air
> a speck of dust
> I have no obligations
> and I float
> like a tiny cloud
> a cloud
> no one holds it responsible
> a cloud moves
> a cloud is displaced
> by the wind
> in the sky
> it has a colour
> white grey black
> it has a shape
> that's all
> it needs nothing else
> and that is why
> looking at clouds
> is appeasing[128]

Yes, one can be a speck of dust, one can be a cloud. It's possible, but you have to get there. Not everyone can do it, because even though being a speck of dust is not so crazy, being nothing but a speck of dust, nothing but a cloud, definitely requires some acquaintance with madness.

In Wim Wenders' film about Pina Baush, a dancer says that Pina once told her: "You have to be crazier" – and this advice completely changed her way of dancing. You must not be afraid of being even crazier, if you want to become nothing.

And what does one become, when one becomes nothing? One becomes pure space: a space of shelter, a place of transit – it depends. This flexibility opens onto infinity and is frightening.

To be nothing, to be a place, requires the suspension of all self-esteem. I have already spoken of this absence of pride when describing the Underground Man and Svidrigailov. I pointed out that this lack of pride came from their indifference to everything, from their insensitivity. I also said that this way of being can exert fascination, and that this fascination can constitute a way of acquiring a hold on others, the foundation of the pathological relation the pervert demands.

The Sonyas of the world are a whole other story. For these women, lack of concern with themselves allows all possible identifications, is the source of the interest they take in others, the place from which all horizons can come into view, the basis of absolute hospitality, welcoming the other's difference and singularity.

Let us remember what Raskolnikov thinks of Sonya: "He was afraid of Sonia too. Sonia stood before him as an irrevocable sentence. *He must go his own way or hers.* At that moment especially he did not feel equal to seeing her".[129]

Why is Sonya's selflessness so frightening? And why does it create distance? Why is it daunting? Because by abandoning all the trappings of the ego, Sonya becomes a space that can *contain* everything. Be careful when you are told "You can tell this person *everything*", because such a person may be able to *hear everything*. There is a similarity between Sonya's attitude, that of a good primary maternal figure, and the attitude required of the analyst in his work.

Therapists know that being able to *hear everything* does not involve having no desire or paying no attention to the meaning of what one thinks or feels. Complete availability does not prevent an ethical requirement, or the respect of limits and of the *framework* in which the encounter with the other takes place. A psychoanalyst has his metapsychology; Sonya has her religion – to each his theory.[130]

The usual conception of a good primary mother figure emphasises her protective qualities. This aspect is present and should be pointed out. But the sphere in which a good primitive mother functions brings us to the most mysterious facets of the construction of a human being and a subject. There is no passion here, only what I call *the pure desire for the desire of the other.*

One day I had the intuition that *the first identification is identification to a place*: a protective place in which what dominates is *the pure desire for the desire of the other*, the desire that the subject may emerge in his absolute singularity, that he be unique. Sonya is the place where Raskolnikov can deposit his impulses, his thoughts, his inadequacies, his plans, his attempts at desire. But there is a price to pay: that of accepting that this disorganised and fragmented deposit be *processed, questioned*, that is, *interpreted*, by the frame of thought of the subject who receives it. Sonya's frame of thought is governed, as it is in every good primary mother figure, by the *pure desire for the desire of the other.* This means, *necessarily*, that the interpretations have to be taken into consideration, which *requires* that the representations of ideals deposited in this psychic space be seen in the light of *the pure desire for the desire of the one who deposits them.* For this to happen, these representations of ideals must be considered before their final organisation – the presumption being that they go back to the moment when they emerged. As long as Raskolnikov refuses this regression, he uses hate to attack the impulse which drove him to make Sonya his witness.

The encounter between Sonya and Raskolnikov

Dostoevsky waits until he has written one third of his book before giving Raskolnikov a glimpse of Sonya at her dying father's bedside. In fact, Marmeladov dies in her arms. Sonya was wearing attire to suit her work: a gaudy silk dress and a straw hat with a bright feather – so unsuitable in those circumstances. Despite her frightened expression, once can see that she is "rather pretty, with fair hair and wonderful blue eyes".[131] She is eighteen, of small stature and thin.

When a little girl, one of the daughters of Marmeladov's widow, runs after him as he is leaving the deceased man's house to ask for his address, he is happy. He *knows* that Sonya sent her.

He sees Sonya again when she comes to his lodgings. He introduces her to his mother, to his sister and to Razumikhin. He is visibly excited to see her, and becomes flushed when he speaks to her. Noticing this, his mother tells Dunya: "So he must [care for] her".[132] He also regains his good humour and can show his affection when he teases his friend Razumikhin about being in love with Dunya. But how did Raskolnikov's love come to be, since he had only seen Sonya twice? It is certainly not explained by her delicacy – and courage – when she says:

> "You gave us everything yesterday," Sonia said suddenly, in reply, in a loud rapid whisper, and again she looked down in confusion. *Her lips and chin were trembling once more.* She had been struck at once by Raskolnikov's poor surroundings, and now these words broke out spontaneously.[133]

This is *when Sonya started to fall in love with Raskolnikov*. For him, this happened before – let us remember his happiness when the little girl, sent by Sonya, ran after him to ask for his address.

It is likely that our hero began to love Sonya after hearing the things Marmeladov said about his daughter, this child so greatly loved by her father. That a father could cherish his child so much is certainly a fundamental unconscious element in Raskolnikov's love for Sonya. [Bear in mind that in his dream about the beating of the horse, Raskolnikov's father is portrayed as absent or indifferent.] This possibility of love is confirmed when they meet for the first time, when Marmeladov is on his deathbed. But what exactly in Sonya provides this confirmation? Raskolnikov became aware that

> her blue eyes were so clear, and when they lighted up, there was such a kindliness and simplicity in her expression that one could not help being attracted. Her face, and her whole figure indeed, had another peculiar characteristic. In spite of her eighteen years, she looked almost a little girl – almost a child. And in some of her gestures, this childishness seemed almost [comical].

Thus, it is this promise of childhood that attracts him and makes him fall in love with Sonya – childhood, the place of all new beginnings. But he pushes away this love for a long time, and only accepts it after tremendous hesitation; in the meantime, he acts just as Razumikhin described: "He does not like showing his feelings and would rather do a cruel thing than open his heart freely".[134]

When Raskolnikov first visits Sonya at her apartment, he imagines three possible explanations for the way she endures her suffering: she could be suicidal, she could be mad, or she could draw pleasure from depravity. When he understands her infinite tolerance and generosity, qualities he had already sensed in her, which he secretly wanted to discredit, *he drops down to the ground before her and kisses her foot*, saying: "I did not bow down to you, I bowed down to all the suffering of humanity".[135] After this, he asks her to read from the Bible the passage about Lazarus.

And yet, throughout this visit, Raskolnikov wonders whether Sonya is mad. In his attitude towards the young woman there is the same cruelty as that shown by the Underground Man towards Liza. Like the Underground Man, he torments her, predicts a terrible future for her, and showers her with frightening conjectures. Raskolnikov even conjures up a scene involving a murderer and a prostitute, in a seedy decor. But thanks to the young woman, who, unlike Liza, is neither bitter nor mistrustful, the two tormented characters become humanised, find each other and recognise each other as soul mates. Afraid of dropping his guard, Raskolnikov continues to speak in a sharp, even brutal, tone. But in the end, his need, his sensitivity and his honesty express themselves with one voice:

> I have only you now. [...] Let us go on together. [...] I've come to you. [...] *If you remain alone you'll go out of your mind like me.* You are like a mad creature already. So we must go together on the same road! Let us go![136]

Later, Raskolnikov decides to visit Sonya again, to confess the murder. He goes to see her as soon as he leaves the memorial meal given by Katerina Ivanovna for Marmeladov, where he passionately defended the young woman against the slanderous accusations made by Luzhin, the novel's detestable character *par excellence*. In his spirited and earnest speech, Raskolnikov even declared his love for Sonya openly when he said: "[her] honour and happiness are very precious to me".[137]

Dostoevsky emphasises that his hero *had to* confess the murder to Sonya. This "clinical" remark indicates clearly that Raskolnikov understands the necessity and urgency of speaking to another, if he wants to avoid going mad: "he felt at the very time not only that he could not help telling her, but also that he could not put off the telling. *He did not yet know why it must be so*, he only *felt* it, and the agonizing sense of his impotence before the inevitable almost crushed him".[138]

Why does he feel *crushed*? Because speaking to another means abandoning your illusions of omnipotence. There is also the risk that the other will not understand, or will find what you say strange, exaggerated or even crazy. Raskolnikov knew all this. This is why, when he reached Sonya's house, "he felt a suddenly impotence and fear".[139]

He starts by creating a diversion, to attempt establishing complicity with Sonya. He asks her if she would be able to eliminate Luzhin, the swine, to spare Katerina Ivanovna suffering. She replies: "How could it happen that it should depend on my decision – who has made me a judge to decide who is to live and who is not to live?"[140] This answer is essential for understanding her reaction once Raskolnikov has confessed being the moneylender's assassin.

The narration goes on to describe Raskolnikov's psychic pain when he breaks his silence, when he abandons his omnipotence, when he shares his secret, and when he faces the fear of being rejected or considered mad. With good reason, Dostoevsky presents this scene as one in which lovers declare their love, an encounter between two beings eager for honesty and truth, who play for the highest stakes.

At the very moment when Raskolnikov is about to confess,

> a strange surprising sensation of a sort of bitter hatred for Sonia passed through his heart. As it were wondering and frightened of this sensation, he raised his head and looked intently at her; but he met her uneasy and painfully anxious eyes fixed on him; there was love in them; his hatred vanished like a phantom.[141]

This sudden transformation of hatred into love, which characterises what Freud calls the primary process, is a common occurrence in extreme situations – and being in love is an extreme situation. At the very moment when the psychic need for absolute acceptance by the other becomes primordial, attacking the link is a surreptitious attempt to destroy the encounter and thereby avoid the danger – which always exists – of being rejected. The love he sees in Sonya's eyes gives Raskolnikov strength and leads him back to his desire to speak. As he starts to speak, the reality of the actual murder comes back to him:

> His sensations at that moment were terribly like they were at the moment when he had stood over the old woman with the axe in his hand and felt that "he must not lose another minute". [...] He could not utter a word.

Sonya, like any loving beloved, went over and "sat down [...] beside him [...] not taking her eyes off him". Then, "[a] pang of terror passed through Sonia's heart".[142] Raskolnikov has deposited in Sonya's being the horror he feels but cannot name. This is the particular moment in burgeoning love when the lovers become a single subject composed of two people. Such an entity sometimes emerges in the analytic process as well.

Their exchange continues in this fashion: Raskolnikov deposits in Sonya's being the horror he feels but cannot name, and she supports him, allowing him to put it into words. She gives her supports ingenuously, for she cannot have guessed anything. "and yet now, as soon as he told her, it suddenly fancied that she had really foreseen *this* very thing".[143]

What follows is so extraordinary that it must be quoted at length:

> All of a sudden she started as though she had been stabbed, uttered a cry and fell on her knees before him, she did not know why. "What have you done – what *have you* done *to yourself*?" [Sonya falls to her knees as Raskolnikov had done during his first visit] she said in despair, and jumping up, she flung herself

on his neck, threw her arms round him and held him tightly. [This violence indicates that Sonya is now in a different position. No longer simply a container, she has become her own person.]

Raskolnikov drew back and looked at her with a mournful smile. "You are a strange girl, Sonia – you kiss me and hug me when I tell you *about that* [...] You don't think what you are doing".

— "There is no one, no one in the whole world now so unhappy as you!" [Not only does Sonya take in unnamable affects, she formulates a living definition of Raskolnikov (what psychoanalysts call an identificatory statement). Here, for the first time, Sonya uses the familiar form of address "you". (And she will go back to the formal form later in the conversation.) Sonya's (Dostoevsky's) remarkable intuition impels her to speak to the child, to speak of the mistreated part of him.]

[A]nd she suddenly broke into violent hysterical weeping.[144]

Raskolnikov no longer alone

A feeling long unfamiliar to him flooded his heart and softened it at once. He did not struggle against it. Two tears started into his eyes and hung on his eyelashes.

"Then you won't leave me, Sonia?" he said, looking at her almost with hope.

"No, no, never, nowhere!" cried Sonia. "I will follow *you*, I will follow you everywhere. [...] Why, why didn't I know *you* before! Why didn't you come before?" [Here again, she has an astounding intuition – probably accurate – that if she had known him before, the crime may not have taken place.] "Together, together!" she repeated, as it were unconsciously, and she hugged him again. "I'll follow *you* to Siberia! [...] How could *you*, you, a man like you? [...] How could you bring yourself to it?"[145]

Raskolnikov explains his theory of *ordinary and extraordinary men*. But before that, he says:

"I asked you for one thing, I came to you for one thing – not to leave me. You won't leave me, Sonia? [...] And can you love such a mean wretch?"

"But aren't you suffering too?" cried Sonia. Again a wave of the same feeling surged into his heart, and again for an instant softened it.[146]

Sonya promises him that although she does not understand anything yet, she will find the strength to understand: "speak, speak, I shall understand, I shall understand *in myself!*"[147] [Sonya is convinced – remarkably – that a position of ignorance provides the best chance for understanding the beloved.]

Raskolnikov speaks haphazardly, telling her about his poverty, his solitude, his fruitless inner monologues, the lengthy silence in which he has lived: "'I haven't talked to anyone for so long, Sonia.' [...] Sonia saw how he was suffering".[148]

Then he expounded his theories, which were very complex for Sonya. She said nothing, but heard what he said. She "felt that this gloomy creed had become his faith and [law]".[149] Dostoevsky takes great care to show that Sonya understands by means of her particular conceptual framework. This is how her great intelligence is revealed.

And then, perhaps because she asks no questions and only listens with an attitude of respect and openness that only love or friendship make possible, he is able to tell her, and no doubt himself, for the first time and in a deeply felt manner, what had remained unthinkable until then: "I only wanted to have the daring, Sonia! That was the whole cause of it!"[150] Thus, he had given himself a challenge in the hope of gaining self-esteem. An act of daring to overcome the difficulty he had in trying to love himself, to compensate for the loneliness of the child he once was, and for the absence of someone to talk to. This act of daring, this challenge he gave himself, is in fact a desperate attempt to bring himself to life – a rebirth whose impetus is rooted in the most archaic fibres of the being.

He went on: "I wanted to murder without casuistry, to murder for my own sake, for myself alone!"[151] This is the first time Raskolnikov presents his project as *a gratuitous act* – something perfectly coherent with his theory of the extraordinary man, who can commit a meaningless act. "I wanted to find out then and quickly: whether I was a louse like everybody else or a man"[152] – a reminder that we cannot escape the meaning of our deeds. The urgency to which Dostoevsky refers (*find out quickly*) points to the hero's excited and feverish state, to a pressing need for immediate release, to the impulsive nature of Raskolnikov's act. "Listen, when I went to the old woman's I only went *to try*... You [should know] that!"[153] He does not say this as a justification. Contrary to the characters in Sartre's *The Roads to Freedom*, whose direct ancestor he is, for Raskolnikov the fact that he wanted *to experiment* is an aggravating factor. What he says next proves it: "Did I murder the old woman? *I murdered myself, not her! I crushed myself once for all, for ever* [this is the real reason he comes to Sonya. He is dead and he wants to come back to life. This is why he had asked Sonya to read the biblical passage about Lazarus, when he first visited her.] *But it was the devil that killed the old woman, not I*".[154] These last two sentences help us understand the perplexing statement Raskolnikov keeps repeating, in which he denies being the perpetrator of the crime, while admitting that he has committed a murder. What I find important to point out, is that the meaning of such a split is rooted in affect, and that the discovery of the affect can reduce the split.

> "What suffering!" A wail of anguish broke from Sonia.
>
> "Well, what am I to do now?" he asked, suddenly raising his head and looking at her with a face hideously distorted by despair.[155]

Sonya does not judge Raskolnikov. On the contrary, she recognises and understands his suffering at once, and even guesses, as I said earlier, that it is the suffering of a child. But she does not hesitate to call his act a crime, an insult to the living, to humanity. In other words, Sonya does not identify Raskolnikov to his madness; she considers his action insane. And she tells him exactly what she thinks he should do to deserve to reenter the human community. Her recommendations are simple, even childish, but Raskolnikov – who will consent to follow them out of love for Sonya – knows that they are *symbolic gestures* that initiate a process in which his frame of thought, and literally the whole meaning of his life, will be overturned.

To this is added a huge complicating factor – common in the initial stage of falling in love. Raskolnikov experiences it, as lovers always do, very painfully:

> He looked at Sonia and felt how great was her love for him, and, strange to say he felt it suddenly burdensome and painful to be so loved. Yes, it was a strange and awful sensation! [...] now, when all her heart turned towards him, he suddenly felt that he was immeasurably unhappier than before.[156]

Why this unhappiness, why this pain? Because the play of love presupposes that the one who loves recognises in the beloved qualities that the latter is not aware of having, or that he denies. This in turn means that he consents to being reinvented and expected to leave behind the usual framework of his self-representation. Sometimes, this inevitable idealisation of the beloved by the lover, instead of nurturing the desire for the desire of the other, can be experienced as persecutory, as a burden. The range of responses to the feeling of persecution goes from attacking the link by resorting to hate, to demanding symbiosis which turns the other into an extension of one's own internal world. Another response to the fear of being so greatly loved is massive inhibition of any show of emotion; impotence in men and frigidity in women are the most common symptoms of this response.

Young therapists are often surprised when a patient wants to stop the analysis just after moving away from the "trauma zone", when conditions are in place for things to improve. Since patients are very aware of their analysts' emotions, they can feel persecuted by the joy of the latter in response to partial results achieved in analysis. They are afraid of not living up to the expectations and hopes associated with the analyst's joy. Freud once remarked that he was not sadistic enough to want the Good of his patients. This bit of irony can serve as a warning against premature enthusiasm: one cannot say just anything to anyone at any time.

Epilogue: Coming out of madness, leaving pain behind, encountering the other

The Epilogue of *Crime and Punishment* is short – something which has often been criticised. But life in a prison camp had already been the subject of Dostoevsky's *Notes from a Dead House* (sometimes translated as *The House of the Dead*).

Dostoevsky was twenty-eight when he was arrested, at four in the morning on an April day, by the Tsarist police, for having read aloud, on two occasions, an open letter addressed to Gogol after the latter began to defend the political status quo. The letter was written by an influential Russian intellectual. Dostoevsky was condemned to "the degradation and confiscation" of all his personal property, and to the death sentence. To be clear, he was sentenced to death for having read the letter to a small group of progressive-minded young intellectuals who met regularly to discuss books banned by the autocratic regime; the group was falsely denounced by an informer as a gathering of dangerous conspirators preparing an imaginary plot.[157]

At the trial, Dostoevsky admitted the charges but pleaded not guilty: he stated that Belinsky's letter was "a literary monument", that literature relies on freedom of press, and that the printing press he bought with several of his friends was intended solely to allow them to print a few copies of their own literary works.

Three days after the verdict, the military tribunal which had tried him commuted the sentence to eight years of hard labour. Two days later, the Tsar himself changed the sentence to four years and ordered the staging of a horrific mock execution: the prisoners – the entire Petrashevsky group had been arrested – were to believe until the last minute that they would be executed. They were brought before a firing squad, their eyes were covered, they heard the order to aim and only then were they told about the pardon granted by the Tsar, and had their sentences read. One of the prisoners went mad.

Ten years later, Dostoevsky described this experience in *The Idiot*:

> But the chief and worst pain may not be in the bodily suffering but in one's knowing for certain that [...] now, at [this] very moment [...] one will cease to be [...] and that that's bound to happen; the worst part of it is that it's *certain*. [...] Perhaps there is some man who has been sentenced to death, been exposed to the torture and has then been told, "you can go, you are pardoned". Perhaps such a man could tell us. It was of this torture and of this agony that Christ spoke, too. No, you can't treat a man like that![158]

The *House of the Dead* (translated literally, "The Dead House") recounts the four years Dostoevsky spent in a prison camp. The book passes on to the reader two essential conclusions about life: that "man is a creature that can get accustomed to anything", and that "it is very hard to understand a man, even after long years!"[159] The second conclusion implies a third: that a degree of amoralism is needed if one is to understand what another man is capable of feeling, of imagining and of doing, and to what extent the inhuman is part of the human.

The prison camp was in Siberia. It housed common criminals and people accused of military crimes. There were two hundred and fifty prisoners in all.

> Probably more than half of them actually could read and write. [...] The divisions were distinguished from one another by their dress: some had half their jackets brown and half grey, and the same with their trousers – one leg dark brown and one grey. [...] Our heads were shaved in different ways too; some had half the head shaved lengthways and others transversely. [...] The majority were corrupt and horribly depraved. [...] [Even] the terror of whole villages and towns [...] looking about him, soon realized that he had come to

the wrong place, that there was no one he could impress here, and he gradually [...] fell in with the general tone. This general tone was apparent externally in a certain peculiar personal dignity of which almost every inmate of the prison was acutely conscious. It was as though the status of convict [...] was a sort of rank, and an honourable one too. There was no sign of shame and repentance!

[...] backbiting, intrigues, womanish slander, envy, quarrelling, hatred were always conspicuous in this hellish life. [...] Yet surely it would have been possible [...] to have detected something [...] which would have borne witness to some inner anguish and suffering in those hearts. But it was not there, it certainly was not there.

Of course, prisons and penal servitude do not reform the criminal; they only punish him. [...] [This system] drains the man's vital sap, enervates his soul, cows and enfeebles it, and then holds up the morally withered mummy, half imbecile, as a model of penitence and reformation.

Only in prison I have heard stories of the most terrible, the most unnatural actions, of the most monstrous murders, told with the most spontaneous, childishly merry laughter. I am particularly unable to forget one *parricide*.

[...] on rare occasions [...] some prisoner would grow talkative, and another would listen coldly and gloomily. [...] I remember how a robber began once when he was drunk [...] telling how he *had murdered a boy of five*, how he had enticed him first with a toy, led him away to an empty shed, and there had murdered him.

Work, occupation, were not formally forbidden; but it was strictly forbidden to have [...] any tools. [...] But [people] worked by stealth. [...] Many convicts came to the prison knowing nothing, but they learned from others, and afterwards went back into the world skilled workmen. There were cobblers there, shoemakers, tailors, cabinet-makers, locksmiths, woodcarvers and gilders. [...] They got orders for work from the town.

I could never have imagined [...] how terrible and agonizing it would be, never once for a single minute to be alone for [all the] years of my imprisonment.[160]

In his Siberian prison, Raskolnikov was ashamed.

But it was not his shaven head and his fetters he was ashamed of: *his pride had been stung to the quick. It was wounded pride that made him ill.* [...] His exasperated conscience found no *particularly terrible fault in his past,* except a simple *blunder* which might happen to anyone. *He was ashamed just because he, Raskolnikov* [...] *must humble himself and submit to "the idiocy" of a sentence, if he were anyhow to be at peace.* [...] *"In what way," he asked himself, "was my theory stupider than others that have swarmed and clashed from the beginning of the world? One has only to look at the thing quite independently, broadly and uninfluenced by commonplace ideas and my idea will by no means seem so* [...] *strange.* [...] *Why does my action strike them as so*

> *horrible?* [...] *Is it because it was a crime? What is meant by crime? My conscience is at rest. Of course, it was a legal crime, of course the letter of the law was broken and blood was shed.* [.... *Of course, in that case many of the benefactors of mankind who snatched power for themselves instead of inheriting it ought to have been punished at their first steps. But those men succeeded* and so *they were right,* and I didn't, *and so I had no right to have taken that step.*[161]

It is clear that Raskolnikov, when he begins his life in the prison camp, believes that his crime is not really a crime, and that he was right to carry out the plan his ideas suggested to him. But now his ideas do not hold the same place they did before he consented to give himself up, out of love for Sonya – a love he still tries to resist. Before he gave himself up, his beliefs made him the founder of a new symbolic order, the one who overturns the old order. Now that he has accepted to be judged, he can despise his judges as much as he likes, but he cannot deny the existence of the world which judges his act.

In his new setting, his old convictions become delusional rationalisations. Raskolnikov falls ill, very ill. "*He held aloof from everyone* [...] *his fellow prisoners did not like him* [...] *he kept silent for days at a time and was becoming very pale*".[162]

Like the Underground Man, he has no regrets. The indifference he so fervently wished for has now rendered him unable to feel anything:

> And if only fate would have sent him repentance – burning repentance that would have torn his heart and robbed him of sleep, that repentance, the awful *agony of which brings visions of hanging or drowning!* Oh, he would have been glad of it! Tears and agonies would at least have been life. But he did not repent of his crime.[163]

The other prisoners did not like him.

> He was disliked and avoided by everyone; they even began to hate him at last. [...] A quarrel broke out, he did not know how. All fell on him at once in a fury. "You're an infidel! You don't believe in God," they shouted. "You ought to be killed!" He had never talked to them about God, nor his beliefs, but they wanted to kill him as an infidel. He said nothing.[164]

Raskolnikov has become a ghost. In his notes, while writing *Crime and Punishment,* Dostoevsky had written these words, to be spoken by Raskolnikov when he confesses to Sonya: "Did I murder the old woman? I murdered myself, not her! I crushed myself once for all, for ever".[165]

Like any ghost, zombie or one of the living-dead, he cares neither about life nor about death:

> One of the prisoners rushed at him in a perfect frenzy. Raskolnikov awaited him calmly and silently; his eyebrows did not quiver, his face did not flinch.

> The guard succeeded in intervening between him and his assailant, or there would have been bloodshed.[166]

Raskolnikov falls ill and is taken to the prison hospital. There, he can finally abandon himself to suffering which "*brings visions of hanging or drowning*".[167]

His love for Sonya – he loved Sonya before she loved him – demanded a price: that he consent to consider his act a murder, and admit that after killing the moneylender and Lizaveta, he carried two ghosts in himself, which made him a corpse, psychically speaking (*Did I murder the old woman? I murdered myself, not her!*). But admitting this *requires* a change in the *frame of thought*. As we may remember, his *act* sprang from convictions intended to establish a set of new premises for a new understanding of the world. Recognising his failure is painful. But admitting that there still is life after this failure means invalidating his action and proposing (once again!) the creation of a new frame of thought. Abandoning all convictions, accepting the loss of all points of reference and all support, is a Herculean task. It is an enormous psychic effort, compounded by the pain of knowing that one's old convictions have become delusional certainties.

It is the strength of Sonya's love – Sonya, a speck of dust, Sonya pure subject, pure receptivity to the other – which allows Raskolnikov to enter this "illness" known as psychotic regression. Here, "illness" refers to the abandoning of all ideals, of everything representative of the ego function. During his "illness", nightmares are the therapeutic tools serving to get through psychosis. They illustrate the fragmentation of the ego, murder, cannibalistic impulses.

This confirms the hypothesis of British psychoanalyst D.W. Winnicott, a brilliant clinician, who understood that psychosis is closer to psychic health than are the ideals of normality. Let us note that Dostoevsky's idea of madness is the same as Freud's and Winnicott's. Dostoevsky had already understood the indistinction between the normal and the pathological. He lets Zossimov, the young doctor who tends Raskolnikov, express this idea. In response to a comment made by Dunya, Zossimov says:

> There is some truth in your observation. [...] In that sense we are certainly all not infrequently like madmen, but with the slight difference that the deranged are somewhat madder. [...] A normal man, it is true, hardly exists. Among dozens – perhaps hundreds of thousands – hardly one is to be met with.[168]

But let us return to Raskolnikov's "illness". In this context, his nightmares are part of the process of adopting a new frame of thought. But first, nightmares must illustrate the fragmentation of the ego and elaborate a critique of his old convictions about the murder of the moneylender. These nightmares must also deal with the two corpses he carries inside him.

Let us look at the content of the nightmare. As a reaction to the theory of extraordinary men: "But never, never had people considered themselves so intelligent and unshakable in the truth as did these infected ones. Never had they thought their judgments, their scientific conclusions, their moral convictions and beliefs more unshakable". As an illustration of the fragmenting of the ego: "*All were excited and did not understand one another. Each thought that he alone had the truth and was wretched looking at the others*".[169]

The psychic work set in motion by the nightmares will succeed in putting an end to the eroticisation of thought (eroticisation of thought refers to the great tension associated with any imaginary scenario, tension which requires discharge through action: eroticisation renders the "circuit" between thought and action very short). When thought is no longer eroticised, daydreaming becomes possible. Raskolnikov dreams of Sonya, thinks of Sonya.[170] *To love is to think*, says the great Portuguese poet Fernando Pessoa. At the end of his "illness", Raskolnikov's psychic being can inhabit his body again; he is no longer a ghost.

> He had even fancied that day that all the convicts who had been his enemies *looked at him differently; he had even entered into talk with them and they answered him in a friendly way*. [...] But he could not think for long together of anything that evening, and he could not have analysed anything consciously; *he was simply feeling. Life had stepped into the place of theory and something quite different would work itself out in his mind.*[171]

Dostoevsky considers Raskolnikov's emergence from psychosis a resurrection. This is Sonya's perspective as well. Raskolnikov escapes from the world of the dead and from the hold of the corpses of the moneylender and Lizaveta, and this is crucial. But the most important thing, I believe, is that *for the first time in his life*, he desires the desire of the other. This is why he thinks of his beloved constantly, why he dreams of her. In short, Sonya was right to have faith.

Raskolnikov's mood changes, his fluctuating emotions, his wide range of subjective positions, his resistance to listening and depending on another; and then comes the recognition of the link and its consequences: regression and a new organisation of desire – all these things taken together are what could be called the catastrophic advent of love. When this takes place in the course of a psychoanalytic treatment, it is called transference.

Let us give Dostoevsky the last word:

> But that is the beginning of a new story – the story of the gradual renewal of a man, the story of his gradual regeneration, of his passing *from one world into another, of his initiation into a new unknown life*.[172]

I said earlier that the double is a fundamental element in Dostoevskian narration. It structures the relations between characters in a very definite manner. So much so, that it can serve as the key to deciphering a novel, an incomplete but enlightening element based on the question: who is the double of whom?

We will now examine the work of reference illustrating this narrative element in Dostoevsky's work.

Notes

1 Kaplan, L., "L'Expérience du meurtre", in *Les Outils*, p.43.
2 Gauchet, M. (1999), *The Disenchantment of the World*, Burge, O. (trans.), Princeton University Press.
3 See *Letters to a Young Psychoanalyst*, letter 28: "Loup Verlet. Psychoanalysis as a Revolution of the Conceptual Framework".
4 Winnicott has said of psychic health that it is closer to madness than to normalcy.
5 Vidal-Naquet, P. (1990), Preface to *Tragédies de Sophocle*, Gallimard, p.12 and p.17.
6 Aristotle (1981), *The Politics*, Sinclair, T.A. (trans.), Penguin Classics.
7 Letter sent by Dostoevsky to M. A. Katkov, September 12, 1865.
8 Frank, J. (2012), *Dostoevsky: A Writer in His Time,* Princeton University Press, p. 478.
9 Dostoevsky, F. (1960), *Notes from Underground*, p. 96.
10 Dostoevsky, F. (2000), *Crime and Punishment*, Wordsworth Classics, Garnett, C. (trans.), p. 3. Dostoevsky's emphasis, then mine.
11 There is one other clear indication given by Dostoevsky of Raskolnikov's thinking about the murder before he commits it: "he decided that in his own case there could not be such a morbid reaction, that his reason and will would remain unimpaired at the time of carrying out his design, for the single reason that his design was 'not a crime'. [...] *We will omit all the process by means of which he arrived at this last conclusion*" (pp. 63–64). My emphasis.
12 Dostoevsky, F., *Crime and Punishment*, p. 45.
13 Ibid., pp. 10–11.
14 Ibid., p. 14.
15 Ibid.
16 Ibid., p.11.
17 Ibid., p. 21.
18 See "True Love" in *Letters to a Young Psychoanalyst.*
19 "Le hazard et la réalité", in Topique, N° 63, 1997.
20 Dostoevsky, F., *Crime and Punishment*, p. 97.
21 Ibid., pp. 47–48.
22 Ibid., p. 53.
23 Ibid., pp. 54.
24 The conversation between Razumikhin and Zossimov, his young doctor friend who treats Raskolnikov, about a common acquaintance, reveals Razumikhin's character and sensitivity. Ibid., pp. 116–117.
25 Dostoevsky, F., *Crime and Punishment*, pp. 46–47.
26 Ibid., p. 45.
27 Ibid., pp. 91–92.
28 Ibid., p. 97.
29 Ibid.
30 Ibid., p. 98.
31 Ibid., pp. 99–100.
32 In *Letters to a Young Psychoanalyst.*
33 Dostoevsky, F., *Crime and Punishment*, p. 116.
34 Dostoevsky, F., *Crime and Punishment*, p. 120. My emphasis.
35 Ibid., p. 127.
36 Ibid., pp. 128–129.
37 Ibid., p. 129.
38 Ibid., pp. 131–132.
39 Ibid., p. 185.
40 Ibid., pp. 220. My emphasis.
41 Ibid., pp. 258–59. My emphasis.
42 Ibid., pp. 222–223. Dostoevsky's emphasis.
43 See above, section on Raskolnikov.

44 Dostoevsky, F., *Crime and Punishment*, p. 225. My emphasis.
45 Ibid., p. 214, pp. 216–217. My emphasis.
46 As Razumikhin observes, commenting on the meeting with Porfiry; p. 229.
47 Dostoevsky, F., *Crime and Punishment*, pp. 226–227. My emphasis.
48 Ibid., pp. 284–285.
49 Ibid., p. 287.
50 Ibid., p. 295.
51 Ibid., p. 336.
52 Ibid., p. 290.
53 Ibid., p. 387.
54 Ibid., p. 290.
55 Ibid., p. 379.
56 Ibid., p. 294.
57 Ibid., p. 379.
58 Ibid., p. 380. My emphasis.
59 Ibid., pp. 386–387. My emphasis.
60 Ibid., pp. 385–386. My emphasis.
61 See *Letters to a Young Psychoanalyst*, "The Celestina Superego and the Dulcinea Superego", op. cit.
62 Dostoevsky, F. (1915), "Akulka's Husband", in *The House of the Dead*, Garnett, C. (trans.), London: Heinemann, p. 208.
63 Dostoevsky, F., *Crime and Punishment*, p. 389.
64 See also Winnicott, D.W. (2005), "Dreaming, Fantasizing and Living", in *Playing and Reality*, Routledge Classics: "Suicide brings no solution, only cessation of struggle", p. 35.
65 This is what Raskolnikov tells Sonya. Svidrigailov's account of this exchange – given that his cynicism and envy guarantee objectivity – testifies to the persistence in Raskolnikov of the need to identify what is at stake when he struggles with his torments.
66 Dostoevsky, F., *Crime and Punishment*, p. 239.
67 Part III ends with Svidrigailov entering Raskolnikov's room and introducing himself. Yet Part IV starts as we have described.
68 Dostoevsky, F., *Crime and Punishment*, p. 241.
69 Ibid., p. 239.
70 Ibid., pp. 241–242.
71 Ibid., p. 243.
72 Ibid., p. 244. My emphasis.
73 Ibid., p. 245.
74 Ibid., p. 246. My emphasis.
75 Ibid.
76 Ibid., p. 246. My emphasis.
77 Ibid.
78 Ibid., p. 246. My emphasis.
79 Ibid., p. 247.
80 Ibid., p. 241.
81 Ibid., p. 249.
82 Ibid., pp. 250–251.
83 Ibid., p. 389–390. My emphasis.
84 Ibid., p. 393.
85 Ibid., p. 394.
86 Ibid., p. 394.
87 Ibid.
88 Ibid., p. 395.
89 See above, chapter on *Notes from Underground*.
90 Dostoevsky, F., *Crime and Punishment*, pp. 395–396. My emphasis.
91 Ibid., p. 397.
92 Ibid.

93 This theme is examined in chapter VIII of my book *De l'Amour à la pensée*, L'Harmattan, 1994.
94 Dostoevsky, F., *Crime and Punishment*, p. 398.
95 Her hatred of Dunya is only a projection of homosexual attachment, intolerable for the ego.
96 Dostoevsky, F., *Crime and Punishment*, p. 399. Dostoevsky's emphasis.
97 Ibid., p. 400.
98 Ibid., p. 404.
99 Ibid., p. 409.
100 Ibid.
101 Ibid., p. 398, pp. 400–401. My emphasis.
102 Ibid., p. 402.
103 Ibid., p. 400.
104 Ibid., p. 401–402. My emphasis.
105 This could provide an opportunity to think about the relation between the *instinct for mastery* and *denial.*
106 Dostoevsky, F., *Crime and Punishment*, p. 418.
107 Ibid., p. 418. One of my patients took a lover she described as a virile man, with whom she had a good enough sex life, in any case, better than she could have with her paralysed companion. Her lover made all the decisions and never asked for her opinion. He was often very cold and miserly but could also be very considerate to her. She tolerated this control he wanted over everything, since it stayed within the limits of her relatively restricted relationship with him. But the first time they took an extended trip together, these traits became unbearable to her and she told him so in a fit of anger. He was very happy to see her angry and told her a secret: he had always dreamed of being mistreated and humiliated by a woman during the sexual encounter. Would she be willing to do this? Very surprised but touched by his honesty which she correctly interpreted as proof of his love, she asked him why he did not see prostitutes. He answered that this was the first time he had expressed this desire, and he confided it to her because he was sure she would not exceed the limits of what he could endure. He also confessed his fear: that if she accepted, he would never be able to do without her. What is extremely unusual here is that the man formulated his idea of love both in terms of eroticisation of hate (perverse fantasies) and in terms of control (his certainty that he would become dependent on her). Usually, only one of these aspects is openly revealed, as was the case for a woman who accepted the proposal of a man who threatened to seduce and kill her mother, unless she married him. She stayed married to him all her life, and they had three children.
108 Svidrigailov thought that the soldier's face wore the "perpetual look of peevish dejection which is so sourly printed on all faces of the Jewish race" (ibid., p. 430). Earlier, he had told Raskolnikov: "Jews have sprung up and are amassing money" (ibid., p. 405). There is much to say about Dostoevsky's fundamental antisemitism, but that is another subject. We refer the reader to Goldstein, D.I. (1981), *Dostoevsky and the Jews*, University of Texas Press.
109 Dostoevsky, F., *Crime and Punishment*, p. 435.
110 Ibid., p. 431.
111 Ibid., p. 436.
112 Ibid., pp. 435–436. My emphasis.
113 Ibid., p. 437. My emphasis.
114 Ibid., p. 436. My emphasis.
115 Ibid., p. 437.
116 Ibid., p. 438. Dostoevsky's emphasis, and mine.
117 Ibid., p. 439.
118 Ibid.
119 Ibid.
120 Ibid., p. 443.

121 Ibid., p. 207.
122 Ibid., p. 439. My emphasis.
123 Ibid., p. 458. My emphasis.
124 Ibid., p. 207.
125 Ibid., p. 332.
126 Ibid., p. 454. My emphasis.
127 See the chapter titled "True Love" in my book *Letters to a Young Psychoanalyst*, Routledge, 2016.
128 Kaplan, L. (2008), *Toute ma vie j'ai été une femme*, Paris: POL.
129 Dostoevky, F., *Crime and Punishment*, p. 389.
130 In Sonya's case, religion is not something that makes her dogmatic and inflexible; it is, rather, the foundation of the freedom to accept the other without moralising.
131 Dostoevky, F., *Crime and Punishment*, pp. 158–159.
132 Ibid., p. 207.
133 Ibid., p. 205. My emphasis.
134 Ibid., p. 184.
135 Ibid., p. 274. My emphasis.
136 Ibid., p. 280. Dostoevsky's emphasis and mine.
137 Ibid., p. 339.
138 Ibid., p. 342. My emphasis and Dostoevsky's.
139 Ibid.
140 Ibid., p. 344.
141 Ibid.
142 Ibid.
143 Ibid., p. 346. Dostoevsky's emphasis.
144 Ibid., pp. 346–347. Dostoevsky's emphasis and mine.
145 Ibid., p. 347. My emphasis.
146 Ibid., p. 349.
147 Ibid.
148 Ibid., p. 351.
149 Ibid., p. 352.
150 Ibid.
151 Ibid., p. 353.
152 Ibid.
153 Ibid., Dostoevsky's emphasis.
154 Ibid., My emphasis.
155 Ibid., p.354.
156 Ibid., p. 355. My emphasis.
157 In his masterful biography of Dostoevsky, Joseph Frank disagrees with this "innocent" version of events: "Nikolay Speshnev [...] whom Dostoevsky at this time called his 'Mephistopheles', [was] probably the prototype of the character of Stavrogin in *The Devils*". Speshnev, a rich, highly educated aristocrat, irresistible to women, was the head of the Petrashevsky circle, a secret revolutionary society comprised of seven members, including Dostoevsky (who never admitted this compromising affiliation). *Dostoevsky: The Mantle of the Prophet, 1871–1881,* Princeton University Press, 2003, p. 7. My emphasis.
158 Dostoevsky, F. (1996), *The Idiot*, Garnett, C. (trans.), Wordsworth Classics, pp. 18–19. Dostoevsky's emphasis.
159 Dostoevsky, F. (1915), *The House of the Dead*, Garnett, C. (trans.), London: Heinemann, p. 7 and p. 71.
160 Dostoevsky, F., *The House of the Dead,* pp. 9–14; p. 8.
161 Dostoevsky, F., *Crime and Punishment*, pp. 456–457. My emphasis and Dostoevsky's.
162 Ibid., p. 455. My emphasis.
163 Ibid., p. 456. My emphasis.
164 Ibid., p. 458.

165 Ibid., p. 353.
166 Ibid., p. 458.
167 Ibid., p. 456. My emphasis.
168 Ibid., p. 194. My emphasis.
169 Ibid., p. 459. My emphasis.
170 Ibid., p. 461.
171 Ibid., My emphasis.
172 Ibid., p. 462. My emphasis.

3

THE DOUBLE

The Double is Dostoevsky's second novel. It precedes *Notes from Underground* and *Crime and Punishment.* It was also written before the author's deportation to Siberia – an encounter with catastrophe and with humanity that profoundly marked the rest of Dostoevsky's work.

This story establishes the foundation of a key element in the subjectivity of the major characters in future works, and sets the basis for a certain narrative organisation.

The economy of anxiety and shame

Critical reaction to the book was rather negative, and Dostoevsky himself was unhappy with the literary result. But he was certain of the significance of the story and of its innovative character. He attests to this in a letter sent to his brother in 1859: "Why lose a remarkable idea whose social value is considerable, that I was the first to discover and of which I was the herald."[1] And in 1877, four years before his death, he asserted again in *A Writer's Diary*: "Most decidedly, I did not succeed with that novel; however, its idea was rather lucid, and I have never expressed in my writing anything more serious."[2] What exactly was this serious idea? The idea that a human being is not constituted solely of the conscious.

The Underground Man is despicable, he is an assassin. He knows it and declares it openly. He summons the other only to confess how despicable he is, and to confirm that he needs no one, that the other is futile and without interest. The Underground Man is alone in the world. Alone and in anguish. But he does not reject his anguish like an intrusive foreign element; on the contrary, he cherishes it and even puts it on display. He displays it like a defect, like an obscenity – but beware! He asserts and demonstrates that this defect is the very essence of our humanity – and this is why this piece of writing is the foundation of modernity in literature: here, anguish is no longer one *response* among others to the demands of the world.

The Underground Man is not embarrassed by his feelings, he does not hide his actions. His foremost concern is the difficulty he has with his desire. He does not feel guilty about the (perverse) manner in which he resolves his conflict – which he considers *one* way of avoiding anguish (and in this, he is right); he admits that there are other ways: each person has his own.

The economy of anguish is a central concern for Goliadkin, the protagonist of *The Double*. But it is central in a very particular fashion: the fact is that Goliadkin hates anguish with a passion, he wants nothing to do with it and he certainly does not want to feel it. In a way, Mr. Goliadkin resembles those others to whom the Underground Man addresses his commentary, those for whom two and two make four, and *basta*. But not exactly; Mr. Goliadkin would like to be able to say that two and two make four and *basta*, were it not for the fact that the enormity of his anguish – rendered greater because denied – makes everything impossible. Everything: any emotion, any thought. In short, Goliadkin is *ashamed* of everything having personally to do with him. One does not know why Mr. Goliadkin allows himself no trace of intimacy, why every emotion terrifies him – one simply observes it. But because Goliadkin refuses intimacy and the anguish that goes with it, both confront him from the outside, embodied by a double.

Goliadkin teaches us that shame is a mechanism in its own right, rooted in the sensation of displeasure, the initial modality used by the rudimentary psyche to distinguish itself from the surrounding world. Expelling everything unpleasant makes it possible to establish a primary distinction between what is me and what is not me.

Another thing that Mr. Goliadkin teaches us is that the mechanism of shame needs no representation to do its work: in order to expel everything which is foreign, there is no need to name what one evicts, but only to feel burdened by it. This *emptying mechanism* is, of course, very dangerous: if the psyche expels all disturbing sensations, it can end up emptying itself of all sensoriality – and the body that goes with it. In the early stages of life, it is the mother who helps the budding psyche of the *infans* to tolerate the unpleasant; she lessens the intensity of the baby's bodily sensations, so that they can come to be considered familiar, not dangerous. This modulation of intensity allows the psyche to integrate a whole set of experiences and, as a result, to strengthen and consolidate the feeling of its own existence.

For the reader, Mr. Goliadkin's company is unbearably suffocating because the character is constantly involved in a feverish endeavour of evacuation. This endless work of rejecting all psychic events (sensations or inklings of a thought), and his shame at the possibility of *inscription*, are both so foreign to our usual manner of functioning that we become weary and take upon ourselves the terror that fills him, since he throws it off and passes it on to us. I said "inklings of a thought" because Mr. Goliadkin does not have actual thoughts, but rather pictogrammes of thoughts – which he treats like perceptions located outside his psychic world.[3]

Horror, love and the void

When we meet Mr. Goliadkin at the start of the story, this particular mode of functioning is immediately apparent. We do not know the reasons for such a catastrophe, but we can already see its devastating effects. He has just awakened, and we are confronted at once with the horror produced by his surroundings: "The dirty green, smoke-begrimed dusty walls of his little room [...] *looked at him* familiarly. Finally, the gray autumn day, dull and dirty, *peeped* into his room *through the dingy window pane with* [...] *a hostile, sour grimace...*".[4] In short, the real world is looking at him, harassing him, persecuting him. Of course, nothing else is possible; in fact, there is almost no more Goliadkin, there is only a great whirl and the desire to eject this shameful whirl with everything it contains – affects, inklings of thought or of existence and the faint traces of a man once named Mr. Goliadkin.

Why are we so horrified and plunged into the darkest depths by Goliadkin's experience? No doubt because encountering it awakens affects associated with experiences that *must* remain buried and have to do with terror. The terror linked with instances of obliteration, like those when a child is mistreated by a parent, or when someone is subjected to a terrorist regime – situations in which the real, in its totality, becomes threatening and persecutory, since nothing is left to guarantee the meaning of life, and there is no "other" who can confirm the mere continuity of existence: if the referent becomes an assassin, everyone embodies a potential threat of destruction.

During puberty and adolescence, such experiences of obliteration can occur, particularly if the mother has not played her role as intensity regulator for a long enough time in early childhood. In addition to reviewing the affective history he has had up to that point, while temporarily suspending all identificatory models, the young person must accomplish the monumental task of naming and integrating the sensory upheavals, sensual and erotic, which emerge so powerfully at this time. This disturbing accumulation of intimate feelings, often experienced while being subject to shame, ashamed both of oneself and of one's body, sometimes leads to a desperate attempt to evict oneself entirely – with the same consequences as those experienced by Mr. Goliadkin.

Let us come back to him. What has put him in such a state? His meeting with the physician gives us some clues. First, at the time of his previous visit, he was already quite unwell, and caused the doctor to be very concerned. It is probably for this reason that the latter is not very pleased to see him again. Then, during the consultation and despite his incoherent remarks, the reader can guess the cause of all his troubles: Mr. Goliadkin is secretly in love. To put it briefly, we could say that it is because he cannot bear to be in love that Mr. Goliadkin goes mad.

The Underground Man, as we remember, chose to destroy Liza because he could not bear the *living life* she embodied. Mr. Goliadkin is unable to make any choices. The sudden emergence of passion for a woman has immediately triggered convulsions in his very small inner world, in which exaltation and shame erupted at the same time. These feelings reached a peak with the jealousy born of knowing that his beloved has been promised to another man; the exaltation generated a sequence if images of himself as a man of the world, valiant and bold, fearless and without reproach, who tells everyone, except himself, the kinds of truth no one wants to hear. Living up to these images becomes imperative, and this requirement intensifies the feeling of shame to an unbearable degree.

The need to adopt these images, these clichés, is an injunction coming from an internal persecutor, who springs forth from the depths of his torment – an archaic and ferocious persecutor who augments the shame as he continues his attack. There is no space between these clichés and sensitivity; in other words, the imagination does not process these ready-made images, and they certainly don't enter the realm of daydreams. Dostoevsky gives us a precise description of the situation when Mr. Goliadnik's valet tries on the livery rented by his master:

> "— They've brought the livery, sir."
> "— Put it on, and come here."

When he had put on the livery, Petrushka, with a stupid smile on his face, went to his master. His costume was incredibly strange. He had on a much-worn green livery, with frayed gold braid on it, apparently made for a man a yard taller than [him]. In his hand he had a hat trimmed with the same gold braid and with a feather in it, and at his hip hung a footman's sword in a leather sheath. Finally, to complete the picture, Petrushka, who always liked to be in *négligé*, was barefooted now as well: "*Mr. Golyadkin looked at Petrushka from all sides and was apparently satisfied*".[5]

The void, which fills the space between the ready-made images and some small residue of personal existence, forces Goliadkin to dive into it like a man falling from a precipice. These images are too big for him, like his servant's livery; the result is conduct so ridiculous that it only serves to deepen the disaster of his life.

But shame has a cause even more powerful than ridicule: sexuality. Goliadkin is ashamed of the sexual feelings he has for his beloved (I have already spoken of the problematic relation to sexuality we see in Dostoevsky's characters). Mr. Goliadkin's torment becomes obvious while he waits for the meeting his fantasy has promised. To dissipate his sexual excitement, he foresees lecturing his Dulcinea:

> But, to begin with, allow me to tell you, as a friend, that [...] I would have given you and your parents, too, a good thrashing for letting you read French books; for French books teach you no good. There's a poison in them [...] a pernicious poison, madame! Or do you imagine, allow me to ask you, do you imagine that we shall elope with impunity, or something of that sort [...] that we shall have a hut on the shore of the sea and so on; and that we shall begin billing and cooing and talking about our feelings, and that we shall spend our lives in happiness and content; and then there would be the little ones. [...] And how do I come in? Why have you mixed me up in your caprices? [...] And I must own I've never been a beauty to look at.[6]

Out of time, out of the body

The theme of the Father, central in Dostoevsky's work, is also present in Mr. Goliadkin's universe. Traces of it let the reader suppose that before his collapse the question of the father constituted a wish, an expectation, a request: "I [...] look upon my benevolent superior as a father and blindly trust my fate to him".[7] And a little further: "I put my fate in your hands. [...] I look upon you [...] as my father, do not abandon me [...] save my dignity, my honour, my name".[8] A few years later, when Dostoevsky wrote *Notes from Underground*, recourse to the father or to a humanist law had become impossible: "We [...] have long ceased to be born of living fathers, and we like this more and more. We're acquiring a taste for it. Soon we'll contrive to be born somehow from an idea".[9]

After his visit to the doctor, Mr. Goliadkin pretends to be a millionaire, before he is denied access to the home of his beloved's parents, where a few days earlier he had insulted the young woman's fiancé in public – no doubt imagining this to be an elegant way of declaring his love openly. Instead, his act of bravado was met with outrage.

After all the commotion,

> his brain was in the utmost confusion and chaos. For a long time he paced the room in agitation; at last he sat down in a chair, propped his brow in his hands and began doing his very utmost to consider and settle something relating to his present position.[10]

Here, Dostoevsky creates a distortion in the time dimension. A distortion of the greatest import.

The passage quoted above brings Chapter III to an end. Chapter IV starts: "That day [...] was being celebrated by a brilliant and sumptuous dinner-party, such as had not been seen for many a long day".[11] The reader might think that Mr. Goliadkin is remembering an event that occurred recently. But this is not the case. The dinner in question takes place at a time subsequent to the occasion on which we last saw our hero sitting with his head in his hands. In fact, it is a reception where Mr. Goliadkin, the hero of some heroic scenario, finds himself in the midst of guests, before his beloved and his superiors, until the moment when, "looking about him – he almost [went dead]. [...] Every one stood still, every one was silent, every one was waiting".[12] After reading these painful and grotesque passages, it becomes clear that by distorting the text Dostoevsky indicates that his character *is outside of time*, that the present, the past and the future are all compressed in one dimension. Mr. Goliadkin refers to this phenomenon once, much later in the story, when he tries to determine when his beloved wrote him the imaginary letter – a hallucination – he received a short time before his final collapse: "Perhaps she wrote a letter to me yesterday. [...] Or it was tomorrow in the letter, that is, that I".[13]

Let us look more closely at the phenomenon of hallucination. In keeping with my reading of the novella, I would suggest considering everything Mr. Goliadkin thinks and feels as part of a hallucinatory process. I include in this hypothesis the letter he thinks he received from the woman he loves. As it happens, in *The House of the Dead*, Dostoevsky describes the delusional hallucination of a prisoner, a hallucination astonishingly similar to Mr. Goliadkin's fantasy love relationship.

In the prison hospital, one often saw prisoners condemned to receive lashes, who devised all manner of stratagems to delay the carrying out of the punishment. The doctors were very understanding, accommodating and respectful of these dissemblers. But at times, the prospect of the corporal punishment caused the prisoner to go mad:

> I remember another strange madman. There was brought in one summer day a healthy and very clumsy-looking man of forty-five, with a face horribly disfigured by smallpox, with little red eyes buried in fat, and a very gloomy and sullen expression. They put him next to me. He turned out to be a very quiet fellow, he spoke to no one, but sat as though he were thinking about something. It began to get dark and suddenly he turned to me. He began telling me without the slightest preface, but as though he were telling me a great secret, that he was in a few days to have received two thousand "sticks", but that now it would not come off because the daughter of Colonel G. had taken up his case. I looked at him in perplexity and answered that I should not have thought that the colonel's daughter could have done anything in such a case. I had no suspicions at the time; he had been brought in not as a lunatic but as an ordinary patient. I asked him what was the matter with him. He answered that he did not know, that he had been brought here for some reason, that he was quite well, but that the colonel's daughter was in love with him; that a fortnight ago she had happened to drive past the lock-up at the moment when he was looking out of the grated window. She had fallen in love with him as soon as she saw him. Since then on various pretexts she had been three times in the lock-up; the first time she came with her father to see her brother who was then an officer on duty there; another time she came with her mother to give them alms, and as she passed him she whispered that she loved him and would save him. It was amazing with what exact details he told me all this nonsense, which, of course, was all the creation of his poor sick brain. He believed devoutly that he would escape corporal punishment. He spoke calmly and confidently of this young lady's passionate love for him, and although the whole story was so absurd, it was uncanny to hear such a romantic tale of a love-sick maiden from a man nearly fifty of such a dejected, woebegone and hideous countenance. It is strange what the fear of punishment had done to that timid soul. Perhaps he had really seen some one from the window, and the insanity, begotten of terror and growing upon him every hour, had at once found its outlet and taken shape.[14]

We cannot help but admire the clinical description, as well as the hypotheses the author formulates about the genesis of delusion. When reading *The Double*, one is struck by the resemblance between Mr. Goliadkin's fate and that of Dostoevsky's prison-mate in Siberia. This fact is even more troubling considering that the author met the prisoner several years after writing the novella.

Let us come back to *The Double*. When he left the reception, Mr. Goliadkin

> looked as if he wanted to hide somewhere from himself. [...] Mr. Golyadkin did not want only to run away from himself, but to be obliterated, to cease to be. [...] Mr. Golyadkin reached such a pitch of despair, was no harassed, so tortured, so exhausted, and so weakened in what feeble faculties were left him.[15]

This is when the first delusion appears in the story. And immediately afterwards, there is a second fantasy. This one is preceded by the sound of a cannon shot, which in St. Petersburg gave the alarm in case of a flood, since the catastrophic events of 1824.[16] With this sound, the last remaining psychic dams burst, and Mr. Goliadkin is propelled into the reality of the world: Mr. Goliadkin Jr. is born and fills the universe – in anticipation of a time when the whole space would be filled with an infinity of Mr. Goliadkins.

Throughout the story, from the beginning to the definitive dissolution of the person of Goliadkin, the narrator plays an essential role. His contribution is made with great subtlety: his perspective is always that of the narrator, whose words, expressions and linguistic idiosyncrasies he duplicates. This aesthetic choice aims to produce a specific effect. It imprisons the narration in Mr. Goliadkin's psychic world: the reader suffocates just as Goliadkin does. Another consequence of this duplication of the character's perspective is that the novel takes place over a timeless duration, a duration crowded with the accumulation of shame, emptiness and absence, anguish and agitation, terror and trembling, impulsiveness and powerlessness, false deeds and false words, prudishness and aberration, indecision and rage, sideways glances and regrets, seething and fatigue, coldness and exhaustion, excitement and deep sorrow – a duration cluttered with washed-up dreams and desolation.[17]

Once his Double comes on the scene there is no longer any difference between what Mr. Goliadkin feels and reality, between reality and his imaginings, between reality and his inventions or fears. Everything becomes persecution and his entire relation to the world is a hallucination: he lives in a dream or a nightmare he considers a real experience.[18]

The Double and its fates

The relationship between Mr. Goliadkin Sr. and Mr. Goladkin Jr., without its hallucinatory aspect, was to become the paradigm of the *internal* persecutor of all the major characters that followed; this means that the persecutor is part of the character's psychic world, in conversation with another part of this psyche. Raskolnokiv often converses with his internal persecutor, and we have looked closely at one of these typical exchanges in *Notes from Underground*:

"You are a scoundrel," a thought flashed through my mind, "if you laugh at this now!"

"No matter!" I cried, answering myself. "Now everything is lost!"[19]

After the first horror-filled moments of the encounter, Mr. Goliadkin hallucinates that he takes Mr. Goliadkin Jr. home with him. The first evening they sped together is full of sentimental outpourings: Mr. Goliadkin Jr. composes a poem for Mr. Goliadkin Sr. who, "[with] tears in his eyes [says:] 'You and I will take to each other like fish to the water'".[20] A sinister scene depicting a tuneless serenade, in which a mouth twisted with pain soundlessly sings the amorphous geometry of shadows. The two Mr. Goliadkins and reality congregate, hanging on to the gigantic nipple of the void.

This macabre pantomime, in which the double, instead of representing the disintegration of the person, and consequently death, is taken to be a figure of integration, was to play a fundamental role in Dostoevsky's work. It would change into a series of coupled characters, both opposed and complementary, serving to structure the narration. Within these couples, one character is the repressed part of the other, whom he confronts with the truth he is trying to hide from himself: Raskolnikov is the repressed portion of Porfiry; Svidrigailov is the repressed portion of Raskolnikov (in *Crime and Punishment*); Rogozhin is the repressed part of Prince Myshkin (in *The Idiot*). Smerdyakov is the repressed part of Ivan (in *The Brothers Karamazov*), etc.

But Mr. Goliadkin Jr. clearly does not represent the repressed portion of Mr. Goliadkin Sr. Indeed, how can anything be represented when reality no longer exists? After the brief sentimental episode described above, Mr. Goliadkin Jr. becomes the internal persecutor, projected into the outside world – an imaginary persecutor, fierce, sadistic and contemptuous, who will end up bursting into tiny pieces, in an explosion that contaminates all the air we breathe, and transforms our hero into a compact speck of silent pain suffused with horror.

Notes

1 Frank, J. (2012), *Dostoevsky: A Writer in His Time*, Princeton University Press, p 254.
2 Dostoevsky, F. (2004), *The Double: Two Versions*, Translated with an Introduction by Evelyn Harden, New York: Ardis Publishers, in "Translator's Introduction".
3 Regarding the concept of pictogrammes, see Piera Aulagnier's theory in *The Violence of Interpretation*, Sheridan, A. (trans.), Taylor & Francis, 2001.
4 Dostoevsky, F. (1945), *The Double* in *The Short Novels of Dostoevsky*, Garnett, C. (trans.), New York: Dial Press, p. 477. My emphasis.
5 Ibid., p. 479. My emphasis.
6 Ibid., pp. 605–606. My emphasis.
7 Ibid., p. 577.
8 Ibid., p. 596.
9 Dostoevsky, F. (1993), *Notes from Underground*, , p.130.
10 Dostoevsky, F., *The Double*, p. 498.
11 Ibid.
12 Ibid., p. 504.

13 Ibid., p. 603. My emphasis.
14 Dostoevsky, F., *The House of the Dead*, pp. 208–209.
15 Dostoevsky, F., *The Double*, pp. 510–511.
16 Ibid., p. 512.
17 I fail to see why, in his book on Dostoevsky's poetics, an essential work for the understanding of Dostoevsky's aesthetics, Mikhail Bakhtine identifies the narrator with Mr. Goliadkin Jr. See Bakhtine, M. (1984), *Problems of Doestoesvky's Poetics*, University of Minnesota Press.
18 Dostoevsky's treatment of Mr. Goliadkin's hallucinations raised some difficulties for André Green, who wrote a psychoanalytic essay on *The Double*. I quote: "What is tragic in what befalls Mr. Goliadkin is that none of his colleagues, nor his servant, is surprised by the existence of the Double. Of course, they do not think it quite proper that there should be two of them, but no one is surprised by the arrival of the second Goliadkin, although the latter evicts the former to the point of banishing him from society by having him locked up in an asylum – at public expense." Thus, the author of the essay considers Mr. Goliadkin Jr. a real character – he considers that all the other characters share in the hero's delusion. André Green, like Mikhail Bakhtine (quoted above), distinguishes three separate voices: that of the protagonist, that of the Double, and that of the narrator, corresponding respectively to the ego, the superego and the id of Freudian theory. What is interesting here is how applying the conceptual framework of neurosis to traumatic reality renders thinking incomprehensible. See André Green, Preface of Dostoevsky's *Le Double*, Gallimard, 1980.
19 Dostoevsky, F., *Notes from Underground*, p. 96.
20 Dostoevsky, F., *The Double*, p. 532.

4

THE IDIOT

I. Prince Myshkin

The book begins with Prince Myshkin's return to St. Petersburg on a train; his return voyage started in Switzerland and led to Berlin and Warsaw before its final destination. On the train, the prince meets Rogozhin, a young man about twenty-seven years old, of medium height and robust build, with curly, almost black hair, the orphaned son of a millionaire who has died very recently. Rogozhin confesses his passion for Nastasya Filippovna – describing her as a vision glimpsed on the street, who bewitched him.

The prince is twenty-six or twenty-seven years old, slightly taller than average, with very fair, thick hair: "His eyes were large, blue and dreamy; there was something gentle, though heavy-looking in their expression, something of that strange look from which some people can recognise at the first glance a victim of epilepsy".[1]

Before they part, Rogozhin asks the prince:

> "And women, prince, are you very keen on them? Let me know [right off]!"
>
> "I, n-no! You see. [...] Perhaps you don't know that, owing to my illness, I know nothing of women".[2]

The reader has been warned.

From the train station, the prince goes directly to the home of General Epanchin, a wealthy man whose wife was born Princess Myshkin. The prince's attire causes the servant who lets him in to regard him with suspicion, and to hesitate before announcing him to the general. They wait for the arrival of the secretary, Gavrila Ardalionovich – Ganya – and while they wait, defying all convention, the prince enters into conversation with the servant.

The meeting with the general goes very well. He is touched by the prince's simplicity and learns that he has been orphaned at an early age and placed in the care of a tutor with whom the general is acquainted. Seeing his talents as a calligrapher, the general offers him a position and finds lodgings for him, in rooms rented out by Ganya's mother. Then the general sends Myshkin to see his wife, a distant member of the young man's family. But before he leaves, the prince has a chance to hear a strange conversation concerning Nastasya Filippovna; the reader senses that there is something shady in the matters discussed.

The general's wife, Elizaveta Prokofyevna, and her three daughters are in the midst of great excitement. The reader learns that there are plans for a marriage between the eldest daughter, Alexandra, and Totsky, Nastasya Filippovna's so-called "protector". The meaning of the conversation overhead by the prince in the general's office between Ganya and the general becomes clear: in order to marry without the risk of a scandal, Totsky must obtain Nastasya's agreement. That very evening, the evening of the day when Myshkin arrives in St. Petersburg, Nastasya must give her answer: will she, or will she not marry Ganya. This, then, is what is being planned. But before the prince leaves the general's house, we learn that Ganya is in love with Aglaya, the youngest and most beautiful of the Epanchin sisters. And if we add into the mix the general's passion for Nastasya – rumour has it that he plans to give her a string of pearls for her birthday – the situation becomes ambiguous at best and sordid at worst.

Against this background, Nastasya Filippovna's portrait stands out in all its singularity and force. Having lost both parents at the age of twelve, she was brought up under the protection of Totsky, who was touched by the young girl's sweetness and intelligence. A governess was brought in to teach her French and the sciences. Then, at sixteen, she was taken to live in a comfortable cottage, where Totsky came to spend the summers for the next four years. On one occasion, when Nastasya learned about her benefactor's rumoured marriage plans, she travelled to St. Petersburg to tell Totsky that she intended to prevent it, to show him her contempt and her hatred. She announced that

> it was a matter of absolute indifference to her if he married at once any one he chose, but she had come [to St. Petersburg] to prevent him making that marriage, and would not allow it from spite, simply because she chose not to, and that therefore so it must be – "If only that I may have a good laugh at you, for I too want to laugh now".[3]

After this, it is not difficult to imagine what was happening in the cottage during the four years when Totsky visited his beautiful, young protégée regularly every summer.

Interestingly, Myshkin and Nastasya have both lost their parents in childhood. But there is a bond between her and Rogozhin, due to their shared trauma. (In Myshkin's case, the trauma has been cut away, and encrypted in his epilepsy.) But of the three of them, she is the only one who has a past, a story. About Myshkin, the reader knows only that he has just been released from a clinic; as for Rogozhin, the only story in his life is his passion for Nastasya.

Dostoevsky does not take a stand one way or the other regarding Totsky's argument that his protégée's extravagant attitude is nothing more than "a chaotic ferment [...] in mind and heart, something like romantic indignation"[4] – in short, a hysterical reaction. But Totsky's cowardice alone is not enough to justify his fear that Nastasya, having come to "[value] nothing and herself least of all [...] [she] was quite capable of facing hopeless ruin and disgrace, prison and Siberia, only to humiliate the man for whom she cherished such an inhuman [loathing] ".[5]

Cowardice alone is not enough to explain that, like a child, accompanied by his friend, General Epanchin, he goes to her to ask for permission to marry; on that occasion, she tells him, before a witness, that the money he is offering to give her as a dowry when she would marry is "simply a compensation for her ruined life".[6] In fact, not much further, all doubt is completely erased when Ganya, speaking to the Prince about Nastasya, declares that she despises him "because take her, another man's mistress, so openly for her money".[7]

Thinking and psychosis

General Epanchin is obviously very happy to introduce Prince Myshkin to his wife and his daughters. The Prince's arrival could serve as a diversion, and perhaps prevent his wife from asking about the string of pearls he intends to give Nastasya Filippovna as a present – he has good reason to believe that she will broach the subject.

Although very reluctant at first to play hostess to this poor relative – and an idiot to boot – the general's wife is finally enchanted to have met the prince. As they are parting, she tells him: "Good-bye for the present, dear prince. Come and see us often. [...] I believe it's simply for my sake God has brought you to Petersburg from Switzerland".[8]

Elizaveta Prokofyevna's brutal frankness, made possible by her rank and the carefree attitude produced by generations of material comfort, is no doubt appreciated by the prince, who hates social niceties. The prince also makes a good impression on the girls, although in their case other feelings colour this impression. Myshkin fascinates them by his ability to express his feelings and opinions without shame, and by his choice of subjects for discussion. But there is another reason as well.

From the start of the story, when Rogozhin meets Myshkin, Dostoevsky insists on a character trait that endears the prince to everyone he meets (or makes him fascinating): a total absence of pride.

As I was reflecting on *Notes from Underground*, it occurred to me that this work draws attention to the conditions allowing thought to exist: all thinking begins where pride is left behind. I commented at the time that it is impossible to think and also protect oneself from the consequences of one's thoughts. One does not put a thought into words in order to be loved or admired; the intent is to share the thought with others, to submit it to their assessment, to send it out into the world. In addition, an absence of pride makes it possible to perceive with great acuity the most subtle nuances of sensitivity in oneself and in others.

This, then, is the first thread we can follow: Myshkin thinks, but to what purpose?

This is the central question guiding the research I will undertake with you. An investigation of this kind is not conducted out of time, it takes place at a certain moment of a specific era. This means that it is inscribed in the historicity of the field of reflection to which it pertains, and can draw on results obtained previously in this field.

In the preceding chapters, I submitted a hypothesis I believe has been suitably proven: perversion is a defence against psychosis. The demonstration of this hypothesis is based on a metapsychological discussion of what I identify as Dostoevsky's analysis of the human psyche. To conduct this discussion, we have read and reread carefully *Notes from Underground* and *Crime and Punishment*. And we recognised, just as Porfiry did, that dislodging this defence requires transferential and countertransferential strategies, and great effort.

Based on this hypothesis, I will try to give the research a more ambitious scope. The research question could be formulated as follows: how does working with psychotic patients make it possible to perceive differently what thinking means?

As you know, Freud saw a continuity between the normal and the pathological, between psychic health and pathological processes; in his view, the latter highlighted elements of the psyche that were part of its ordinary functioning. The mechanism of *negation* is a clear example of this continuity.

Freud has taught us that when the content of a repressed thought is disqualified by consciousness, its recognition becomes possible and the ego can eventually accept it. Saying "I do not desire (a certain thing)" allows the desire for this thing to exist in the ego-support domain.

Negation is not simply a rhetorical operation through which a desire can be expressed thanks to a negative formulation; the process includes the replacement of one affect by another, and pleasure takes the form of displeasure – I say that I do not like the object of my desire, and by doing so, I tell myself what my desire is.

I wonder whether the psychotic defences – hallucinations, delusions and dissociation – are not means to gain access to an aspect of the functioning of all thought processes, previously unknown and as revealing as the process of negation. What similarity is there between psychotic defences and prolonged coexistence, at the same level of thinking, of psychic investments and various sensations? What relation is there between this type of defence and the emergence of an idea, an intuition or a form previously non-existent? For instance, when we wake up in the middle of the night with an idea that allows us to get to work on a project – like Descartes who woke up thinking "I think, therefore I am". Such dazzling thoughts occur during sleep, when primary or originary processes dominate. Indeed, upon awakening, the certainty of having found a new idea comes from the intense feeling of joy we feel, and the more easily we embrace this feeling, the more precise the idea becomes.

Thinking means finding the modalities illustrating the encounter with the real – the real of the world, the real of the other, the real of emotions – but what interests me most is the aimless drifting of thought while it seeks these modalities, a path which is not that of rationality, and is not located within the framework in which the unconscious aspect of what is thinkable is defined based on its relation to repression.

Negation is a strategy which, by reversing the quality of emotional response, protects the ego, in order to allow the thought about a desire to exist in consciousness. This is another thread to follow: thinking akin to psychotic defences does not burden itself with the ego and shows no particular regard for repressed content. Therefore, this process may be more tolerant and more receptive to the scandal of the real, and could take shape based on the dominant affective response present when the encounter with the event coming from the sphere of the unexpected takes place.

Because his own ego does not stand in the way, Prince Myshkin has an extraordinary ability to identify with the emotions of others, to guess his interlocutor's feelings and name them; while he is waiting with the valet for the secretary to arrive, he can guess what the valet is thinking. He also expresses clearly the reason for the general's embarrassment, as well as his opinion of Rogozhin. Gazing at Nastasya Filippovna's portrait, he speaks of *a wonderful face* and adds that although "*the face is cheerful* [...] *she has passed through terrible suffering*". Later, alone with the portrait again, when the "impression it had made had scarcely left him", just before kissing the painting,

> he was [...] even more struck by the face, which was extraordinary from its beauty and from something else in it. [I find it noteworthy that Dostoevsky speaks of an impression. This word interests me because it is neither affect nor thought; referring to sensation, it designates the region in which divination originates.] There was a look of unbounded pride and contempt, almost hatred, in that face, and at the same time something confiding, something wonderfully simple-hearted. The contrast of these two elements roused a feeling almost of compassion. Her dazzling beauty was positively unbearable – the beauty of a pale face, almost sunken cheeks and glowing eyes – a strange beauty![9]

This type of detailed description of emotional states is one of Dostoevsky's brilliant talents. One last example of prophesy, among many others: when Ganya asks him if Rogozhin would marry Nastasya Filippovna, Myshkin says yes, adding: "he'd marry her and in a week perhaps murder her".[10] And Myshkin will see to it that things go just as he has predicted.

Myshkin drives all those who arouse his affections crazy: he either nurtures the anguish he senses in them, or he provokes it or increases it. But this is not my first concern. Of course, he has "resolved to be [...] open with every one,"[11] to always tell anyone what he thinks, any time, just as he told Ganya, whom he just met: "I can't marry any one, I am an invalid".[12] This "frankness" can be considered, with reason, to be a rationalisation of the prince's perversion. But I would like to consider in a positive light the prince's ability to instantly capture the other's essence, which is a mode of thinking, based on an exacerbated receptivity to the other's sensitivity, feelings and sensoriality.

The General and his daughters

Aglaya does not beat about the bush regarding the perverse traits of the prince, as soon as they meet – although this does not prevent her from falling madly in love with him. She tells him:

> And your philosophy is exactly the same as [...] an official's wife, a widow, [who] calls on us, a sort of sponger. [Let us remember that this conversation is taking place at the General's dinner table, where the prince is a guest.] Her whole purpose in life is cheapness; only to live as cheaply as possible; the only thing she talks about is kopecks – and, mind you, she has money, she's a sly fox. Your immense life in prison is exactly the same, and maybe also your four-year happiness in the village, for which you sold your city of Naples, and not without profit, it seems, though it was only a matter of kopecks.[13]
>
> With your quietism one might fill a hundred years of life with happiness. If one shows you an execution or if one holds out one's finger to you, you will draw equally edifying reflections from both and be quite satisfied. Life is easy like that.[14]

It is surprising how quickly Aglaya understands that Myshkin's remarkable freedom of speech is not solely a result of lack of pride – even the valet noticed it[15]– but also denotes a lack of true interest in anything. With deep sincerity, Myshkin displays his boredom everywhere. And boredom is a form of hate.

But since he is as disinterested in himself as he is in everything else, since he pays no attention to himself and has an ego like a sieve, he is able to identify to an incredible degree with another person; he identifies without moral judgment and so completely that it is impossible not to consider this mode of encounter a promise. This is a complete misunderstanding since, given that Myshkin takes no interest in anything, he is incapable of making a decision. For him, the other is a mere curiosity, which interests him in contrast to the emptiness of his desire. The prince is only a transcriber, a great calligrapher, able to lend his soul like a magnifying mirror to those he meets. Yes, Aglaya is right about him: a finger or an execution, it's all the same as long as it offers him a distraction. Indeed, Aglaya will be the first to fall victim to this morose sincerity.

The prince tells her:

> You are exceedingly beautiful, Aglaia Ivanovna. You are so beautiful that one is afraid to look at you. [...] It's difficult to judge beauty; I am not ready yet.

> Beauty is a riddle. [...] Extremely [beautiful], [said] the prince with warmth, looking enthusiastically at Aglaia. [And he added:] Almost as beautiful as Nastasya Filippovna.[16]

The tremendous violence of this statement is a major reason for the three girls' hesitation to express an opinion about this new person entering their lives. This violence is often present in what the prince says. For instance, he tells Ganya, just after the latter apologies for slapping him:

> "I shall never again look on you as a scoundrel now," said Myshkin. "Just now I thought of you as quite wicked, and you have so rejoiced me all of a sudden. It's a lesson to me not to judge without experience. Now I see that you can't be considered wicked, nor even a very demoralised man. *In my opinion you are simply one of the most ordinary men that could possibly be, only perhaps very weak and not at all original*".[17]

During his first visit to the home of the general's wife, the latter asks him to feel free to talk about any subject he chooses. This is an important detail, since Myshkin chooses mostly horrible topics of discussion. He starts with the last moments in the life of a man condemned to death, and goes on to describe the face of another condemned man. We must keep in mind that he is speaking to three beautiful young girls brimming with life, and to their mother, his hostess. He speaks first to Adelaida:

> One thought came into my mind just now [...] when you asked me for a subject for a picture, to suggest that you should paint the face of the condemned man the moment before the blade falls, when he's still standing on the scaffold before he lies down on the plank. [The prince had already described this moment at length while he was with the valet, waiting to be received by the General.] Why not? [...] It's practically the minute before death [...] that moment when he has just mounted the ladder and has just stepped on to the scaffold. Then he glanced in my direction. I looked at his face and I understood it all. [...] But how can describe it? [Let us note in passing that to paint such a portrait Alexandra would have to travel to France to witness an execution – which is what Myshkin invites her to do.] I thought at the time that a picture of it would be good. You know one has to imagine everything that has been before – everything, everything. He has been in prison awaiting execution for a week at least; he has been reckoning on the usual formalities, on the sentence being forwarded somewhere for signature and not coming back again for a week. But now by some chance this business was over sooner. At five o'clock in the morning he was asleep. It was at the end of October; at five o'clock it was still cold and dark. The superintendent of the prison came in quietly with his guard and touched him carefully on the shoulder. He sat up, leaning on his elbow, saw the light, asked: "What's the matter?"

> "The execution is at ten o'clock".
>
> He was half awake and couldn't take it in, and began objecting that the sentence wouldn't be ready for a week. [...] The next three or four hours are spent on the usual things: seeing the priest, breakfast at which he is given wine, coffee and beef (isn't that a mockery? Only think how cruel it is! Yet on the other hand, would you believe it, these innocent people act in good faith and are convinced that it's humane); then the toilette (do you know what a criminal's toilette is?); and at last they take him through the town to the scaffold. [...] I think that he too must have thought he had an endless time left to live. [...] There were crowds of people, there was noise and shouting; ten thousand faces, ten thousand eyes. [...] There is a ladder to the scaffold. Suddenly at the front of the ladder he began to cry, and he was a strong manly fellow, he had been a great criminal, I was told. [...] At the foot of the ladder he was very pale, and when he was at the top and standing on the scaffold, he became as white as paper, as white as writing paper. His legs must have grown weak and wooden, and I expect he felt sick – as though something were choking him and that made a sort of tickling in his throat. Have you ever felt that when you were frightened, or in awful moments when all your reason is left, but it has no power? [...] When that weakness was beginning, the priest with a rapid movement hastily put the cross to his lips – a little plain silver cross. [...] And so it was till he was laid the plank. [...] It's strange that people rarely faint at these last seconds! On the contrary, the brain is extraordinarily lively and must be working at a tremendous rate – at a tremendous rate, like a machine at full speed. I fancy that there is a continual throbbing of ideas of all sorts, always unfinished and perhaps absurd too, quite irrelevant ideas: "That man is looking at me. He has a wart on his forehead. [...] One of the executioner's buttons is rusty". and yet all the while one knows and remembers everything. There is this one point which can never be forgotten, and one can't faint, and everything moves and turns about it, about that point. And only think that it must be like that up to the last quarter of a second, when his head lies on the block and he waits and [...] *knows*, and suddenly hears above him the clang of the iron! He must hear that! *If I were lying there, I should listen on purpose and hear!* It may last only the tenth part of a second, but one would be sure to hear it. And only fancy, it's still disputed whether, when the head is cut off, it knows for a second after that is has been cut off! What an idea! And what if it knows it for five seconds! Paint the scaffold so that only the last step can be distinctly seen in the foreground and the criminal having just stepped on it; his head, his face white as paper; the priest holding up the cross, the man greedily putting forward his blue lips and looking – and *aware of everything*. The cross and the head – that's the picture.[18]

At this point, the middle sister, Adelaida, interjects, in a somewhat comical manner:

> "And now tell us how you were in love".

> "I haven't been in love," answered Myshkin as gently and gravely as before. "I [...] have been happy in a different way.[19]

Death and the truth

Myshkin now tells the story of a young woman he met while in Switzerland. Suffering from tuberculosis, seduced and then abandoned by a man for whom she left her mother's house, she returned to her village disgraced; she wandered, ill, hungry and barefoot, through the streets of the village. Here, we are reminded of Dostoevsky's distaste for sexuality; the accent is placed on the prince's compassion for this humiliated creature abandoned by everyone. He lavished attention on her, gave her money, kissed her tenderly and helped her gain the affection of the village children. He observed her as she sat sick and alone, outside the village, in a pasture.

> She used to sit a little apart. There was a ledge jutting out in an overhanging, almost vertical rock there. She used to sit out of sight on the stone, right in the corner, and she sat there almost without moving all day, from early morning till the cattle went home. She was by then so weak from consumption that she sat most of the time with her eyes shut and her head leaning against the rock and dozed, breathing painfully. Her face was as thin as a skeleton's, and the sweat stood out on her brow and temples.[20]

During this first visit to the Epanchin family, which lasts no more than a few hours, Myshkin tells three stories. Three stories about death: the thought of death, the link between love and death, and the link between sexuality and death, all of which occupy a dominant place in Myshkin's psychic world. The exchange between him and the general's wife about Nastasya Filippovna's portrait is highly revealing in this regard:

> "That's the sort of beauty you appreciate, then?"
> "Yes, it is," answered Myshkin with some effort.
> "You mean, just that sort of beauty?"
> "Just that sort".
> "Why?"
> "In that face [...] *there is so much suffering*".[21]

If we add to this the fact that Myshkin *knows nothing about the real woman* depicted in the portrait – and that this fact does not worry him at all – we have here the two essential traits of perversion, as Freud defined it: the denial of the difference between the sexes, and the disavowal of castration. The painful emotions associated with denial of the difference between the sexes and with castration are replaced, for Myshkin, by the pleasure drawn from a *feeling of ambiguity*. We often find this enjoyment of ambiguity in Dostoevskian characters – think of Svidrigailov, in *Crime and Punishment*, whom we have already examined.

What I would like to emphasise here is the priority given to an economy of the emotions – the seeking of ambiguous pleasure – over the economy of a representational framework – with its associated concerns with desire and meaning. Indeed, let us remember that it is the absence of pride and of ego-support demands that allows Myshkin to identify so completely with another person. But his way of formulating his thoughts is also, no doubt, greatly influenced by the question of death, and specifically that of being a trauma survivor. Myshkin fears nothing because he has placed himself beyond risk, all risk, including that of death. He speaks from this place and assumes that the person who loves him can join him there. The result can be a revelation – if it reveals to the other something about himself – or the destruction of the psychic balance of the other, with the risk of madness that this involves. In the first case, when a truth-revealing effect is produced, it may be taken as a promise, a promise that creates a bond and the expectation of some continuity – of the meaning and of the story – something of which the prince is absolutely incapable.

An example of this kind of truth is Myshkin's remark to Aglaya about her beauty – "[You're] almost like Nastasya Filippovna" – which she evidently took to be an interpretation. But this interpretation is crucial enough to cause her, a few minutes later, to give the prince the note sent by Ganya. The latter is astonished to learn that – and wants to understand how – the prince has been able to gain his beloved's trust so quickly and so completely. This is a mystery to him. And the whole scene is a mystery to the reader if he does not grasp the interpretation given by Aglaya to the prince's remark about her beauty.

As for the prince, he is obviously unable to understand why Aglaya suddenly places her trust in him. He can't possibly do this because he can never fathom the imaginary consequences of the things he tells others, and less still reflect on the imaginary conditions necessary for revealing to the other an intimate aspect of himself of which he is as yet unaware.

Taking into account the imaginary reverberations of what one says is essential in any therapy, and particularly in psychoanalysis, where the aim is to act on unconscious configurations through transference. It is easy to discern the importance of imaginary after-effects when one is in love – and every analysis is a love story. For instance, telling someone who loves us that we will call at a certain time sets in place a very precise imaginary organisation in that person's relation to temporality. If the call is not made at the specified time, the energy spent by the lover to restructure his realm of imagination and relocate himself in time can be exhausting. This surreptitious ill-treatment becomes obvious, and even ferocious, in the affective relationships between adolescents and their parents.

In the scene we have been discussing, before telling Aglaya that she is not as beautiful as Nastasya – which is the equivalent of an interpretation – the prince had already commented on her exceptional beauty. These two contradictory statements – contradictory within the limits of what a woman's ego can withstand – will provide Aglaya, against all odds, with a new, satisfying image of herself: in addition to recognising her beauty, Myshkin credits her with being able to hear the truth.

We have now undertaken the ambitious task of understanding what it means to make an interpretation. To begin with, let us note that our first impression – which is right – that Myshkin's statement is violent, does not extend to the diversity of messages heard by Aglaya. In other words, the weight of the phenomenological dimension is not sufficient to determine the unconscious consequences of a statement. One can never be sure of how someone hears what he has been told.

Thus, the fact that Myshkin's statement was taken by Aglaya to be an interpretation reveals a fundamental attribute of interpretation: the fact that it does not concern the ego. In this particular case, even in its formulation the statement does not take the ego into consideration. Remember: what the prince tells Ganya, in the example I quoted above, can be described in the same way. This being said, examples of interpretation are rare in the course of an analysis.

Four examples: I am thinking of Françoise Dolto, who received a phone call during a work session with a colleague, and told the caller, after listening for a little while: "You have my complete respect". Then she calmly explained to her colleague: "It was a patient who said he was going to commit suicide". This is interpretation in a setting of transference. Dolto interpreted the violence of the call, rather than the content of the message.

Second example: Gisela Pankow, who told the patient who had come from Germany to kill her: "After all, it's not my fault that your mother chose your brother as a lover, and not you". This interpretation names the unconscious position given to the interlocutor.

Third example: an analyst listening for the thousandth time to the story of the tortures inflicted on the patient by his father: "Your father is a paedophile". An interpretation of the unconscious position of the analysand's father; this interpretation changes the patient's representation of his father, allowing the patient to position himself differently in the unfolding of his story.

Fourth example: the same analyst saying to a patient whose abusive, beloved father died suddenly when she was a small child, and who keeps repeating that she is unable to love: "I am very sorry that I am not willing to die so you can finally admit, out of remorse, how much you love me". In this transference-related interpretation, unconscious idealisation is revealed to be present, along with overt sadism.

Transmitting the unknown

For the moment, I suggest we set aside the various psychic mechanisms at work when the psychoanalyst's interpretation takes form. It would also be best not to concern ourselves here with the difference between, an intrusive and traumatic interpretation and an interpretation in the context of transference which sets in motion psychic elaboration. (We have to admit that any interpretation which conjectures the subject to an extent beyond that made possible by the deciphering of a fantasy could be traumatising – like the interpretation mentioned above, heard by Ganya.) If we examine the four examples I gave earlier – as well as those illustrated by Myshkin's relation to Aglaya and Ganya – we can advance the following hypothesis: interpretation aims to transform the psychic position of the subject. This transformation would make thinkable that which was previously unknown or out of reach. The interpretation, which allows thinking to venture into a territory previously beyond its reach, changes the relation to the unknown; which can then become an object of desire in itself. But transforming the unknown into the thinkable can produce suffering because this shift radically changes the position of the subject: in his relation to himself, to the world, to his past, to present circumstances and to his plans for the future. To desire the unknown involves accepting a certain degree of displeasure inexorably tied to this quest, a displeasure mitigated by the promise of an achievement: the promise of widening the field of the thinkable, of having greater power over one's own psychic responses.

Several Dostoevskian characters, like Prince Myshkin, impart the desire for the unknown. The interest and the pleasure that the prince takes in death, cruelty, suffering and sickness go beyond their morbid character. Myshkin makes it possible for his interlocutors and for the reader to take into their psychic space, for a time, affects and feelings previously unknown to them. No doubt, this context, in which the prince tells Aglaya that she is not the most beautiful woman on earth, is essential in order for his statement to produce an effect of interpretation; Myshkin's statement frees Aglaya from the prison of her beauty, allowing her to contemplate the rest of her life in view of the reality of death. Parenthetically, very beautiful women always feel imprisoned by their beauty, which cuts them off from the world. If love does not free them, they become the servants of an image which eventually turns into a mask behind which hate, pain and emptiness mingle. Alternatively, and very often, in order to live while waiting for love, the woman refuses to be an object of contemplation, and this refusal of her beauty allows her to draw the strength she needs to live fully.

But let us return to Myshkin. The reason for emphasising the effects on Aglaya of what Myshkin tells her is that this scene illustrates the positive effect of full presence in the encounter with the other. Still, as I have shown, the prince cannot help making interpretations, but is unable to recognise himself as the one who carries out this act.

Now, let us try to consider, in a person who knows that he is interpreting, this positive quality of clear-sightedness, of perceiving the other person's being. Freud and Ferenczi both spoke of "guessing transference". Defined in these terms, interpretation invokes something broader: the radical consequences in a subject's life of a true encounter with another subject.

Does encountering the other without regard for the interest of one's ego, accepting at a deep level the emotional upheaval caused by this presence, presuppose that one has survived one's own death? Two psychoanalysts who built their theoretical edifice around affect as a central element answer "yes" to this question: Aulagnier considers that the psychoanalyst – about whom it is justified to presume that he has an unusual quality of presence – always has a score to settle with the *death drive*. As for Bion, he used to say of himself: "I died in the Ardennes". So be it.

But in that case, what are the essential points that survivors of catastrophe can teach us about the ability to identify so incredibly well and so entirely with the other without losing one's own identity, and without recourse to the boredom and disinterest characterising the pervert?

Once again, it is the state of being in love which can best guide us towards a tentative answer. In terms of sensibilities, being in love is an extreme situation in which affect and primary processes have the upper hand over the transformational effect of representations. Love also causes the limits of the ego to disappear, and the crossing of the limits is always signalled in extremely dazzling flashes which indicate the widening of the field of the possible, as a prelude to the reorganisation of the functioning of the psychic apparatus.

But contrary to madness, the excessive aspect of the experience of being in love is rooted in desire, the boundless desire for the full intensity of life. This desire for intensity finds support by leaning on the edge of death, whose shadow produces an urgent and vigorous reaction to inevitable finitude. The bedrock of investments in the unknown, whether it be thoughts, sensations or feelings – the state of being in love shuns no paradoxes in its peculiar manner of treating the presence of the other in the world, and in the internal reality of the lover: respect goes hand in hand with the greatest intransigence, the seeking of joy can be associated with great tolerance for pain, the foregoing of trying to know everything, to better focus on oneself – is associated with a readily available and living capacity to remember, the experience of clear-sightedness is coupled with a passion for secrecy, and friendship coexists with the greatest selfishness.[22]

II. Nastasya Filippovna

The Little Girls

Prince Myshkin has a talent I have not yet mentioned: he introduces others to language, teaches them the importance of words, teaches them what speaking means.

The first example of this occurs following the scene where, after the prince stopped Ganya from hitting his sister Varya, Ganya slaps Myshkin violently. Then the young man goes to Myshkin's room to apologise. Varya is there; against all expectations, she speaks to her brother sincerely and with affection. This is no doubt due to the influence of the prince, who during the entire previous episode, which was very brutal, never stopped talking: about what was happening and what he was thinking.

The scene in which the prince is slapped in the face is also the one in which Nastasia Filippovna makes her entrance for the first time in the novel; she has come to call on Ganya's family. She is portrayed as the agent of trauma, and this trauma takes the form of shame. Varya asks her brother "are you dragging me […] to beg her pardon for having insulted your mother and for having come here to disgrace your family, you base creature?"[23]

Nastasya storms into the house, obviously determined to provoke Ganya who, clearly unable to hold his own, is rejected and humiliated. Ivolgin, pathetic figure of a failed father, cannot oppose her either. It is the prince who stops her, by speaking to her directly.

Nastasya carries with her a devastated world, full of devastation and rubble over which she reigns triumphantly. She turns everything she encounters into a landscape of ruins. Having transformed her terrible experience of embittered love into a call for revenge addressed to the firmament and the unchained elements, she respects nothing and destroys everything lying in her path.

Trauma is her speciality. This is well understood by Ferdyshchenko, the buffoon, terrible figure of a vulgar, unscrupulous scoundrel, a freeloader in Nastasya's home, who takes on the task of entertaining her guests by dispensing venom and insults. On the evening of the birthday festivities, when Nastasya has promised to say whether she will marry Ganya, while everyone seems to be waiting – no one knows for what – Ferdyshchenko suggests that they all play a game: that each person tell *the worst thing he has done in his life*. In short, a game of trauma, trauma combined with the shame of evildoing. Each guest has to tell his story of evildoing. Tell me your shameful trauma and I will tell you who you are.[24]

Having survived a psychic cataclysm which almost destroyed her, Nastasya Filippovna inflicts on men the violence that Totsky inflicted on her. She displays to anyone who cares to look the wound of her gaping vulva, a gash as great as the wound she has carried in her soul since the day when her sexuality was torn away from the anchor of tenderness and love.

Men, all men, are paralysed, unable to find the answer to the enigma Nastasya personifies in brilliant style, highlighted by a tinge of scandal. Each one falls prey to the extremely erotic terms of the challenge she sets for him: can he, if only for a moment, become Jupiter coupled with Priapus, to satisfy the sensuousness she flaunts?[25] While this sombre parade of powerless men files past her, she does her best to escape the anguish caused by the frigidity of her own feelings. She stops to listen to the prince because he speaks to the abandoned little girl he sees in her. Nastasya complements him on this talent when he first visits her: "you are first-rate at guessing".[26]

Nastasya Filippovna, a major character in Dostoevsky's work, brings to mind another important figure in the world of psychoanalysts: Dora, the little girl who, at the age of fourteen, was subjected to the advances of the husband of her father's mistress, a sinister sexual trade-off between two very proper gentlemen. Contrary to Prince Myshkin, Freud did not guess, during the analysis, the reasons for the young girl's distress. But, thanks to this error, he discovered the central tool of analytic work, transference, which, in fact, has to be guessed.

The reasons for Freud's error are various, and they deserve closer attention. Freud met Dora the year *The Interpretation of Dreams* was published (1900). He had just abandoned his *neurotica*, the theory claiming that hysterical symptoms are the consequence of a traumatic sexual experience inflicted on the child by an adult in his intimate circle – most often, the father. After abandoning this theory, he came to consider fantasy alone as the actual cause of neurotic disorders. The agent of trauma is eliminated, but at the same time – as Ferenczi would observe – the other as such ceases to be included in the constitution of the psychic apparatus. From that point on, this apparatus is considered a monad, closed in on itself; based on this vision, the functioning of the psyche is autarchic. As to how the monad comes into being, Freud admits that the role of the mother is crucial:

> an organization which was a slave to the pleasure principle and neglected the reality of the external world could not survive. [...] The employment of a fiction like this is, however, justified when one considers that the infant – provided one included with it the care it receives from its mother – does almost realize a psychical system of this kind.[27]

But this way of seeing things implies taking for granted that the mother always fills her maternal function, and always provides a good primary environment. Just as Ferenczi had done, Winnicott would question the validity of this presumption, and would reflect on the conditions needed for a mother to offer the best care to her infant.[28]

When Freud met Dora – whose real name was Ida – he had introduced the concept of the monad, had set aside the other as the agent of trauma, fantasy reigned supreme and his monumental *Interpretation of Dreams* had been completed. Now, he planned to apply the method used for dream interpretation to neurotic symptoms: look for the fantasy masked by the symptom; decipher the meaning of the fantasy and see the symptom disappear once the meaning is uncovered.

Dora seems to lend herself well to the enactment of his plan. She is eighteen when she meets Freud. She was fourteen – no longer a child – when the traumatic events occurred. This "authorised" Freud to presume that she had extensive knowledge of sexuality, and an adequate ability to recognise fantasmatic functioning. Thus, Freud looked for infantile sources to explain the impasses in which she was caught; given that her father was very present in her life, Freud looked for Oedipal elements underlying her conflicts.

But Dora did not agree with an analysis that focused on various displacements of psychical investments and identifications. In her case, following their progression would only have made sense if the analyst had accepted to deal with the trauma in its present reality: trauma always exists in the present, it is never forgotten and never cured by repression; trauma demands to be recognised, named, accepted and seen for what it is – and at the time when he was faced with Dora's trauma, Freud was unable to recognise its existence in the present.

Love and sexuality

Dora teaches us that when a traumatic intrusion renders love and sexuality incompatible, the subject is plunged into a place of hell. Nastasya Filippovna, Dora's remarkable predecessor, says:

> "And why have I wasted [...] five years in [this hatred]! [...] But afterwards, thank God, I thought he wasn't worth such [hate]! And I suddenly felt so disgusted with him then that, if he had besought me, I wouldn't have married him. [...] Did you really think I meant it? [...] Ruin a child like that? That's more in Afanasy Ivanovitch's line: he is fond of children! [...] I've been Totsky's concubine. [...] I am proud myself perhaps, although I am a shameless hussy. You called me perfection this evening; a fine sort of perfection who, simply to boast of trampling on a million and a princedom, is going into the gutter! What sort of wife should I make you after that? Afanasy Ivanovitch, I really have flung away a million, you know? How could you think I should be glad to marry Ganya for the sake of your seventy-five thousand? [...] Look, prince, your betrothed takes the money because she is a low woman, and you wanted to marry her! But why are you crying? Are you sorry? You ought to laugh as I do". – Nastasya Filippovna went on, though there were two large tears glistening on her cheeks. – "Trust to time; it will pass! [...] What's the matter with you, Katya dear? [...] I've made an honest girl like you wait on a low creature like me. [...] It's better so, prince, it's really better; you'd have despised me later on, and we should not have been happy. Don't swear, I don't believe it! And how stupid it would have been! [...] No, better part as friends, or no good would have come of it, for I am something of a dreamer myself, you know. Haven't I dreamed of you myself? You are right, I dreamed of you long ago, when I lived five years all alone in his country home. I used to think and dream, think and dream and I was always imagining some one like you, kind, good and honest, and so stupid that he would come forward all of a sudden and say, 'You are not to blame, Nastasya Filippovna, and I adore you!' I used to dream like that, till I nearly went out of my mind. [...] And then this man would come, stay two months in the year, bringing shame, dishonour, corruption, degradation, and go away. So that a thousand times I wanted to fling myself into the pond, but I was a poor creature, I hadn't the courage".[29]

The woman bereft of love is, at the same time, a woman whose sexuality is crippled: one of the living dead. Another Nastasya speaks, a hundred and fifty years later:

> I made myself beautiful. I wanted him to look at me. I like that. It makes me feel good when he looks at me. And I want to take him in my arms, I want him to make love to me. When I think of him I see pictures in my head. I see myself sitting on top of him, his face against my chest, the two of us locked together. So we go to his place. And suddenly, when he starts to undress me, I become frightened. I am afraid that he will touch me. As if my body was an abscess filled with pus that would burst at the slightest contact. But if he stops, if he speaks to me, tells me stories and talks about his love for me, I want him again. I hold him very tight, I unbutton his shirt, I caress his chest. He kisses me, he is a real man, not a ghost. I take his penis in my mouth, I like that, we

> undress quickly, we kiss, I want to devour him and want him to swallow me, I am happy. I am not a little girl any more. And, again, suddenly something goes wrong. Suddenly I find him old, I find myself disgusting and everything seems too heavy. I tell myself that I am in a bed rubbing myself against a man who is rubbing himself against me. I feel clammy. I stink. I forgot to put on make-up. I am afraid that my blemishes will show.
>
> *I think: he finds me beautiful. I try to concentrate on this idea so that the rubbing will stop and the magic will come back. But nothing works. I think: he finds me beautiful because he's stupid. He is fucking me. I pretend and I wait for it to be over. I am dead.*[30]

When sexuality breaks into the psychic space by destroying all the bonds of love that tie the subject to life, life comes to a standstill, is impoverished and decays. Dissociated from the person and no longer serving the interests of the ego which rejects it, sexuality becomes persecutory, shameful, guilty. It no longer enriches life but is intrusive and fills all the spaces to the point of saturation: eating or fucking – it's all the same. Once it has disqualified love, sexuality remains frozen, cut off from sensations.

Nastasya Filippovna knows, unconsciously, that her contempt for herself is really directed towards Totsky. It is who deposited in her being his own guilt and disgust, which now fill her. She has eroticised her pride, and now displays her catastrophe like a trophy and a weapon of war, and defies anyone to judge her. Because Ganya is flippant enough to treat her with disdain, she directs the full force of her hatred against him. After calling him a "shameless" man,[31] she dares him to pull out of the flames the packet of a hundred thousand roubles she has thrown into the fireplace. The ultimate humiliation. He does not try to save the money, but as he is about to leave, he faints, crashing to the floor.

> "It's all his! The whole roll is his! Do you hear, friends?" Nastasya Fillipovna declared, laying the roll of notes beside Ganya. "He wouldn't do it, he stood the test, so his vanity is even greater than his love of money. […] But for this he might have murdered some one".[32]

Aglaya is the one who understands Nastasya best. She understands that Nastasya is incapable of love:

> because you were too proud […] no, not proud, that's a mistake, but too vain […] that's not it, either, it's your self-love which amounts almost to. […] You can love nothing but your shame and the continual thought that you've been brought to shame and humiliated.[33]

Contrary to what unfolded between Freud and Dora, Prince Myshkin is able to embrace all of Nastasya's distress. He even tells her so:

> you have suffered and have come pure out of that hell, and that is a great deal. Why, then, are you ashamed? […] I won't let any one say a word about you.

> [...] I [...] understand the meaning of honour, and I am sure I spoke the truth. You wanted to ruin yourself just now irrevocably; for you'd never have forgiven yourself for it afterwards. *But you are not to blame for anything.* [...] Few people would do what you have done. [...] You are proud, Nastasya Filippovna, but *perhaps you are so unhappy as really to think yourself to blame.* [One would think that Dostoevsky has read Ferenczi's *Confusion of Tongues.*] I shall respect you all my life.[34]

Trauma and transference

But why was Freud unable to "take in" all of Dora's distress? Because, after he abandoned his former theory, his *neurotica,* which claimed that behind each hysterical patient there is a seducer who caused the trauma, Freud did not take an interest in real trauma. I would summarise his thinking as follows: I do not need to deal with the trauma because I will have access to its effects through the fantasies – since these effects will necessarily influence the manner in which these fantasies are produced as a consequence of the trauma. This was in keeping with fantasy theory. But – and this is a substantial reservation – Freud "overlooked" the fact that, conceptualised in this manner, fantasy as a staging of desire, is a pleasant construct at some level of the psychic apparatus and, as such, is unable to include pain, fright and trauma - induced psychic sideration. (It was not until 1920, with the publication of *Beyond the Pleasure Principle*, which discussed traumatic dreams, that Freud recognised that fantasy has no usefulness for understanding and processing psychic pain.) But – and here the same reserve applies – in order to recognise pain, fright and sideration, the trauma must be seen as existing in the present, and transference must be seen as the agent which reveals it and is able to call it forth. The problem is that Freud preferred to avoid the question of transference. (While Ferenczi, supported and encouraged by Freud, placed transference not only at the centre of experience, but also at the centre of analytic theory.)

Freud's reluctance, not to say refusal, to be caught up in transference is a crucial factor in his position vis-à-vis trauma. It is no doubt the main reason preventing him from recognising the importance of Ferenczi's *Confusion of Tongues*. Of course, this text resonated with his former theory of seduction as it applied to hysteria, but I see this argument as a way to agree with Freud's own rationalisation: that what prevented him from reading *Confusion of Tongues* was the fact that he had no experience with this practice and did not wish to have it, due to the involvement in transference that it demands.

Freud's difficulties with transference were twofold. First, they were theoretical: after the *Interpretation of Dreams*, the entire metapsychology was already in place when Dora caused Freud to discover transference as an unforeseen complication; Freud recognised transference in his work with Dora, but there was no place left for it in the theoretical edifice already constructed out of concrete and steel – and at such great expense of energy! It was to be Piera Aulagnier's concept of the original, and her innovative concept of transference, that granted transference a metapsychological status.[35] The second difficulty is that Freud was not analysed; he only had an experience of self-analysis, relying on his relationship with Fliess. Another factor, identified by Philippe Réfabert, is the psychotic transference on the part of Fliess in this relationship, to which Freud chose to submit. In my present perspective, this element is obviously one which merits attention. We may understand Freud to be saying: I have already been subjected to psychotic transference, and have dealt with it without analysis, with only my self-analysis, and it almost killed me. So now, it's too much for me, go and see Sandor – and for maternal transference also, which is part of Dora's analysis, because I paid a price for that too with Fliess and I won't do it again – since I was never analysed and only conducted self-analysis.[36]

The prince can embrace all of Nastasya's distress. But he cannot do anything about it; he can in no way help Nastasya to change her subjective position. Why? I said earlier that, fundamentally, the prince does not take any interest in anything, he has no desire. The reasons for this are many. For the moment, I simply wish to point out the similarity between this position and that of certain therapists, who are full of good intentions, fully empathetic with the suffering of their patients and totally unable to do anything other than sympathise and feel sorry for them. In the same way, the prince does not go so far as to involve his own desire in the plight of this woman he admires. Incapable of desiring, what he offers her is his life. But for a woman like Nastasya, who knows better than anyone that happiness in love relationships cannot be built on sacrifice, what he offers is not good enough.

Still, the prince is not wrong: he speaks to the child, the child whose hopes were betrayed. If only he would have felt desire, or would have persisted, he would certainly have won Nastasya's heart and perhaps been able to help her to live.

Endowed with the talent of a brilliant clinician, Dostoevsky understood, as Freud would some years later, that in Nastasya's case, pregenital functioning is predominant, and that it is in this mode that she experiences all sexually-tinged emotions. Dostoevsky also understood that the partially destroyed sphere of illusions is what made Nastasya say that she had been dishonoured, offended, inflamed and debauched. This is what she says to her friend Darya about illusions:

> "You say, take the hundred thousand and get rid of him, if it's horrid [she is referring to Rogozhin]. And it really is horrid. [...] I might have been married long ago, and not to Ganya either; but that would have been just as horrid too. And why have I wasted [...] five years in [this hatred]! [...] No, I'd better be in my proper place, in the streets!"[37]

Nastasya is dishonoured and suicidal: "a thousand times I wanted to fling myself into the pond, but I was a poor creature, I hadn't the courage." Dostoevsky also understood that for Nastasya auto-eroticism serves as a defence against genital sexuality, whose traumatic character makes it invasive. When sexuality is traumatic, it cannot enrich the sphere of the ego; as a result, it becomes dissociated from the ego. Nastasya's sexuality, not integrated into the ego, wavers back and forth between two pitfalls: if she tries to integrate it, she fears destruction, since she is very reliant on it as a means of aggressive defence. But if she wants to eliminate it, the unreality of existence and the prospect of suicide immediately loom on the horizon.

The theory of repression does not provide an explanation for the fact that Nastasya Filippovna transposes everything into the realm of sexuality, that for her everything becomes sexual, but without anything ever being achieved, either in the realm of pleasure or in that of thought. Knowing that for Nastasya sexuality and the ego are dissociated leads us to suppose that three types of logic exist: that rooted in the ego, which applies to psychic needs of the ego (in the realm of the ego, sexuality is a psychic need); reasoning based on the pleasure principle, applying to repression and conflicts between drives and the field of identifications; and reasoning stemming from external encroachments, which in Nastasya's case are closely intertwined with sexuality.

In a situation like this, the analyst, like the prince, must take into account the needs of the ego and those of sexuality mixed with destructiveness. He must treat the ego while waiting for the right conditions to integrate sexuality in a beneficial manner. The aim is well-being – the well-being of sexuality. To treat the psychic needs of the ego means to treat wounds of love; this is why in such a context, very often treating the ego is the equivalent of taking care of the subject:

> Myshkin was sitting by Nastasya Filippovna, with his eyes fastened upon her, stroking her head and cheeks with both hands, *as though she were a little child.* He sighed in response to her laughter and was ready to cry at her tears. He said nothing, but listened intently to her broken, excited, incoherent babble. He scarcely took it in [...] and as soon as he fancied she was beginning to grieve again, or to weep, to reproach him or complain, he began at once stroking her head again, and tenderly passing his hands over her cheeks, *soothing and comforting her like a child.*[38]

Why didn't Nastasya Filippovna accept the marriage proposal made by the prince? We have answered this question in part by saying that Nastasya recognised a sacrificial aspect in Myshkin's compassion. We can even add that the prince feels no passionate love for her, nor is he romantically in love: he admires who this woman is, and takes on the mission of protecting her. He loves her out of compassion, but is not interested in sexuality and has no desire to know what a woman is.

But Nastasya knows life well. After five dreary years spent tyrannising Totsky and many other men, and being very unhappy, she could have chosen to live a peaceful life, if only for a time, with the man she recognises to be *the first man she has met* whose sincerity cannot be doubted.[39] Of course, at the end of Part One, looking back on what happened on the occasion of the birthday celebration, Dostoevsky suggests that Nastasya committed suicide before the man who disgraced her to avenge this outrage. So be it. But in the course of that evening,

Totsky had not enjoyed himself: he had been unmasked as a paedophile, and had been called a villain, a coward and a miser.

I believe Nastasya Filippovna refused the prince's proposal because she could not and would not set aside her concerns about sexuality. To live with the prince would have meant giving up these concerns, accepting to cut away a part of herself. Yet she loves the prince. As Rogozhin tells Myshkin: "One might almost believe that your pity is greater than my love. [...] She ran away from you then, because she realised how much she loved you. It was too much for her to stay with you".[40]

Nastasya is made to suffer by the dissociation she experiences between love and sex; she lives her life on the edge of this fracture. This is why Rogozhin is the right choice for her.

He disgusts her because she is certain that with him sexuality will occupy centre stage. But he is passionately in love; he loves and desires her at the same time. Truly. For him she is a queen. This kind of love provides an assurance: she will never be disdained. The intensity of this love attracts her, the strength of this sensuality is a promise: she would be dispensed, to some degree, of bearing the entire responsibility for her desire, and would carry less guilt for her pleasure – in certain types of love affairs, the man serves this purpose.

Nastasya Filippovna finds Rogozhin intelligent, she may even feel affection for him. He tells Myshkin: "And never, never before had she talked to me like that, so that I was positively amazed. For the first time I breathed like a living man".[41] But Nastasya knows that living with Rogozhin means being locked in his world, and that he will never find peace. Rogozhin loves and desires her passionately, she is everything to him, he wants all of her, can't tolerate the least distance, the least difference. But neither can he bear the thought that she may be completely absorbed in his person. She must remain outside, in the world, beautiful and desirable. Rogozhin is mad about Nastasya, and his love makes him madly jealous. This is the second thing that makes Rogozhin a good choice: he will be her murderer.

Since she knows that marrying Rogozhin will lead to her death, she puts off the marriage, goes to Moscow to stay with the prince, and takes flight on other occasions. But she never abandons the project, and does not forget to torment her fiancé: she takes lovers, causes public outrage and has endless escapades.

Myshkin's love

What part of responsibility does the prince have in all this? He does, in fact, ask himself this question: "'Am I to blame for all this?' he muttered to himself, almost unconscious of his own words". Pursuing his reflection, he even came to understand that Nastasya inspires something

> *deeper than mere passion.* And does her face inspire no more than passion? Can that face indeed inspire passion now? *It* [*inspires*] *grief, it clutches the whole soul,* it

> [...] and a poignant, agonising memory suddenly passed through Myshkin's heart. Yes, agonising. He remembered how he had suffered not long ago when first he had noticed *in her symptoms of insanity*. Then he had been almost in despair. *And how could he have left her when she ran away from him to Rogozhin? He ought to have run after her himself without waiting for news of her.*[42]

For the prince, to love a woman means to love her suffering; only a woman who suffers can inspire his love. Thus, it is not inconceivable that he contributed to what he calls Nastasya's insanity. He asked her to marry him, he invited her into his home. She accepted his invitation; then she left. Rogozhin is convinced that she ran away because she was afraid of her passion for the prince. But this is only one aspect of the explanation: the consequence of something else. Why was she unable to stay and take the risk of living this passion? And, indeed, how could the prince abandon her. What happened between Myshkin and Nastasya during her visit? The prince's conversation with Aglaya gives us some important clues.

Myshkin agrees to meet Aglaya at seven in the morning in the park next to her house. It is early, and while waiting for her he falls asleep and has a dream in which a criminal "had just committed an awful crime". Not the most pleasant preliminary to their meeting. And it continues: when he sees Aglaya, the prince says that he had the impression he had seen another woman there – obviously Nastasya. After a moment of silence, he speaks of Ippolit's suicide attempt. After such an unseemly start to their conversation, Aglaya, a young woman barely out of adolescence, does what she can: she offers her friendship, invites the prince to travel around the world, rambles. Finally, she comes to what is really on her mind: "I'm certain you came here fully persuaded that I am in love with you and was making a tryst with you". Very embarrassed, the prince admits that the previous day he "was afraid of that".

Aglaya, whose lower lip started to tremble, went on: "You suspected perhaps that I invited you here to ensnare you, so that we might be found here afterwards, and that you might be forced to marry me". Myshkin doesn't understand any of this. To create a diversion, he treats Aglaya like a child: "Aglaia Ivanovna! Aren't you ashamed? How could such a nasty idea arise in your pure, innocent heart?" Aglaya is aghast at what she just said, but she does not give up. She does not deny her desire: "'I'm not ashamed at all,' she muttered. 'How do you know that my heart is so innocent? How dared you send me a love letter, that time?'" The prince is astonished. Yet, he in fact wrote in his letter:

> I felt an irresistible desire to remind you, just you, of my existence. [...] Of all three [of you] I saw only you. I need you – I need you very much. I have nothing to write to you about myself, have nothing to tell. [...] I have a great desire that you should be happy.

We can all agree that to consider this a love letter one had to be – as the prince said – insane. In fact, he insists:

> "A love-letter? My letter – a love-letter? That letter was most respectful; that letter was the outpouring of my heart at the bitterest moment of my life!"
>
> "Oh, very well, very well," she interrupted Aglaya, who was now starting to learn what madness human desire can create.[43]

There is no doubt that Myshkin shares some traits with the Underground Man, who killed Liza.

After this, their conversation is nothing but confusion. Aglaya doesn't know what to make of this scatterbrain who says one thing and then the opposite. He speaks of Nastasya, to whom he had spoken of Aglaya. (This is no doubt why Nastasya thinks he should marry Aglaya.) Myshkin says he feels only *pity* for Nastasya but maintains that he stays away because "In her pride she will never forgive me for my love – and we shall both come to ruin". A little earlier he was saying that Nastasya had gone so far as to "[accuse] me bitterly of setting myself up above her (though I had no thought of such a thing)", and then said that with no man did she ask to be "elevated to anyone's level". Then Aglaya speaks of Nastsya's love for the prince – as Rogozhin had done earlier. She is surprised that the prince does not acknowledge this. Nor does he want to acknowledge Nastasya's jealousy, or the jealousy Aglaya is unable to hide. By the end of this conversation, Aglaya had been rendered … would insane be too strong a word? In any case, she is disturbed enough to declare that she will marry Ganya. This meeting with the prince only lasted an hour. One can imagine what it would he like to live with this man for weeks and months. It would surely be enough to drive someone … insane.[44] The prince must be aware of the destructive repercussions of his blindness. A few months after his separation from Nastasya, he was telling himself that it had always seemed to him that "that woman was bound to appear at the last moment, and tear asunder his fate like a rotten thread".[45]

Myshkin's blindness, his lack of desire for the other, is certainly the result of the fact that sexuality is excluded as a cause – the epileptic attack being the equivalent of orgasm: "Yes, for this moment [of the seizure] one might give one's whole life!" because "that moment was really worth the whole of life".[46] Aglaya points out another characteristic of this deficiency of desire: "*You have no tenderness, nothing but truth, and so you judge unjustly*".[47] (I have already commented on the violence often associated with what the prince says.[48])

The truth is that Myshkin doesn't like himself, but wants others to like him. This explains his cruelty, what Aglaya calls his unfairness. He asks Nastasya to marry him, lives with her in his house, cannot bear it when she leaves, writes a love letter to Aglaya – but protests afterwards: what, was that a love letter? – offers his compassions, exaltation, but cannot bear that another should dream of him. This is why he forfeits Nastasya's and then Aglaya's love – while refusing, like the good pervert that he is, to take responsibility for it.

But accumulating these denials ultimately exhausts him:

> A terrible longing came upon him to leave everything here [as he left Nastasya?] and to go back to the place from which he had come, to go away into the distance to some remote region, to go away at once without even saying good-bye to any one.[49]

Ippolit had seen through this incoherent behaviour displayed by the prince:

> Then let me tell you, if I hate anyone here […] it's you, *Jesuitical, treacly soul*, idiot, philanthropic millionaire; I hate you more than every one and everything in the world! I understood and hated you long ago, when first I heard of you; I hated you with all the hatred of my soul. […] *This has all been your contriving*. You led me on to breaking down! *You drove a dying man to shame*! You, you, you are to blame for my abject cowardice! I would kill you if I were going to remain alive! I don't want your benevolence, I won't take anything – anything, do you hear? – from anyone! *I was in delirium, and don't you dare to triumph!* [50]

Insanity

After Aglaya's meeting with the prince in the park, insanity takes hold of all the characters, as if it was brought on by the prince's impending epileptic seizure. Contrary to his first fit of epilepsy, which had made him acutely aware of Rogozhin's presence and his murderous intention, before this attack he experienced a sensation which "gripped him to the heart […] everything seemed opening out before him".[51] This expansion caused him to ask for Aglaya's hand in marriage, and to ask her parents to give a reception to officially introduce her unlikely fiancé. During the reception, the elated prince spoke with exaltation, becoming more and more flushed, coming closer and closer to an epileptic seizure.

But before this resolution, the prince reads Nastasya's letters to Aglaya. Here Dostoevsky shows his extraordinary talent as a clinician: he understands the importance of feminine homosexuality in the structuring of femininity. Nastasya declares her love for Aglaya, but it is too late. She says:

> I have almost ceased to exist and I know it. God knows what in my stead lives within me. […] [Rogozkin's] house is gloomy, and there is a secret in it. I'm sure that he has, hidden in hs box, a *razor*, wrapped in silk like that murderer in Moscow, he too lived in the same house with his mother [like Rogozhin], and kept a razor wrapped in silk to cut a throat with. […] I know he loves me so much that he can't help hating me. […] I should kill him from terror. […] But he will kill me first.[52]

Then there is Myshkin's meeting with Nastasya. The reader is convinced of her love for him, her deep and absolute love, this love which, finding no dwelling place in a desiring other, drives her completely insane. She comes to see the prince, with Rogozhin, before complying with his request: to leave and stop sending letters to Aglaya. She must have believed that for Aglaya – and thanks to her own encouragement – the prince was finally willing to risk feeling desire. Of course, her pain knew no bounds:

> She sank on her knees before him on the spot, in the street, like one demented. He stepped back in horror, and she tried to catch his hand to kiss it, and, just as in his dream that night, the tears glistened on her long eyelashes.
>
> "Are you happy? Happy?" she asked. "Only say one word to me, are you happy now? To-day, this minute? Have you been with her? What did she say?" She did not get up. She did not hear him. She questioned him hurriedly, and was in haste to speak, as though she were being pursued. "*I'm going tomorrow, as you told me.* I won't […] it's the last time I shall see you. The last time! Now it's absolutely the last time!"
>
> "Calm yourself, stand up!" he said in despair.
>
> She looked greedily at him, clutching at his hands.
>
> "Good-bye," she said at last, she got up and went quickly away from him, almost running.[53]

This is the second time Nastasya leaves Myshkin. He is very troubled by her suffering; his torment is obvious. But, probably like the first time she left, he said nothing to her, made no move to stop her from leaving, took no action. He is not a man, but merely an unsubstantial phantom.

Since his meeting with Aglaya in the park, and contrary to what he made us expect from the moment we met him, emotions no longer serve to sharpen Myshkin's perceptions, to guess what is real. Drawing on Piera Aulagnier's hypothesis, which defines the pictogramme as being the affect of representation and the representation of affect, I would say that following his meeting with Aglaya the prince harbours a jumble of emotions and a whole array of muddled representations.

The conversation between Nastasya and Aglaya constitutes a high point unfolding before Myshkin's eyes. Ippolite tells him about the meeting planned between the two women and gives him important advice of which he will fail to make use.

First, Ippolite gives him his interpretation of Aglaya's attachment to him: "Was it because I wounded her vanity by hinting that she enjoyed Nastasya Flilippovna's 'leavings'?" Then he gives Myshkin some advice: "Mind you take steps at once, *if you deserve to be called a man*". Then he speaks of a woman's desire, and generally of desire:

> Look here, Prince, nobody jumps out of windows, but when the house is on fire the grandest gentleman or lady is ready to jump out of the window. When it's a case of necessity, there's no help for it, and our young lady will even go to see Nastasya Filippovna. […] I fancy you take Aglaia Ivanovna for a young lady or a boarding-school miss.[54]

When Aglaya came to take Myshkin with her, on her mission, "he followed her like a slave. [...] He divined how strong her determination was. It was beyond him to check this wild impulse".[55]

Now, what is enacted centre stage is the element which constitutes the backbone of his availability to everything, of his immense receptivity, and of his tolerance of any excess, of any vice. Suddenly, the void appears, a total absence of desire, the inability to make any decision, lack of imagination, numbness, stupidity and laziness.

Now, the prince finds himself caught between these two women he has driven insane, rivals who pass back and forth between them the wounds he inflicted, who insult each other, who display their pain, their scars, their hatred. It is not by choice that the prince stays with Aglaya, but because Nastasya knows that his emptiness will always prevent him from confronting the force of desire, of her desire, of suffering, her suffering – suffering which fascinates him, in which he is engulfed. As for Aglaya, she is too fresh, too alive. Aware that to triumph over her rival would mean finding herself with a spineless man, Nastasya comes full circle. Confining herself to the space of the slimy delights of this world of ghosts, consenting to disappear in the transparent and shapeless distortions of this space, her only wish is deliverance. Her wish shall be granted: Rogozhin, the prince's enforcer, is present at the meeting. Nastasya's slaying is only the enactment in reality of the murder already carried out by the prince.

Notes

1 Dostoevsky, F. (1996), *The Idiot*, Garnett, C. (trans.), Wordsworth Classics, p. 2.
2 Ibid., p.10.
3 Ibid., pp. 36–37.
4 Ibid., p. 37.
5 Ibid., pp. 37–38.
6 Ibid., p. 42.
7 Ibid., p. 112.
8 Ibid., p. 75.
9 Ibid., p. 72.
10 Ibid., p. 31.
11 Ibid., p. 67.
12 Ibid., p. 31.
13 Ibid., p. 52.
14 Ibid., p. 55.
15 Ibid., p. 16.
16 Ibid., pp. 69–70.
17 Ibid., p. 113. My emphasis.
18 Ibid., pp. 58–59. Dostoevsky's emphasis, then mine.
19 Ibid., pp. 59–60.
20 Ibid., p. 65.
21 Ibid., p. 73. My emphasis.
22 The reader can refer to my discussion of the metapsychology of love in *Letters to a Young Psychoanalyst*, letter 33: "True Love".
23 Dostoevsky, F., *The Idiot*, p. 107.

24 I have borrowed this formulation from Leslie Kaplan's play *Toute ma vie j'ai été une femme* (All my life I have been a woman), Paris: POL, 2008.
25 François Perrier wrote: "In her offensive language, the hysterical woman maintains a position of double dissatisfaction. Given her phallic position, when she refers to a masculine ego ideal, she finds it lacking in her father: *she can only be raped, and only by Jupiter. She finds it intolerable that man owes the emergence of his desire to the assumption of symbolic castration*" (my emphasis), in *Structure hystérique et dialogue analytique*, Paris: Albin Michel, 2008, p. 236. The psychic deadlocks with which the prince struggles could be taken for the recognition of the limits imposed by castration. Indeed, Aglaya makes this mistaken interpretation.
26 Dostoevsky, F., *The Idiot*, p. 129.
27 Freud, S. (1911), *Formulations Regarding the Two Principles in Mental Functioning*, S.E., 12: 2186226. London: Hogarth.
28 See my book *De l'amour à la pensée*, which provides a detailed discussion of the consequences of this change of perspective; Paris: L'Harmattan, 1994.
29 Dostoevsky, F., *The Idiot*, pp. 152 and 158–160.
30 See *Letters to a Young Psychoanalyst*, Letter 20.
31 Dostoevsky, F., *The Idiot*, p. 151.
32 Ibid., p. 163.
33 Ibid., pp. 531–532.
34 Ibid., pp. 153 and 157.
35 I discuss this at length in *Letters to a Young Psychoanalyst*, Letter 16.
36 Sylwan, B. and Réfabert, P. (2010), "Fliess et Freud, un transfert psychotique", in *Freud, Fliess, Ferenczi. Des phantômes qui hantent la psychanalyse* (The Ghosts of Psychoanalysis), Paris: Hermann.
37 Dostoevsky, F., *The Idiot*, p. 152.
38 Ibid., p. 536.
39 Ibid., p. 163: "Good-bye, prince. You are the first man I have seen in my life!"
40 Ibid., pp. 197 and 200.
41 Ibid., p. 199.
42 Ibid., pp. 208 and 213–214.
43 Ibid., p. 403. The prince's letter to Aglaya: p. 174.
44 Ibid., pp. 408 and 407.
45 Ibid., p. 528.
46 Ibid., p. 210.
47 Ibid., p. 399. My emphasis.
48 When he tells Ganya: "*In my opinion you are simply one of the most ordinary men that could possibly be, only perhaps very weak and not at all original*". Ibid., p. 113.
49 Ibid., p. 287.
50 Ibid., p. 279. My emphasis.
51 Ibid., p. 513.
52 Ibid., p. 426. Dostoevsky's emphasis.
53 Ibid., p. 428. My emphasis.
54 Ibid., pp. 526–528. My emphasis.
55 Ibid., p. 529.

5

DEMONS

Dependence and reparation

Dostoevsky teaches us that dependence was first a primary psychic need for any subject, before constituting a risk. This need is as great as the primary need to heal the loved one. What psychoanalysis teaches us, is that the greater the unwellness, the more pressing is the need to heal the other, to be his therapist. The range of pathological reparation extends from the intrusive solicitude of the hysteric to the totalitarian tyranny of the crazy-making mother.

When the pathology is very serious, the need to be the therapist of the other, which in time becomes a true therapeutic skill, emerges in early childhood, due to the inadequacy of the primary maternal environment. The baby feels the inadequacy (or absence) of the mother in dealing with his basic psychic needs, and conceives of the possibility of repairing her shortcomings, so that she may be able to carry out the function she normally should fill. For this to happen, the child must first develop an extraordinary ability to identify with the psychic needs of the other – specifically the mother: the surprising ability to feel in her place the deprivation she cannot feel and can certainly not name.

All this brings us to the question of divination, which I formulated in my discussion of *The Idiot*. In that novel, the fact that the prince is unencumbered by ego-support needs grants him an unusual capacity to identify with the other's feelings, as well as an exceptional power to *sense* the feelings of his interlocutor, and to name them. We should add that in the realm of the *originary* (Aulagnier) and of the *factory of the self* (Oury), thoughts are indistinguishable from sensations – recall the thought/sensation experienced by the prince at the sight of Nastasya Filippovna's portrait, or when he predicted Rogozhin's murderous act.

I have suggested that this dazzling ability to grasp the other's being is a function of the thought process, like the thought process that leads the baby to become his mother's therapist. In this process, the thinkable relies on intensified receptivity to the sensitivity, the feelings and the sensoriality of the other. This exacerbated receptivity to the full presence of the other shows that the entire psychic apparatus has become an organ of perception of external reality. The subject *sees* the whole presence of the other, *sees* the entire density of the world. I am reminded of Rainer Maria Rilke's phrase, so often analysed from various perspectives: "With all eyes the creature sees the open". But to better illustrate my meaning, we could separate Rilke's idea into four parts: the subject *hears* with all ears, feels with the subtlest *touch, smells* with flaring nostrils and *tastes* with all his mouths the full presence of the other and the density of the world.

As I said, Dostoevsky teaches us that dependence with its risk is a primary psychic need for everyone, a need as great as the primary need to heal the loved one. Since this need is fundamental and universal, it is not a pathological trait. It can be the source of great generosity and attentiveness shown to others, particularly when the subject is aware of the possibility of a reversal of roles, which would allow him to depend on the other and benefit from his care. Dostoevsky also highlights various types of reaction formation due to the horror of dependence: hatred (of oneself and of the other), cynicism, self-destruction and murder – and *Demons* is a remarkable illustration of this phenomenon, as are the Underground Man, Svidrigailov in *Crime and Punishment*, Rogozhin, Nastasya and the prince in *The Idiot.*

We know that this great ability to identify with the psychic needs of the other becomes even more acute in critically ill people. This brings us to consider the strange situation where a seriously ill person has to care for another person. For instance, when someone very ill – very fragile – is entrusted with the care of a handicapped person, such as someone paralysed by a stroke, or a very old and weak person. Because the possibilities of improvement are very slim, the degree of investment on the part of the caregiver is very limited from the start. This keeps in check fantasies of all-powerful therapeutic intervention, causing the caregiver to focus on the satisfaction of his masochistic needs. His energy is therefore invested in long-term meticulous work, which requires patience and self-sacrifice.

Another very frequent occurrence is a couple made up of a hysteric and a seriously disturbed person. This situation can serve to illustrate Lacan's aphorism: *The hysteric seeks a master to rule over,* where the all-powerful caregiver must pay the emotional cost of the great deception inflicted by his inability to keep the impossible promise of total reparation of the other's deprivations. In a therapeutic context, such a couple enters a one-way guru/follower relation. But if the need to heal the other is accompanied by a paranoid tendency, the resulting personality type can efficiently free subjects stuck in very harmful defensive positions reinforced by the pain and the dangers associated with primary deprivation: drugs, alcohol, delinquency.

If we set aside these extremes in order to consider the forms this phenomenon takes in therapeutic work, we encounter much greater complexity.

When the therapist's function is built *above all* on the primary desire to bring reparation, the dynamics set in place encounter various difficulties, manifesting in ways we have, in some cases, identified. (I say *above all* because we generally suppose that the therapist's position results from the integration of several other levels of desire.)

Let us take as an example a patient with obvious primary affective deprivation – in other words, lack of love. The massive transference present from the start of the therapeutic work and the great dependency associated with it satisfy to a great extent the therapist's primary need to make reparation. At this point in the process, there is a complementarity of fantasmatic scenarios: the therapist palliates his own mother's unmet needs, while the patient has a mother who recognises his psychic needs. Problems arise when the answers offered to the patient's needs prove to be inadequate. The aggression and even persecution unleashed by this disappointment is experienced by the therapist as a lack of gratitude.

This brings us to the question of the consequences of the therapist's expectation of gratitude from his patient. In the context we are examining, one of the most common consequences of such an expectation is that the patient feels guilty for his aggressive reaction – terrible guilt – and denies his disappointment. By doing this, he repeats what he did with his mother in his childhood.

The difficulty experienced by some therapists in admitting their errors in the clinical handling of transference is part of the problem I am discussing. Aside from the fact that the unconscious demand for gratitude interferes with the ability to accept the patient's aggression, it also indicates the therapist's refusal to let his patient help him find the appropriate interpretation, or to find the best way to handle a complex situation they are facing together.

This incapacity on the part of the therapist is, in fact, an unconscious refusal to recognise his own primary need to be helped. This refusal prevents the patient from using his ability to bring about reparation of the other's deprivations. Worse still, the therapist's refusal prevents the patient from living creatively and usefully the experience of being the therapist of someone on whom he depends – keeping in mind that he experienced his relation to his inadequate mother as therapeutic failure.

Not accepting to be helped – in other words, treated – by his patient lends the therapeutic process persecutory overtones which lead to denial of feelings: feelings of abandonment and pain in the patient, and feelings of hate and impatience in the therapist. The latter's fear of losing control of the relation reinforces certainties that lead to a practice based on domination. As a result, the analyst becomes unable to accept and integrate in the therapeutic process the transgressions and the acting out – always aggressive – without which no subjective change is possible for a deprived or traumatised patient. The absence of surprises in transference reproduces, for both protagonists, the boredom and heaviness they experienced with their mothers. The primary need to be helpful to the other does not suffice for freeing the patient from the aspect of the real which imprisons him. In my work as a guide to young colleagues learning therapeutic practice, I always had more difficulty with those who were certain of their ability to help, to be available, tolerant and accepting, and to exert a containing function. This certainty maintains, in these young colleagues, an illusion of unlimited benevolence. It is easier to awaken the primary need to provide care in those who have doubts about their ability to treat, than to make those who believe in boundless benevolence recognise the need for a setting – in other words, for limits – in order to conduct therapeutic work. Speaking for myself, I am always wary of the satisfaction I feel about the therapeutic effects achieved in an analysis, although I am very happy when I can resolve the transferential difficulties that arise.

The need for illness

The primary need to be helpful is not sufficient for exercising the profession of therapist; there is also the often overlooked primary need to be very ill. This need is based on another primary belief: that we are never loved as well as we should be. In fact, one can only ever be certain of loving, never of being loved – a disparity which sustains the desire for love.

This universal primary need to be ill is evident in the great pleasure associated with the first experience of psychic suffering. For the child, the impression of having a suffering of his own circumscribes for the first time his own space of solitude, and will constitute the source of all future subjectivation. The ability to suffer reveals the existence of an inner world (which explains the associated pleasure), and links certain contradictory dualities essential for the construction of psychic life: pain and pleasure, love and hate, destruction and reparation, aggression and tenderness, separation and coming together, all-powerfulness and disillusion, life and death.

In the psyche, this initial experience of suffering can take the form of a desire to regress. To clarify the concept of regression, I will quote the words of a child – a pre-teen – who, before relating her existential problems to her parents, forewarns them: "I know you can help me to find answers, but right now I just want to complain". In addition, this first experience of suffering is the root of that most important feeling we call sadness. The difference between melancholy and sadness is that the latter is in no way related to guilt. Genuine sadness does not spring from regret; it is combined with a sense of the world. This is why being sad is a preliminary condition for the joy of thinking. It can also be seen as being the expression of the intertwining of the life and death drives, theorised by Freud in 1920. To conclude, let us turn to the Brazilian poet Cassiano Ricardo who, like all poets, knows how to condense what I have been explaining at length: "Perfection, when it exists, is imperfect in that it is sad".

The primary need to be ill can therefore greatly reinforce resistance to healing, and undermine the possibility of benefitting from the other's help. If, in addition to the need to be ill, there is destructive primary envy, the situation is even more serious. I am thinking of a woman I saw in analysis, who would leave her companion as soon as he proved his love for her. Unconsciously, she found it completely unbearable to receive the love she craved and demanded of the other. Making room for the love of her beloved in her inner world reopened a primary wound inflicted on her self-esteem when she had been unable to provide reparation to a mother who abandoned her. Her lover's generosity reactivated the feelings of inadequacy and emotional emptiness experienced in childhood, and created envy, which caused her to attack the relation. By doing this, she remained loyal to the suffering inflicted by her mother.

This was even more distressing because she truly loved this man, with whom she shared an intensely passionate sexual relationship. But, after repeated attacks on their love relation, the lover's emotional investment started to diminish; he showed signs of exhaustion announcing an impending break-up. Previously, this woman lived for many years with a very sick man – a situation which had satisfied her masochistic needs fully. Another factor which rendered her inadequate in a love relationship was that despite her love, she could only treat her companion as a narcissistic prop. The disastrous result was that the smallest sign of the autonomous existence of the loved one generated paranoid feelings; the least mismatch between her current fantasy and her lover's behaviour produced the certainty of being excluded and disavowed. This revealed the terrible handicap leading her to reject the new inscriptions of a love relation, based solely on the extreme excitement triggered by fantasies of exclusion. But the fact is that denying what was experienced while a love relationship lasted can lead to madness. Despite her love of life, this woman was truly unable to be happy without feeling devastating guilt, hidden behind resentful envy, to satisfy the primary need to be ill – which set the whole process in motion again and again. She fought a fierce, exhausting battle – but in vain – to resist being stuck in this demonic repetition. In her professional life, she was an excellent educator, with real therapeutic talent, but for whom any negative transference was unbearable.

Where is all this leading?

My reading of *Demons* and *The Brothers Karamazov* will take into account these primary needs of saving the other and of being ill, in my analysis of the construction of Dostoevsky's characters, and my analysis of the dynamics between the couples constituted by the protagonists. In this regard, let us remember that these couples can be made up of doubles, and that the double is a fundamental element in Dostoevskian narration; it plays an essential role in structuring the relationships between characters to such an extent that it can be used as the key to interpreting a novel; this approach, limited but instructive, starts with the question: who is whose double? In these couples of doubles, one of the characters may be the repressed part of the other. In our reading of *Crime and Punishment*, we saw that Raskolnikov was the repressed part of Porfiry, and Svidrigailov that of Raskolnikov. The figure of the double appears very early in Dostoevsky's work. It is, in fact, the title of his second novel, which we discussed earlier, and about which the most respected literary critic of the period, Belinsky, wrote that the main character, "a victim of schizophrenic break-up, might be more suited for a lunatic asylum than literature".

Tenderness and sexuality

But don't you find that there is something wrong with what I have been saying? I am telling you that a psychoanalyst deals with love and nothing else. I say that our work consists in preparing those who come to see us for this salutary catastrophe, or in repairing the ravages, wounds and scars left by the absence of love or by broken-down loves.

Do you agree with all this? The question is worth asking. In France, it has been held for half a century that psychoanalysis deals exclusively with desire. What do you say?

I think that in order to desire, one must first love oneself – which presupposes that one was loved by someone at the beginning of one's life. I think that the more one loves, the better able he is to desire, and that to consider desire independently of love leads to theoretical confusion whose therapeutic consequences can be devastating.

First, the discharge of instinctual energy is equated with fulfilment of desire. Given that the discharge of instinctual energy only involves partial instincts, not to differentiate it from fulfilment of desire results in the tragic conclusion that passion is confined to the sphere of partial drives. But this idea, which excludes from the field of possibilities passion as the triumph of love, and which – like all mediocre ideas – is widespread, eliminates from what is conceivable a major existential element of the psyche – soma/psyche integration, and of the integration of sensoriality and ideals.[1]

First observation: to consider desire independently of love leads to making them contradictory, not to say antinomical. Freud gave a very clear description of this opposition between desire and love in his depiction of male sexuality restricted to the opposing figures of the mother and the whore, in his 1912 text "On the universal tendency to debasement in the sphere of love". In this text, he also points out the logical priority of primary love over desire:

> When striking cases of psychical impotence are exhaustively investigated by means of psycho-analysis, the following information is obtained about the psychosexual processes at work in them. Here again – as very probably **in all neurotic disturbances** – the foundation of the disorder is provided by an inhibition in the developmental history of the libido before it assumes the form which we take to be its normal termination. **Two currents** whose union is necessary to ensure a completely normal attitude in love **have**, in the cases we are considering, **failed to combine**. These two may be distinguished as the *affectionate (tender)* and the *sensual* current.
>
> **The affectionate (tender) current is the older of the two**. It springs from the earliest years of childhood; it is formed on the basis of the interests of

> the self-preservative instinct and is directed to the members of the family and those who look after the child. From the very beginning it carries along with it contributions from the sexual [drives] – components of erotic interest – which can already be seen more or less clearly even in childhood and in any event are uncovered in neurotics by psycho-analysis later on. It corresponds to *the child's primary object-choice.* We learn in this way that the sexual instincts find their first objects by attaching themselves to the valuations made by the ego-instincts, precisely in the way in which the first sexual satisfactions are experienced in attachment to the bodily functions necessary for the preservation of life. The "affection" shown by the child's parents and those who look after him, which seldom fails to betray its erotic nature ("the child is an erotic plaything"), does a very great deal to raise the contributions made by eroticism to the cathexes of his ego-instincts, and to increase them to an amount which is bound to play a part in his later development, especially when certain other circumstances lend their support.[2]

I shall not comment on Freud's choice not to discuss the conditions prior to the emergence of desire in the infant; to comment here would take us too far afield.[3] But I would like to specify that my title, *From Love to Thought,* could just as well have been *From Love to Desire,* since in the book thinking is not dissociated from desire. It would be legitimate to ask whether the dissociation between love and desire, made by most psychoanalysts in France in their metapsychology, has not had other effects than those we already know.

These effects could include the omission of affect from the therapeutic aspect of clinical practice, on the pretext that the unconscious is constructed of signifiers, considered the only means of access to desire. In the 1970s, a certain story that was making the rounds and was considered to condense the essence of psychoanalytic interpretation is very instructive in this regard: when a highly anxious patient threatened to jump from a window, the person acting as his analyst commented: "Splash". But, more generally, I ask myself if this use of the theory did not serve above all as a philosophical system allowing the practitioner to be anesthetised against any feeling and any anguish produced by the encounter with the patient, and with anyone else in his life.[4]

Repetition and invention

Such a melancholy view of psychic processes brings to mind Freud's manner of reducing transference to the repetition of intrapsychic processes. Seeing the psyche as closed in on itself, Freud limited considerably the field of therapeutic intervention the psychoanalyst could explore as a result of transference. Therefore, analysis could not be offered to those who expected to work on pre-existing conditions, so that sexuality and desire could be free of anxiety; nor to those for whom the psychoanalyst is not solely the one who reveals aspects of one's past, but also someone with whom one shares a novel and "enlarging" experience in the present. (Ferenczi was the first to open the way for this kind of work.)

I think that the repetition of this clinical impasse – since it truly is an impasse and a tragedy – stems from a misunderstanding of Lacan's work on the ego. What Lacan objected to, with reason, regarding psychoanalysis in America in the 1950s, was the fact that the ego was seen primarily as playing a role in adapting to reality reduced to its ideological definition. I do not believe that Lacan ever brought into question the *integrative function* of the ego, which makes it possible to create an internal world by the transposition of the care and the love received from one's primary environment. Although Lacan did not address these questions in the elaboration of his theories, I am pointing out that he never rejected their validity. Moreover, he never suggested that a split in the subject was the equivalent of a split in the ego. A split in the subject can be traced back to the unconscious, and much work is required to allow the subject to gain control of his life. Splitting of the ego refers to aspects or moments of a life that have not been integrated. This lack of integration can manifest itself in a mode of perception or of thinking, or in a feeling of annihilation caused by the inability to organise primary experiences of sensoriality.

Gisela Pankow's brilliant discovery was that in psychosis time inhabits space, and experiences of the body are lodged in forms whose existence is unrelated to any meaning that could be shared. Speaking of time that becomes space, and alluding to Winnicott, she points out that "the other who could be loved becomes space, an envelope in which to be safe".[5] As for what is to be done with forms in analysis, she gave us a detailed description of the long process making it possible, simply by taking forms into account, to allow the subject to live in his body again and, as a result, to renew contact with time and acquire a narrative:

> The possibility of opening the world of the schizophrenic depends on the possibility of finding a means of access to his body as he experiences it, and of makng a choice based on a dynamic and ambivalent body image. [...] When human desire emerges, it involves the notion of time, the structuring of a future. [...] It is through recourse to a primitive obsessional model, in search of the point of extreme concentration of its vital energy, that we can access a [proto-fantasy]. [...] We must look for the proto-fantasy (that Pankow calls phantasy) hidden in an obsessional image and, to do so, it is essential to find the dynamic energy hidden in the thing. [...] The therapeutic effect [of this search] confirms that the image exerts its action through its dynamic effect as a [proto-fantasy]: A negativistic patient whose body as she experienced it was destroyed in large part was able to take up her own history when she was confronted with two parts of her body and was able to speak *first* of one and *then* of the other. This means that when she refers to one of these parts of her body, the other can no longer take its place. It is no longer possible to mistake one for the other. And when, some time later, there is reference to the second part of the body, this part cannot be confused with the first. To designate a

> part of the body precisely automatically *excludes* the other part. *This process of exclusion is also a choice.* And when there is a choice, it becomes clear that in the sphere of time, simultaneity in relating to things is no longer possible. [This can offer the possibility of recognising a not-me] *If this act of exclusion can be applied to the entire body, non dissociated,* that is, if the patient can say: "This body external to me is not my body", then it becomes possible to *recognise a not-me,* not only in the sphere of *the living in general,* but also in the relation with the human body. [Of course, these dissociations give rise to unimaginable anguish] *It is therefore a matter of using anguish to transform it into desire,* and desire turned towards a unisexual body. This is the objective of my effort of *dynamic structuration* in psychosis.[6]

This brings us to the role of divination in the therapeutic process. In fact, Gisela Pankow has described in careful detail the conditions in which these lightning flashes burst on the scene. Her observations will help us examine the lightning flashes occurring in Dostoevsky's characters. Let me remind you of what I was saying when we were working on *Crime and Punishment*: the subject in the position of pervert manipulates words and the encounter with the other in a devastating manner. To foresee the devastating after-effects of this manipulation in the sphere of the real, it is necessary to *imagine* these after-effects. The therapist's talent for divination of the real relies on this practice of the imagination.

In this context, I cannot resist recounting once again an event from Gisela Pankow's practice, which concerns the functioning of thinking in a divinatory mode.

It was a Sunday, as usual. When I arrived at her office, she was very pale. She said something terrible had just happened. The brother of a patient she had treated quite a while ago had called and asked to see her. She said:

> Today was the day of the appointment. He arrived, he rang downstairs. I pressed the button to open the street door. He rang again, saying that the door didn't open. I found that strange because someone had come earlier and there had been no problem. [She comments: I immediately felt that there was something aggressive about him.] So I went downstairs, I opened the door, I tried the code and found that it worked, and we took the elevator. [She comments: Of course, I didn't look at him, we were not in the session yet.] I had him come straight into the office. [She comments: When someone comes for the first time, I don't make them wait in the waiting room. You should never make a patient wait the first time, because you don't know the person yet.] He came in, he sat down, I closed the door, I sat down, I took a sheet of paper, I looked at him. And when I looked at him I was certain that he was there to kill me. I asked myself who was going to find my body. I said: "And what will you do with my dead body?" [She comments: Because with a psychotic, you always have to place the focus beyond his desire.] He then took out a gun and said: "I don't know why, but I have to kill you." [She comments: Now that he had spoken, I knew the danger was past.] I said: "Listen,

> you did not come from Germany to kill me; that was not part of our agreement. Your name?" He answered. "Your age?" He answered. I stopped and noticed that he was still very agitated. I said: "After all, it's not my fault that your brother was the one who slept in your mother's bed and not you".

An amazing story, like many that are told by analysts working with psychotic patients. The story is so fascinating, it is easy to find it magical. And yet it is constructed on rigorous reasoning, like a theorem. Of course, there is Pankow's clinical genius, and all her experience. But what impresses me most is the persistence of her search, the way she takes her cues from her hypotheses regarding the patient's unconscious, her refusal to compromise, and her unshakable ethics.[7] Notice that when she asked: "And what will you do with my corpse?" her visitor had not yet said anything!

And now, Demons

From a historical point of view, *Demons*, like *Notes from Underground* and *Crime and Punishment*, is part of Dostoevsky's battle against the nihilism of the 1860s in Russia. On the surface, *Demons* is a novel about transmission. This most obvious reading was important to Dostoevsky. He held those known as the "radicals" directly responsible for the nihilist movement which preached the destruction of all humanist values. His initial intention to write a pamphlet showing this direct relation was born on the occasion of an event which shocked the whole country, with good reason: the murder, by a group of nihilists, of a member of their circle who was opposed to their political views.

This sordid crime revived the trauma inflicted on Russians on 4 April 1866, when a student belonging to a clandestine radical group attempted to assassinate Tsar Alexander II. The brutal repression that followed targeted those who held radical views, seen by conservatives as being directly responsible for this type of action – and even as instigating it.

Dostoevsky held in particular esteem two figures of the intelligentsia, who supported the liberalism of the "radical" movement. The first was Belinsky, the famous literary critic who had praised Dostoevsky's first novel, *Poor Folk*, but had hated *The Double*, and wrote that the character of Goliadkin was better suited to a psychiatric institution than as the hero of a work of fiction. In fact, it was for having read out loud, twice, Belinsky's open letter to Gogol, after the latter joined the ranks of the tsarist autocracy, that Dostoevsky was arrested and sent to Siberia. The relation between the two men ended after Belinsky reviled Christ in front of the writer on several occasions – no doubt to be provocative.[8]

The other member of the intelligentsia who supported the liberalism of the "radical" movement was Ivan Turgenev, author of *Fathers and Sons* (2008). In fact, *Demons* might be considered a sequel of *Fathers and Sons*, one generation later. Dostoevsky, who had liked the book very much, came to despise the writer, whom he ran into by chance several times while in exile. Dostoevsky had no respect for Turgenev's "aristocratic airs and manners, his avowed preference for Europe, the destruction of Russian culture (in his latest book)". This contempt was mixed with indignation about Turgenev's recent attempts to gain favour with the young generation by claiming to share the convictions of (his character) Bazarov in *Fathers and Sons*.[9] In *Demons*, Karmazinov is a wicked, cruel caricature of Turgenev.

From Dostoevsky's point of view, what was scandalous about the radical ideology had less to do with its political aspects – he was, for example, a staunch supporter of the abolition of serfdom – than with its cultural aspects. The Westernisation advocated by the radicals horrified Dostoevsky because it led the Russian people away from belief in Christ. This is why the project of applying the ideas of the Enlightenment to Russia was disastrous. The use of the Gospel of Luke in *Demons* should therefore be understood literally. This is what Dostoevsky wrote in a letter to his friend Apollon Maikov about his novel:

> the facts showed that the disease which had attacked cultured Russians was much more violent than we ourselves had imagined, and that the matter had not ended with the Bielinskys. [...] But then came the miracle testified by St. Luke. The devils had entered into the man and their name was legion, and they asked Him: "Suffer us to enter into the swine", and He suffered them. The devils entered into the swine, and the whole herd ran violently down a steep place to the sea and was drowned. When the people came out to see what was done, they found the man, out of whom the devils were departed, sitting at the feet of Jesus clothed and in his right mind, and those who saw it told them by what means he that was possessed of the devils was healed. Exactly the same has happened with us in Russia. The devils went out of the Russian and entered into a herd of swine. [...] These are drowned or will be drowned, and the healed man, from whom the devils had been cast out, is sitting at the feet of Jesus. [...] And observe, my dear friend: he who loses his people and nationality, loses also the belief of his fathers, and God. Well, if you want to know, – this is precisely the theme of my novel. It is called *The Devils* and it is a description of how these devils entered into a herd of swine.[10]

In *Demons*, Stepan Trofimovich is the composite figure of the radical intellectual. In terms of transmission, Stepan Trofimovich is the father of Pyotr Verkhovensky, a nihilist with certain traits borrowed from the terrorists who murdered the student. Stepan Trofimovich is also the teacher of Nikolai Stavrogin, the demon. In terms of transmission again, Stavrogin is the one who first introduced Kirillov and Shatov to the ideas they now espouse.

A deeper level of meaning is attached to the group of terrorists. Dostoevsky shows how, in a group, the ideal ego that fills the existential void produces alienation, conferring to the discussions between the members of the group a religious functioning. Power and dependence, mixed with hate, vanity and various frustrations produce violence, uncontrolled behaviour, murder.

In order to connect these two levels of the narrative, that of transmission and that of the functioning of power, Dostoevsky had the brilliant idea of setting the action in a provincial town. This micro-universe acts as a magnifying mirror that reveals the workings of political power. Staying within the limits of a small society also makes it possible to bring to light the intertwining between social functions and roles, and the singular subjectivity of the characters – something Dostoevsky does particularly well. The small size of the terrorist group also lets the author present a detailed description of how a narcissistic and psychopathic leader takes control of parasitical subjects whose lives lack meaning – a subject Freud would later develop in *Group Psychology and the Analysis of the Ego.*

A third level of meaning, the one which will be our focus, brings together two ideas present in the thinking of the Underground Man, which we have already examined:

> We [...] have long ceased to be born of living fathers, and we like this more and more. We're acquiring a taste for it. Soon we'll contrive to be born somehow from an idea.[11]

This thought introduces the question which preoccupies Raskolnikov: is it possible to live in a world without God? In *Demons*, three characters examine this question: Kirillov, of course, then Shatov and Stavrogin. This question is related to another: how can one invent a new frame for thought without being an impostor? Is it possible to build a life on an idea dissociated from the roots of our history, without this idea becoming a system and causing us to lose our sense of the world? – a fundamental question for any psychoanalyst. The figure of the impostor is personified by Pyotr Verkhovensky. The question of imposture is Nikolai Stavrogin's torment.

This is the landscape we will explore together, with the help of the major characters in the novel. We shall start with Stepan Trofimovich, who illustrates the psychopathological need to be ill.

Stepan Trofimovich

The radical intellectual

I said earlier that on the surface *Demons* is a novel about transmission. Dostoevsky considered the so-called radicals directly responsible for the nihilist movement which preached the destruction of all humanist values. The murder, by a group of nihilists, of a member of their circle who became critical of their political views was an illustration of this kind of radicalism.

In constructing the plot for *Demons*, Dostoevsky introduces Stepan Trofimovich early, and reveals his essential traits from the start. A composite figure of the radical intellectual, he represents those "superficial people, leading purposeless lives [...] incapable of genuine effort, impotent and dejected. And yet they believe themselves worthy of being placed on a pedestal. To be sure, 'they were honorable in thought and pure in heart'".[12] Dostoevsky goes on to say of this type of man that he

> [p]laces himself unconsciously on a pedestal, in the style of relics to be worshipped [...] and loves it. [...] A *pure* Westernizer [...] who embraced with an equal sympathetic glance [...] the beautiful however it may appear [and] whose traits are aimlessness and lack of firmness in his views".[13]

According to Joseph Frank, Dostoevsky's biographer, the symbolism in *Demons* is based essentially on the idea that a false and perverted "beauty" has replaced the "true beauty" of Christ. Stepan Trofimovich is the archetype which allows Dostoevsky to conceive more clearly of a way to transform his suppressed anger against Russians of his generation and his hatred of the manifestations of nihilism. He builds his character based on a point of view he formulates in a May 1871 letter to his editor, Strakhov:

> If Belinsky [...] and that whole bunch of scum were to take a look now, they would say: "No, that is not what we were dreaming of, that is a deviation; let us wait a bit, and light will appear, progress will ascend to the throne, and humanity will be remade on sound principles and will be happy!" They would never admit that their way can lead at best but to the Commune. [...] They [the members of the Paris Commune] desire the common good, but [...] can only reiterate Rousseau's aphorism that "good" is a fantasy never yet ratified by experience. The burning of Paris is a monstrosity: "It did not succeed, so let the world perish because the Commune is higher than the happiness of the world and of France". [...] to them (and many others) this monstrosity doesn't seem madness, but only *beauty*. The aesthetic idea of modern humanity has become obscured.[14]

But Stepan Trofimovich also has some of the traits of Herzen, the illustrious radical respected by Dostoevsky, who saw him primarily as a poet: "he has been, always and everywhere, *primarily a poet*. [...] The political activist is a poet; the socialist is a poet; the philosopher is a poet in the highest degree!" (letter to Strakhov).[15]

Joseph Frank comments:

> The 'poetic' quality of Herzen's temperament, his inability to commit himself wholeheartedly to whatever intellectual or practical activity he was involved in, will constitute one of the most engaging traits of Stepan Trofimovich's whimsically volatile character. [This trait] also provides the historical background for his stormy relations with Peter Verkhovensky and the nihilist ideas of his offspring.[16]

Joseph Frank summarises brilliantly the relation between Stepan Trofimovich and Russian history (Slonim, 1950); I paraphrase his thoughts:

> The sources for Stepan Trofimovich [...] can be found [...] in the controversies that began in 1858, when the tension between the generations exploded in public. Dostoevsky [...] describe[s] the dislike of the "sons" for [...] pretentious and complacent Westernizers and the aversion of the "fathers" for insolent [...] vulgarity, and for the materialistic coarseness of their heirs of the 1860s. But in the end [he] cannot resist tipping the scales in favour of the love of art imbued with romanticism, characteristic of his own generation: he refuses to deliver human nature into the grasp of the restrictive materialism and determinism of the 1860s.

The campaign against the "superfluous men", liberal and idealistic, of the 1840s (that is, of Dostoevsky's generation) ushered onto the Russian cultural scene a new force, the more radical intellectual group called *raznochintsy*. The spokesmen for this vociferous group, all of them possessed of fanatical inflexibility *instilled by their religious education*, rejected the precepts of orthodoxy in favour of atheism and materialism. They "unleashed a flood of derogatory articles against the generation of the 1840s", written in mocking terms best exemplified by ferocious, passionate satires. This generation was accused of weakness, indecision and an inability to act; "its members were slaves to high-flown principles that only served to bolster their egoism and vanity".[17]

Joseph Frank cites two critical passages referring to this group of intellectuals. This shows how thoroughly Dostoevsky had documented his portrayal of the relations between Pyotr Verkhovensky and his father:

> People of *that* generation [the 1840s] were possessed by lofty but somewhat abstract strivings. They strove toward truth, longed for the good, they were captivated by everything beautiful; but highest of all for them was *principle*. [...] Withdrawing in this way from real life [...] they took on much more than they were capable of performing. Hence their eternally false position [...] their eternal grandiose phrases of self-approval [...] and their eternal failure in any practical activity. Little by little they sank into their passive role, and, of all that had gone before, they preserved only a youthful inflammability, yes, and the habit of conversing with well-bred people. [...] No better outline of Stepan Trofimovich's character profile could be sketched.[18]

And a little further:

> You [Mr. Herzen] are a poet, an artist [...] a storyteller, a novelist, anything you wish but not a politician. [...] Failing to perceive that you have been left behind, you [...] reproach the younger generation with ingratitude to [...] the first high priest of Russian Socialism [...] you, Mr. Herzen, are a dead man.[19]

Herzen did not reply directly to these insults made by a young activist. He wrote to Mikhail Bakunin – who was fascinated by Nechaev, the leader of the terrorist group that assassinated the student. Herzen's position is the same as Dostoevsky's; the latter would attribute this perspective to Stepan Trofimovich:

> [This man] is insolent and a fool; but the worst is that *the majority* of the young Russians *are the same* and we're the ones who have contributed to make them *like this*. [...] This isn't Nihilism. Nihilism is a great phenomenon in the evolution of Russian thought. No. These are the dispossessed noblemen, the retired officer, the village scribe, the local priest and the petty landowner disguised in costumes. [...] Woe to the revolution poor in spirit and weak in a sense of art, which will make of all that has been acquired by time a depressing workshop, and whose sole interest would be subsistence and nothing but subsistence![20]

Remember what Stepan Trofimovich says at the fête:

> The whole difficulty lies in the question which is more beautiful Shakespeare or boots, Raphael or petroleum? [...] [We can see that postmodernism goes back a long way.] "But I maintain," Stepan Trofimovitch shrilled at the utmost pitch of excitement, "I maintain that Shakespeare and Raphael are more precious than the emancipation of the serfs, more precious than Nationalism [...] more precious than the young generation, more precious than chemistry, more precious than almost all humanity because they are the fruit, the real fruit of all humanity and perhaps the highest fruit that can be. A form of beauty already attained, but for the attaining of which I would not perhaps consent to live".[21]

Varvara Petrovna

The lengthy first chapter of *Demons* makes it possible to describe the peaceful life in the provincial town before the arrival of Pyotr Verkhovensky, as well as Stepan Trofimovich's multifaceted personality.

Another very important element in the construction of the novel is the narrator, described as "gossipy, intimate, slightly ironic [...] worried about the social breakdown he observes all around, but concerned to preserve the proprieties and to reduce the shocking events to the proportions of a juicy local scandal".[22]

In the beginning, the narrator introduces Stepan Trofimovich as a self-satisfied man imbued with unwarranted smugness. An intellectual with a pompous style, staunchly believing his own fabulations, he is a rather ridiculous man whose relationship with Varvara Petrovna will show him to be a scared baby, sentimental and irascible, under the affectionate domination of the marvellous hysteric she is:

> But there was one thing he had not discerned up to the end: that was that he had become for her a son, her creation, even, one may say, her invention; he had become flesh of her flesh, and she kept and supported him not simply

> from "envy of his talents" [now that he was no longer a tutor to her son Nikolai Stavrogin]. And how wounded she must have been by such suppositions! An inexhaustible love for him lay concealed in her heart in the midst of continual hatred, jealousy, and contempt. She would not let a speck of dust fall upon him, coddled him up for twenty-two years, would not have slept for nights together if there were the faintest breath against his reputation as a poet, a learned man, and a public character. She had invented him, and had been the first to believe in her own invention. He was, after a fashion, her day-dream. [...] But in return she exacted a great deal from him, sometimes even slavishness. It was incredible how long she harboured resentment.[23]

The following exchange between Varvara Petrovna (who speaks first) and Stepan Trofimovich illustrates the character of the two protagonists well:

> "Without being a Bismarck I'm equal to falseness and stupidity wherever I meet it. The Lembke's falseness, and Praskovya's folly. I don't know when I've met such a flabby woman, and what's more her legs are swollen, and she's a good-natured simpleton, too. What can be more foolish than a good-natured simpleton?"
>
> "A spiteful fool, *ma bonne amie*," Stepan Trofimovitch protested magnanimously.[24] [Let us note the modern tone of the dialogue.]

After presenting this utterly unattractive portrait of Stepan Trofimovich, the narrator describes his social interactions. The reader discovers an affable, intelligent man, not without a sense of humour, quick-witted, likeable – but whose thoughts lack substance, are sentimental and declamatory, chatty.

Stepan Trofimovich is an old dandy, a man of imposing stature. But his passion for cards and wine have left their mark. When she returned from Switzerland, where she visited her son, Varvara Petrovna noticed that her friend had grown decrepit: "You've begun to sputter when you laugh, it's a sign of senility! And what a strange way of laughing you've taken to!"[25]

Our hero is deeply troubled by these words; he knows that he has gained Varvara Petrovna's favour because he is a handsome man, and not only because he is an exile or a scholar.

It is in these circumstances that Varvara Petrovna suddenly decides to have him marry her ward Dasha, Shatov's sister, no doubt because she intuits the passion between her son and Dasha. What Varvara tells Dasha about her protégé on this occasion is instructive:

> He's frivolous, shilly-shally, cruel, egoistic, he has low habits. But mind you think highly of him, in the first place because there are many worse. [...] He's an old woman, but you know, that's all the better for you. Besides, he's a pathetic old woman. He doesn't deserve to be loved by a woman at all, but he deserves to be loved for his helplessness, and you must love him for his

> helplessness. [...] He will complain of you, he'll begin to say things against you behind your back, he'll whisper things against you to any stray person he meets, he'll be for ever whining and whining; he'll write you letters from one room to another, two a day, but he won't be able to get on without you all the same, and that's the chief thing. Make him obey you. If you can't make him you'll be a fool. He'll want to hang himself and threaten to, he will threaten to – don't you believe it. It's nothing but nonsense. Don't believe it; but still keep a sharp look-out, you never can tell, and one day he may hang himself. It does happen with people like that. It's not through strength of will but through weakness that people hang themselves, and so never drive him to an extreme, that's the first rule in married life. Remember, too, that he's a poet.[26]

This is the secret women whisper to one another: that men are children. They are children because they find desire in women hard to bear. This means that most men don't know how to respond to women's phallicism, to the masculine in them. Men find it difficult to tolerate the fact that women think and create, that they are subjects in their own right, and that they participate in the spheres of love, work and sexuality.

Men find it difficult to welcome the encounter with a desiring woman, because for women abandoning oneself to desire presupposes feelings of love. But men are afraid of love. Masculine narcissism makes it difficult to place the other at the centre of one's life, to depend on the other to such an extent. It is easier to separate love from sexuality, the mother from the whore – and when he places the woman in the role of mother, she says the things Varvara Petrovna told Dasha.

But a hysterical woman like Varvara Petrovna teaches us that being passionately loved by a man is not necessarily easy for a woman. If she does not succeed in making him her child, she will try to make him an appendage, an extension of her psychic world. If this does not succeed either, she will try to make him her nursemaid, and will become a temperamental child. It can be very dangerous for a woman to accept this love-and-desire as something coming from the outside, and to love the other without expecting any compensation, simply for the joy of loving another being. To do this, she must accept that her desire is greater than her self-esteem, and that pride is an inanity. But this gift of the encounter, demanding a strong and vital commitment to generosity, can frighten her so much that she may choose to make the other crazy, to kill him.

The plot of *Demons* is thrust into madness once and for all by the planned marriage between Stepan Trofimovich and Dasha. Good society has already been forced to tolerate Nikolai Stavrogin's eccentricities during his last visit to their town. But now, it is Varvara Stavrogin, his mother and the mainstay of this little universe, whose meddling is about to trigger a landslide.

What is Varvara Stavrogin trying to achieve? She is trying to prevent Dasha from becoming her son's wife, for she could not bear such a marriage – totally unsuitable in her view. To attain her goal, she does not hesitate to destroy her bond with Stepan Trofimovich, by reducing their relationship to a financial arrangement.

Despite his sentimental, lukewarm humanism, Stepan Trofimovich does not lack imagination; he understands that he is expected to be the designated cuckold. He does not have the strength to object. But his acceptance of the situation delivers a painful blow to Varvara Stavrogin's female pride. The ensuing whirlwind of injunctions and contradictory emotions culminates with the appearance at Varvara Stavrogin's home of Marya Timofeevna, the half-witted woman Nikolai has married. Through this narrative device, Dostoevsky announces that the apparent tranquillity of provincial life founded on negation is over, and that from then on contempt, horror and murder would fill the whole space of life.

For Stepan Trofimovich, the catastrophe is ushered in by his son Pyotr. Before a witness, who happens to be the narrator, Pyotr calls him a parasite and a coward, and reveals the secret of his impotence – Pyotr could in fact be the offspring of his mother's Polish lover.[27] Pyotr Stepanovich personifies the idea that has haunted Dostoevsky since *Notes from Underground*: "We [...] have long ceased to be born of living fathers, and we like this more and more. We're acquiring a taste for it. Soon we'll contrive to be born somehow from an idea".[28]

The second stage of the catastrophe takes place the first time Varvara Petrovna meets with Stepan Trofimovich after the long-awaited evening when he was to celebrate his engagement to Dasha. On this occasion, he hears the same judgmental words as those spoken by his son: that he is a finished man, a parasite, a coward, belonging to a bygone age, verbose and boring. Because her pride is deeply wounded by his compliance with her request that he marry Dasha, Varvara Petrovna does not hide her contempt, her hate, or her delight in humiliating him.

After this, Stepan Trofimovich attends the fête given by the governor's wife, where he antagonises everyone. Then he leaves town, starting his pilgrimage on the high road, where *he does not meet the Russian people*. And finally, he dies.

Undoubtedly, through his death, Dostoevsky symbolises the death of liberals and the society that supports them. But he also rejects the perspective personified by the nihilists. The political solution he would prefer is not hard to imagine: a strong, authoritarian, repressive government. Let us remember that *Demons* was dedicated to the son of the Tsar, who would become Alexander III.

Daydreaming and stupidity

But beyond these pessimistic observations on the state of affairs in Russia, what does Dostoevsky teach us through his hero, Stepan Trofimovich?

Varvara Petrovna's ruthless portrayal is not to be disputed. She delivers her verdict before her protégé accepts the marriage plan – thus, before what she considers a betrayal. Her judgment is based on the intimate relations between them over twenty-two years. Therefore, it must be well-founded; but we lack elements that would allow a different perspective.

Pyotr's judgment of his father is just as doubtful. Everyone else considers Stepan Trofimovich a child. But the narrator's description of him shows him to be a more complex figure, touching and possessed of some burlesque traits.

At first, the reader finds his fanciful opinions amusing: we see him as a Russian version of Professor Calculus. Or, to be more modern, as a cartoon character whose misfortunes cause hilarity – the greater, the funnier, because we know that he will survive so he can endure other disasters that will make us laugh even more. We are caught up in play: so important for children of all ages – an experience combining harmoniously aggression, sadism and anxiety. But in Stepan Trofimovich's case, this cruel play with delayed effects quickly becomes disconcerting. We go from amusement to irritation, and suddenly we are ill at ease. Why?

The answer lies in the childlike aspect of our hero. People say he is a child. But what kind of child? Think of a young child who sees in a store window a Superman costume worn by a mannequin: a strong, muscular man. The child is fascinated and asks his parents to buy the costume. When he tries it on, he looks in the mirror and is disappointed: the reflection is not what he saw in the store window. He then has two choices: he can either accept the image he sees in the mirror, letting the costume be a disguise, or he can refuse to play.

But there is another kind of child: the child who can't give up his initial fascination. He wants it to smash through reality, so that he can retrieve the figure in the window. He buys the superhero costume but does not see it as a disguise; it actually is what he imagined. For others, he becomes a laughing stock. While the first type of child learns from his experiences, like an artist, the second is a sick child.

Like a man who thinks he is a mountain climber because he bought some equipment at a sports goods store, Stepan Trofimovich thinks he can set out on the road because he has the clothes he needs. The uneasiness the reader feels is caused by this insistence to try and change reality by means that are neither magical nor humorous. Where is the aggressive, mischievous pleasure of cartoons in a situation where there is only monotony and endless repetition, where talking doesn't change anything, where everything is turned into a means of persecution? This imperviousness to everything that comes from the other, this devastating deafness to the outside world, is exhausting. It is the sadism of the stupid.

Stepan Trofimovich reminds us of people who, as children, were unable to name their emotions. Unhappy children. This inability starts very early in their lives. It can take the form of a *prohibition to think* (Piera Aulagnier). Or it can originate in the parents' difficulty in containing and differentiating their own affects. Parents who repress their emotions because they have difficulty facing them are, of course, unable to encourage the expression of emotions in their children. Unconsciously, they demand that their offspring refuse to express any sensitivity. They pass on to them a feeling of shame about emotions.

The inability to name emotions prevents these emotions from subsisting in a person's internal world. Thus, these emotions become "foreign" to the psychic sphere.

As adults, these children with very limited access to fantasy float in the imaginary realm of a display window where they are supposed to find real feelings in rigidified shapes. Because they cannot dream, they are condemned to vague reverie.

In analysis, one characteristic of *daydreaming* is that *it cannot be interpreted*. It is an activity providing a defence against internal reality, which involves dependence on the other and separation from the other (solitude). Internal reality includes fantasy, governed, as Piera Aulagnier theorised, by the principle of the primary: *all pleasure (or displeasure) depends on the desire of the other.* This means that fantasy, as soon as it appears, involves dependence on the other.

Daydreaming, on the contrary, originates in the despair caused by having no more hope of depending on another, and the desperate measure taken as a consequence: negating the other. In this sense, daydreaming is also an element of manic defence: by negating the other, this reverie becomes no more than a sterile exercise of omnipotence on the part of a subject whose world is a desert, whose life is unbearable torment, whose existence is a series of rigidly controlled events without interest. Because there is no solitude, internal space is a space of isolation. Daydreaming prevents dreaming, fantasy, imagination and thinking.

The activity of daydreaming excludes joy. The subject is made aware of this by his feeling of never being there, in whatever he is doing or experiencing; this feeling is also an aspect of the need to control everything, which involves – if all surprises are to be avoided – control of time based on the predetermined organisation of events that will occur in the future. Daydreaming has no symbolic value. It is pure exaltation without any aim, merely the result of increased instinctual tension, not allowing discharge: the participation of the body is limited to the equivalent of psychomotor agitation.

More generally, daydreaming can serve to avoid thinking, and specifically thoughts of displeasure, suffering and pain. Therefore, daydreaming as such does not lend itself to interpretation.

Daydreaming is a secondary dissociative defensive. Its positive function is to fill the spaces between the different unintegrated portions of the subject: between the body and the thinking process, between dreaming and everyday life, between thinking and fantasy. When daydreaming emerges in an analysis, it can guide the psychoanalyst in his understanding of the situations in which the subject's difficulties with symbolisation are rooted, that is, the traumas that require the subject to daydream.

But when daydreaming is transformed, as it is in Stepan Trofimovich's case, from a defence into a symptom and becomes the subject's *way of being* in the world, the monstrous face of madness emerges, in the form of *stupidity*. This madness is a shapeless combination of hate, anguish, negation and vanity. The way of *being* in the world becomes a pose, similar to the stereotype described by Eugen Bleuler (1950) in *Dementia Praecox*, a major work on schizophrenia. The clinical example in *Demons* is the scene where Stepan Trofimovich stands before the mirror, before giving a reading at the fête organised by the governor's wife. He is certain that what others will see is identical to what he strives to place in the display window. This pathetic situation, arousing horror and disgust, is reminiscent of the scene in *The Double* where Golyadkin's valet tries on the rented livery.[29]

In the sphere of the psyche, fabulation is the activity that corresponds to posing. Fabulation, like daydreaming, is an empty, unreal production. The scenario it creates is frozen, static, a caricature. The subject portrays himself as perfect, all-powerful and loved by everyone.

Through Stepan Trofimovich, Dostoevsky teaches us that the *madness of stupidity* goes hand in hand with the impossibility of naming affects, and the denial of their reality. Every affect is a precursor, and must find at once a representation originating in the manic defence process. This representation is an empty form born of the urgent need to reject a budding emotion. The bodily agitation associated with urgency is a sign of the attempt to expel all sensoriality, to reduce the body to silence and, if need be, to abandon it. A stereotypical pose is a compromise solution, where the desperate need to control sensoriality reduces the body to its muscle structure, to voluntary movement.

In Stepan Trofimovich's case, because he is caught in the madness of stupidity, affect breaks in and persecutes him. Since all affect is a burden, there is no access to rhythm. Without rhythm, there can be no well-being, pleasure, play. And since there is no capacity to dream, there can be no representation of the future. Time is closed in on itself. What dominates is panic, the only possible response to anxiety.

Stupidity prevents aesthetic pleasure, which in the case of burlesque performance is based on the playful experience of sadism. This is so because stupidity exposes us to the violence of shapelessness. It prevents us from thinking because it rejects all common referents, so that the statement just made is disqualified at once by the one that follows. For a stupid subject, any bond is dangerous, because it presupposes shared feelings; therefore, all ties are attacked. *The stupid subject is in love with his emotions*; but not the ones he feels, which are dangerous and therefore forbidden, but the ones he invents – whose only reality is in the unreality of his universe. *Stupidity fears meaning*, because meaning moves the particular *towards the universal*. Meaning is submitted to negation, and negation is, in turn, negated. Stupidity is determined to avoid any psychic elaboration, any new inscription.

Stupidity makes the other crazy, because distinct events never add up to a history, and because daydreams and the aims of a very fragile narcissistic structure are stronger than memory. Anger, in these circumstances, is of no avail. The hatred harboured by stupidity has no address. Suddenly, I vanish, but not because the other makes me disappear. I vanish because I suddenly realise that I never existed for this other caught up in stupidity. I alone imagined that I existed, and that this other existed at my side. Stupidity always stares at its navel, which encloses the void of the world.

Even Varvara Petrovna, insane enough and cruel enough to have produced a murderous offspring, Nikolai Stavrogin, has not been immune to the havoc that Stepan Trofimovich's stupidity could wreck. But thanks to her hold over him, the effects of his folly were restricted. Having no decisions to make, able to count on board and lodging, Stepan Trofimovich spreads his fabulations in a limited and rigid sphere, a framework acting as a sort of envelope, a psychic body.

But when Varvara Petrovna abandons him, everything falls apart. He decides to go away.

> Stepan Trofimovitch [...] was walking resolutely on the damp ground. It was evident that he had planned the enterprise to the best of his ability, alone with

his inexperience and lack of practical sense. He wore "travelling dress," that is, a greatcoat with a wide patent-leather belt, fastened with a buckle and a pair of new high boots pulled over his trousers. Probably he had for some time past pictured a traveller as looking like this, and the belt and the high boots with the shining tops like a hussar's, in which he could hardly walk, had been ready some time before. A broad-brimmed hat, a knitted scarf, twisted close round his neck, a stick in his right hand, and an exceedingly small but extremely tightly packed bag in his left, completed his get-up. He had, besides, in the same right hand, an open umbrella. These three objects – the umbrella, the stick, and the bag – had been very awkward to carry for the first mile, and had begun to be heavy [...]

"Can it really be you?" cried Liza.

"*Lise*," cried Stepan Trofimovitch, rushing to her almost in delirium too. "*Chère, chère.* Can you be out, too [...] in such a fog? [...] *Vous êtes malheureuse, n'est-ce pas?* I (You are unhappy, aren't you?) I see, I see. Don't tell me, but don't question me either. *Nous sommes tous malheureux mais il faut les pardonner tous. Pardonnons, Lise* (We are all unhappy, but we must forgive them all. Let us forgive, Liza), and let us be free forever. To be quit of the world and be completely free. *Il faut pardonner, pardonner, et pardonner!*"

"But why are you kneeling down?"

"Because, taking leave of the world, I want to take leave of all my past in your person!" He wept and raised both her hands to his tear-stained eyes. "I kneel to all that was beautiful in my life. I kiss and give thanks! Now I've torn myself in half; left behind a mad visionary who dreamed of soaring to the sky. *Vingt-deux ans* (Twenty-two years)! Here, a shattered, frozen old man. A tutor *chez ce marchand, s'il existe pourtant ce marchand* (in this merchant's house, if only this merchant exists).

"These people! I saw the glow of their [deeds] all night. They were bound to end in this."

His eyes flashed again. "I am fleeing away from madness, from a delirious dream. I am fleeing away to seek for Russia. *Existe-t-elle, la Russie* (does Russia exist)?"[30]

And later, in the cottage, he goes on:

"You see, my friend. [...] You see I [...] *J'aime le peuple, c'est indispensable, mais il me semble que je ne l'avais jamais vu de près. Stasie* [...] *cela va sans dire qu'elle est aussi du peuple, mais le vrai peuple* (I love the people, that is indispensable, but it seems to me that I have never seen them up close. Nastasya [...] it goes without saying that she is also of the people [...] but the true people), that is, the real ones, who are on the high road, it seems to me they care for nothing, but where exactly I am going. [...] But let bygones be bygones. I fancy I am talking at random, but I believe it's from being flustered.

> "*L'Evangile* [...] *voyez-vous désormais nous prêcherons ensemble* (The Gospel [...] you see, from now on we will preach it together) and I will gladly sell your beautiful little books. Yes, I feel that perhaps is an idea, *quelque chose de très nouveau dans ce genre* (something very new of the sort). The peasants are religious, *c'est admis* (granted), but they don't yet know the gospel. I will expound it to them. [...] By verbal explanation one might correct the mistakes in that remarkable book, which I am of course prepared to treat with the utmost respect. I will be of service even on the high road. I've always been of use, I always told *them* so *et à cette chère ingrate* (that dear ingrate [Varvara Petrovna]). [...] Oh, we will forgive, we will forgive, first of all we will forgive all and always. [...] We will hope that we too shall be forgiven. Yes, for all, every one of us, have wronged one another, all are guilty!"
>
> He told her, too, that he had dreamed of gaping jaws full of teeth, and that he had very much disliked it.[31]

Later, as he lies dying, all fear has receded:

> My immortality is necessary if only because God will not be guilty of injustice and extinguish altogether the flame of love for Him once kindled in my heart. And what is more precious than love? Love is higher than existence, love is the crown of existence; and how is it possible that existence should not be under its dominance? If I have once loved Him and rejoiced in my love, is it possible that He should extinguish me and my joy and bring me to nothingness again? If there is a God, then I am immortal. *Voilà ma profession de foi* (There is my profession of faith).[32]

Seeing the disintegration that follows his abandonment by Varvara Petrovna, the reader understands that stupidity was Stepan Trofimovich's last bastion against schizophrenia. Freewheeling anxiety causes fabulations to spin around a shapeless, sentimental, affective heap. But the pain has no contour, it is diluted in a whiny, ineffectual complaint. And the small portion of soma invested in the vanity of image collapses. We understand that vanity was the last vestige of the ruins of this body; this suggests that very long ago, when its foundations were being constructed, there had been an interruption. Forgiveness as a rampart is not a solid enough reaction formation to stop the torrent of hate turned against oneself and against all expressions of life. And so, Stepan Trofimovich dies as he has lived: stupidly.

All this is absolutely true, yet insufficient. It does not do justice to the character. Stepan Trofimovich is a ridiculous radical intellectual, a Professor Calculus, a grotesque, pathetic, fantastical figure. He is a weak, dependent, pitiful man. A boring, stupid, insane man. But Dostoevsky's genius stays away from categories. His characters are not devitalised by knowledge, they are not locked in a particular form. They are always complex, not to be reduced to the concept that produced them, to their narrative function, and less still to the pathology they illustrate. Dostoevsky combines all these aspects. He takes *everything*.

Stepan Trofimovich's manic exaltation is shown to be coupled with the hatred generating it. Daydreaming and fabulation on the verge of delusion are not presented merely as symptoms. They point clearly to the unbearable truth against which they labour. Stepan Trofimovich says: "*J'ai menti toute ma vie* (I lied all my life)", and: "*Je vous aimais toute ma vie* [...] *vingt ans!* (I loved you all my life [...] twenty years!)". Suddenly, for the reader, his mediocre, colourless existence recedes, in the face of universal human tragedy: the tragedy of powerlessness before the inevitability of aging and death. And we are touched by the death of this man with whom we have become almost intimate.

I have pointed out several times Dostoevsky's respect and love for his characters. But neither this love nor Dostoevsky's talent take anything away from the enigma we encounter in the presence of a real book and a real writer: aesthetic emotion always brings us in contact with the real of the world, the real of the other.

Stavrogin

When we speak of the unconscious today, we generally refer to an aspect of the psychic functioning of a subject which has been buried over time, but which, thanks to interpretation in the therapeutic relation, will be revealed to be active repressed material generating misunderstanding and distortion in the perception of the world.

Of course, revealing what has been repressed can completely change a subject's identificatory configuration and, as a result, his relation to the world and to his future. This hypothesis about the role of the unconscious is commonly accepted in our culture: that discovery of the hidden roots of psychic functioning drastically changes our representation of the self and of the world. This essential work on the unconscious is what is generally oversimplified and distorted by those opposed to taking unconscious processes into account. According to them, this work consists of nothing more than establishing a direct correspondence (like drawing a parallel) between what takes place in reality and a set of symbolic meanings that have remained unchanged since Freud: the Oedipus complex, castration, dependence on the mother, refusal of paternal authority, etc.

This oversimplification presents the psychic apparatus as being composed of two levels, with messages travelling between them, and the blurring of certain messages in the course of this transmission. Thus, this distorted perspective leads back to what it tries to deny – namely, the existence of the unconscious. But this confirmation aims at trivialisation, ultimately to discredit the means by which access to the unconscious is gained: psychoanalysis. Given that symbolic meanings remain unchanged, psychoanalysis has completed its work; now, all that has to be done, thanks to this stupid catalogue, is to adjust and regulate the channels of communication.

But there is another way of applying the hypothesis of the unconscious: by working with the boundless possibilities of madness. Here, compartmental oversimplification loses its hold. Here, we are no longer trying to resolve a psychic conflict caused by messages passing from one level of the psychic apparatus to the other. Willingness to work with the excessiveness of madness implies continuous and renewed effort to temporarily close psychic spaces left catastrophically boundless, without recognised limits. Faced with the excessiveness of madness, there are no unalterable facts, and the unconscious does not exist. Faced with the excessive nature of madness, an unconscious has to be constructed.

Nikolai Stavrogin has no unconscious. Several times, as the plot of *The Demons* unfolds, this void becomes obvious. The confession made to Father Tikhon is a critical passage to which I shall return.

Pyotr Stepanovich

Kirillov's suicide is one of the moments in the plot when the reader encounters this void. Kirillov can be identified as the forerunner of Nietzsche: God is dead, and, if God is dead, everything is permitted. Kirillov is one of Stavrogin's disciples, as is Pyotr Stepanovich, who is there at the time of the suicide, when Kirillov goes into the adjoining room to shoot himself in the head. Pyotr Stepanovich waits to hear the shot; he wants to be sure Kirillov has killed himself, to be able to leave reassured – he has just persuaded Kirillov to write a letter confessing to the murder of Shatov. Let us quote this passage:

> Though he had been reading and admiring the wording of it, he had been listening anxiously all the time, and he suddenly flew into a rage. He looked anxiously at his watch; it was getting late and it was fully ten minutes since Kirillov had gone out. [...] Snatching up the candle, he went to the door of the room where Kirillov had shut himself up. He was just at the door when the thought struck him that the candle had burnt out, that it would not last another twenty minutes, and that there was no other in the room. He took hold of the handle and listened warily; he did not hear the slightest sound. He suddenly opened the door and lifted up the candle: something uttered a roar and rushed at him. He slammed the door with all his might and pressed his weight against it; but all sounds died away and again there was deathlike stillness.
>
> He stood for a long while irresolute, with the candle in his hand. He had been able to see very little in the second he held the door open, but he had caught a glimpse of the face of Kirillov standing at the other end of the room by the window, and the savage fury with which the latter had rushed upon him. Pyotr Stepanovitch started, rapidly set the candle on the table, made ready his revolver, and retreated on tiptoe to the farthest corner of the room, so that if Kirillov opened the door and rushed up to the table with the revolver he would still have time to be the first to aim and fire.
>
> Pyotr Stepanovitch had by now lost all faith in the suicide. "He was standing in the middle of the room, thinking," flashed like a whirlwind through Pyotr Stepanovitch's mind, "and the room was dark and horrible too. [...] He roared and rushed at me. There are two possibilities: either I interrupted him

at the very second when he was pulling the trigger or [...] or he was standing planning how to kill me. Yes, that's it, he was planning it. [...] He knows I won't go away without killing him if he funks it himself – so that he would have to kill me first to prevent my killing him. [...] And again, again there is silence. I am really frightened: he may open the door all of a sudden. [...] The nuisance of it is that he believes in God like any priest. [...] He won't shoot himself for anything! There are lots of these people nowadays 'who've come to it of themselves.' A rotten lot! Oh, damn it, the candle, the candle! It'll go out within a quarter of an hour for certain. [...] I must put a stop to it; come what may, I must put a stop to it. [...] Now I can kill him. [...] With that document here no one would think of my killing him. I can put him in such an attitude on the floor with an unloaded revolver in his hand that they'd be certain he'd done it himself. [...] Ach, damn it! how is one to kill him? If I open the door he'll rush out again and shoot me first. Damn it all, he'll be sure to miss!"

He was in agonies, trembling at the necessity of action and his own indecision. At last he took up the candle and again approached the door with the revolver held up in readiness; he put his left hand, in which he held the candle, on the doorhandle. But he managed awkwardly: the handle clanked, there was a rattle and a creak. "He will fire straightway," flashed through Pyotr Stepanovitch's mind. With his foot he flung the door open violently, raised the candle, and held out the revolver; but no shot nor cry came from within. [...] There was no one in the room.

He started. The room led nowhere. There was no exit, no means of escape from it. He lifted the candle higher and looked about him more attentively: there was certainly no one. He called Kirillov's name in a low voice, then again louder; no one answered.

"Can he have got out by the window?" The casement in one window was, in fact, open. "Absurd! He couldn't have got away through the casement." Pyotr Stepanovitch crossed the room and went up to the window. "He couldn't possibly." All at once he turned round quickly and was aghast at something extraordinary.

Against the wall facing the window on the right of the door stood a cupboard. On the right side of this cupboard, in the corner formed by the cupboard and the wall, stood Kirillov, and he was standing in a very strange way; motionless, perfectly erect, with his arms held stiffly at his sides, his head raised and pressed tightly back against the wall in the very corner, he seemed to be trying to conceal and efface himself. Everything seemed to show that he was hiding, yet somehow it was not easy to believe it. Pyotr Stepanovitch was standing a little sideways to the corner, and could only see the projecting parts of the figure. He could not bring himself to move to the left to get a full view of Kirillov and solve the mystery. His heart began beating violently, and he felt a sudden rush of blind fury; he started from where he stood, and, shouting and stamping with his feet, he rushed to the horrible place.

But when he reached Kirillov he stopped short again, still more overcome, horror-stricken. What struck him most was that, in spite of his shout and his furious rush, the figure did not stir, did not move in a single limb – as though it were of stone or of wax. The pallor of the face was unnatural, the black eyes were quite unmoving and were staring away at a point in the distance. Pyotr Stepanovitch lowered the candle and raised it again, lighting up the figure from all points of view and scrutinising it. He suddenly noticed that, although Kirillov was looking straight before him, he could see him and was perhaps watching him out of the corner of his eye. Then the idea occurred to him to hold the candle right up to the wretch's face, to scorch him and see what he would do. He suddenly fancied that Kirillov's chin twitched and that something like a mocking smile passed over his lips – as though he had guessed Pyotr Stepanovitch's thought. He shuddered and, beside himself, clutched violently at Kirillov's shoulder.

Then something happened so hideous and so soon over that Pyotr Stepanovitch could never afterwards recover a coherent impression of it. He had hardly touched Kirillov when the latter bent down quickly and with his head knocked the candle out of Pyotr Stepanovitch's hand; the candlestick fell with a clang on the ground and the candle went out. At the same moment he was conscious of a fearful pain in the little finger of his left hand. He cried out, and all that he could remember was that, beside himself, he hit out with all his might and struck three blows with the revolver on the head of Kirillov, who had bent down to him and had bitten his finger. At last he tore away his finger and rushed headlong to get out of the house, feeling his way in the dark. He was pursued by terrible shouts from the room.

"Directly, directly, directly, directly." Ten times. But he still ran on, and was running into the porch when he suddenly heard a loud shot. Then he stopped short in the dark porch and stood deliberating for five minutes; at last he made his way back into the house. But he had to get the candle. He had only to feel on the floor on the right of the cupboard for the candlestick; but how was he to light the candle? There suddenly came into his mind a vague recollection: he recalled that when he had run into the kitchen the day before to attack Fedka he had noticed in passing a large red box of matches in a corner on a shelf. Feeling with his hands, he made his way to the door on the left leading to the kitchen, found it, crossed the passage, and went down the steps. On the shelf, on the very spot where he had just recalled seeing it, he felt in the dark a full unopened box of matches. He hurriedly went up the steps again without striking a light, and it was only when he was near cupboard, at the spot where he had struck Kirillov with the revolver and been bitten by him, that he remembered his bitten finger, and at the same instant was conscious that it was unbearably painful. Clenching his teeth, he managed somehow to light the candle-end, set it in the candlestick again, and looked about him: near the open casement, with his feet towards the right-hand corner, lay the dead body of Kirillov. The shot had been fired at the right

> temple and the bullet had come out at the top on the left, shattering the skull. There were splashes of blood and brains. The revolver was still in the suicide's hand on the floor. Death must have been instantaneous. After a careful look round, Pyotr Stepanovitch got up and went out on tiptoe, closed the door, left the candle on the table in the outer room, thought a moment, and resolved not to put it out, reflecting that it could not possibly set fire to anything. Looking once more at the document left on the table, he smiled mechanically and then went out of the house, still for some reason walking on tiptoe. He crept through Fedka's hole again and carefully replaced the posts after him.[33]

Why do I quote this remarkable horrific scene in its entirety? Since Kirillov and Pyotr Stepanovich are two contradictory creations of Nikolai Stavrogin, I suggest that we consider this frightful scenario as representing the internal world of this completely unclassifiable man.

The character Nikolai Stavrogin has a long history in Dostoevsky's imagination, a history worth recounting. He is descended from the protagonist of *The Life of a Great Sinner*, one of two novels on atheism Dostoevsky had been planning for years, but never actually wrote.

The Life of a Great Sinner

The great sinner

> is simply a primitive type, subconsciously agitated by his own primitive strength, a strength which is completely spontaneous [...] an extraordinary innate power, hard to bear for those who possess it, a power which asks for and seeks a foundation to stand on and a cause to lead, a power which greatly suffers if it is exposed to the storms of life, yet cannot help stirring up storms before it finds peace. He finally comes to rest in Christ, but his whole life is all storm and disorder.[34]

Such a type

> joyfully throws itself – in its period of searches and wanderings – into monstrous deviations and experiments until it comes to rest on *an idea powerful enough to be fully proportionate to its own immediate primitive strength* – an idea so powerful that it can at last organize its strength and calm it down to a tranquilizing stillness.[35]

Even as a boy, the "great sinner" feels "disrespect toward people around him, but not yet consciously, *solely because of disgust with them.* [...] A savage boy, but who has an immense opinion of himself".[36]

Dostoevsky's intention for the novel was to have the great sinner undergo a sudden conversion, as a result of meeting Father Tikhon, a character based on "the figure of Saint Tikhon Zadonsky, a Russian clergyman of the mid-eighteenth century who was elevated to sainthood in 1860, and left an abundant literary legacy (fifteen volumes)".[37]

In *Treasury of the Spirit*, one of his major works, Saint Tikhon declares that "the son of God came to save sinners, not only such and such, but all, whoever they may be"; this statement is to be found in the chapter "Criminals and Joyous News for Them". Elsewhere, he declares: "There is no kind of sin, and there cannot be any such on earth, that God would not pardon to someone who sincerely repents".[38] (In *The Devils*, Father Tikhon repeats this to Stavrogin after reading his confession.)

I would add that what the monk calls repentance brings to mind the process of reflection, and what Freud calls elaboration. I say this because one of the attributes of Dostoevsky's characters is that they submit *everything* to reflection. And the tragic thing about these characters is that they are unable to admit that thinking *cannot solve everything*.

Dostoevsky writes in his *Notebooks*:

> After the monastery and Tikhon [Stavrogin] again returns into the world to be the *greatest of men* [...] he is the proudest of the proud and treats people with great arrogance. [...] But (and this is the essential) thanks to Tikhon he had been seized by the idea (conviction): that to conquer the entire world it suffices to conquer oneself. Conquer thyself and thou wilt conquer the world.

A few years later, Freud would say something very similar.

Then, Dostoevsky outlines the successive stages in the life of the *Great Sinner*:

> Suddenly, youth and debauchery. [...] A great moral feat and terrible crimes. Mad pride. Out of pride he becomes an anchorite and a wanderer. Travels all over Russia [...] *Traits*. Out of pride [...] he becomes kindly and gracious toward everybody – precisely because he is already immeasurably higher than everyone else.[39]

We can see clearly what an enormous difference it makes in constructing the character Stavrogin – and the structure of the novel – that the confession to Tikhon was prohibited by Tsarist censure. As a result of this omission, some of Stepan Trofimovich's thoughts in the novel are found in Dostoevsky's *Notebooks* as Stavrogin's thoughts after his visit to the monk. Is the character's suicide the result of this prohibition to publish the *Confession*?

The question is worth asking. In any case, on 11 March 1870, a fundamental change was made to the Stavrogin character: no longer believing in his own redemption, he chooses self-destruction. In *The Notebooks*, Dostoevsky describes him as:

> a person who is easily bored. [...] Yet there remains in him the question: what is he himself? The answer for him is "*Nothing*". [...] But his character is a lofty one, and it causes him dissatisfaction ang agony to be nothing in particular. He finds no solid basis [...] within himself .

Just before this, Dostoevsky had written: "*he does not find it necessary to be a Russian*".[40]

This new portrayal of the character leads Dostoevsky to make Stavrogin – now clearly designated – the protagonist of the novel; he is

> the main hero of the novel. He makes friends with Shatov, causes him to become an enthusiastic follower of his doctrine [nihilism], while not believing in it himself. He just observes everything, remaining indifferent [...] even to the murder of Shatov, of which he has knowledge. [...] He seduces a 13-year-old, which creates an uproar. (It just happened by chance, a passing fancy.) He is gentle, modest, quiet, boundlessly proud and bestially cruel. [...] And so, the whole pathos of the novel lies in [Stavrogin]; he is the hero.[41]

Joseph Frank observes that through Stavrogin, Dostoevsky can express all his complex views on the spiritual disease of the literary idols of his youth – a disease he considered to be the cause of the disintegrating European influence on the Russian cultural psyche. What is this "Russian age" (which produced Stavrogin), if not the history of a culture whose most brilliant and most talented representatives have lost touch with their people, and then, inevitably, with their people's faith? At the end of March 1870, the character Stavrogin no longer seeks ideological inspiration from Shatov; instead, Shatov, Kirillov and even Pyotr Verkhovensky look to him for inspiration. Now, the book takes on a different and richer character. Dostoevsky questions his deepest values and convictions. In fact, Stavrogin is endowed with the religious attributes initially intended for the *Great Sinner* after his conversion. Dostoevsky saw this debate as involving the theme of Russia itself, and its Messianic calling in the destiny of humankind.

In a letter to his editor, Dostoevsky comments that although murder is a central theme in his novel, the main character is not Pyotr Verkhovensky, the leader of the terrorists. Murder is

> only accessory and a setting for the actions of another character, who could really be called the main character [...] [Nikolai Stavrogin] – also a sinister character, also a villain. But he seems to me a tragic character. [...] I embarked on the poem about this character because for much too long I have wished to portray him. *In my opinion he is Russian, and a typical character.* [It is important to point out that Dostoevsky clearly recognises the universal character of Stavrogin.] He comes straight from my heart. Of course, this character seldom appears in *all its typicality*.[42]

The dandy

When we read this today, we probably take "all its typicality" to mean that the character is described fully, with his unconscious dimension. But there is another reason for speaking of the typicality, or fullness, of the character. While it is not hard to see that the relation between Stepan Trofimovich and his son illustrates Dostoevsky's conviction that the liberals of his generation are responsible for the emergence of nihilism as a political phenomenon, Stavrogin's lack of firm identity has its roots in an even earlier era. Indeed, the character of Stavrogin displays the traits of the Byronic Russian dandy who haunted the literature of the 1820s and 1830s. This is what Dostoevsky wrote in 1861 about Pushkin's *Evgeny Onegin*:

> Onegin precisely belongs to that epoch of our historical life marked by the very first beginnings of our agonizing consciousness and [...] our agonizing uncertainty as we look around us [...] that epoch when our leading men sharply separated into two camps [Slavophils and Westernizers] and then violently engaged in a civil war. [...] [These two camps] were also a historical manifestation and in the highest degree national. [...] But in Onegin all this had only just begun to be glimpsed. [...] The skepticism of Onegin contained something tragic in its very principle, and sometimes expressed itself with malicious irony.[43]

Onegin, like Stavrogin, was a member of the Russian gentry, for which he had no respect. Stavrogin does not know what to respect, he is lost. At the same time, he doesn't know how to react to the new phenomena around him, whether he should welcome them or laugh at them. He has no ideals, "he does not even know what to respect, though he is firmly convinced that there is something that must be respected and loved". But he has become cynical and does not respect himself, or his thoughts and opinions.

> [H]e does not respect even his own thirst for life and truth. [...] He becomes an egoist, and at the same time ridicules himself because he does not even know how to be that. [...] [He has] an egoism extending to the limits of self-adoration and malicious self-contempt. And always this thirst for truth, and always the same eternal "nothing to do!"[44]

Thus, the character of the Byronic dandy is the first manifestation of the influence of the Enlightenment on Russian mentality and culture. Joseph Frank observes:

> here was the origin of the negation of Russia that had finally culminated in the abhorrent Nechaev, and since for Dostoevsky the idea of Russia was inseparable from that of the Russian Christ and the Orthodox faith, the tragedy of Stavrogin – like that of Onegin – takes the form of a moral-religious crisis. It is the search for an absolute faith that has been surrendered to the blandishments of the European Enlightenment and cannot yet be recaptured despite the torturing need for a "new truth". It is [Stavrogin] who has brought to Russia all the "beauty" of this idolatrous negation, which, if allowed to go unchallenged by the "authentic beauty" of Christ, would light the same torch of destruction in Holy Russia that was already ravaging the West.[45]

The real figure that Stavrogin most resembles might be Nikolai Spechnev, whom Dostoevsky called "a Mephistopheles of [his] own" at the time when he belonged to Petrashevsky's circle, resulting in his imprisonment in Siberia. Spechnev was indeed a Byronic figure comparable to Stavrogin: a rich and cultured aristocrat, irresistible to women. He was also a fervent radical, a committed communist and the head of *a secret revolutionary group comprised of seven members, including Dostoevsky* (the latter hid this compromising affiliation throughout his life).[46]

A Byronic dandy, Stavrogin's good looks are those of a demon, whose inner conflicts cannot be resolved because nothing can appease him. *"Demon" is the name I will give to a subject with no unconscious.* As Herzen wrote referring to Byron's *Cain*, the fascination exerted by Stavrogin is like "still moonlit water, that promises nothing but death in its comfortless, cold, glimmering embraces".[47]

Madness and murder

It is through Stavrogin that madness enters the novel. He is presented to the reader as a living corpse:

> His hair was of a peculiarly intense black, his light-colored eyes were peculiarly light and calm, his complexion was peculiarly soft and white, the red in his cheeks was too bright and clear, his teeth were like pearls and his lips like coral – one would have thought that he must be a paragon of beauty, yet at the same time there seemed something repellent about him. It was said that his face suggested a mask [...] they talked of his extra-ordinary physical strength.[48]

We are given sufficient information about his childhood. His parents separated when he was very young, and Stepan Trofimovich took charge of his education, at the request of Varvara Stavrogin, his mother, left to bring him up alone. Because Stepan Trofimovich was himself a child, he could not be a father figure for little Nicolas.

> More than once he awakened his ten- or eleven-year-old friend at night, simply to pour out his wounded feelings and weep before him, or to tell him some family secret, without realising that this was an outrageous proceeding. They threw themselves into each other's arms and wept.[49]

As for the mother, we have already witnessed her ruthless character and her madness. "She talked little to him and did not often interfere with him, but he was always morbidly conscious of her intent, searching eyes fixed upon him". At sixteen, "he was fragile-looking and pale, strangely quiet and dreamy".[50] To please his mother, he embarked on a military career and, before falling into a life of debauchery, was very well thought of by his superiors. But soon he started to display brutal conduct to the ladies, who succumbed easily to his charm.

When he visited his native province, after a period of silence, he unexpectedly forced a highly respected member of the town's high society to walk along while he was holding him by the nose. This gentleman was in the habit of declaring vehemently: "*No, you can't lead me by the nose!*" Indeed, Dostoevsky apparently understood that in a state of madness words are taken to be the things themselves, and not merely their representation. Stavrogin's outrages continued: he bit the ear of the governor while seeming to whisper a secret, and he kissed the wife of his host passionately at a party. The narrator comments: "It is remarkable that no one in the whole town put down the savage act to madness. They must have been predisposed to expect such actions from Nikolay Vsyevoloditch, even when he was sane".[51]

It was not until four years later that Nikolai Stavrogin returned to his home town. He arrived at his mother's home just as she had received a surprise visit from Marya Timofeevna, the demented woman he had secretly married in the city. Pyotr Trofimovich, the evil doer, had just arrived. In the course of the evening, Shatov strikes Stavrogin in the face because he surmises the latter's marriage to the poor girl, and despises Stavrogin for not admitting it (but the reader may well wonder whether this rage has to do with the fact that Stavrogin seduced Shatov's wife, as well as his sister).

What impressed everyone who witnessed this incident was Stavrogin's impassiveness, not his self-control, after Shatov struck him. Nikolai Stavrogin spent the following week at home, away from people, waiting for his wounds to heal.

This is how the narrator describes him when he returns to his home town after an absence of several years:

> His eyes had the same stern, thoughtful and, as it were, preoccupied air. But one thing struck me. In the old days, though he had been considered handsome, his face was "like a mask". [...] Now – now, I don't know why he impressed me at once as absolutely handsome, incontestably beautiful, so that no one could have said that his face was like a mask. Wasn't it perhaps that he was a little paler and seemed rather thinner than before? Or was there, perhaps, the light of some new idea in his eyes?[52]

Now let us return to Stavrogin as he prepares to go and see Kirillov, and then Shatov, to discuss urgent matters. Pyotr Trofimovich has come to see him, very agitated, bringing the latest gossip going around town, some of which he has started himself. Pyotr suggests, in a round-about manner, that Stavrogin could make use of Fedka, a convict who escaped from Siberia, and had been his serf, to murder Marya Timofeevna, should the need arise. He adds, in passing, that Fedka is ready to do anything for a price. Later, things would be carried out in just this way, at Pyotr Trofimovich's instigation. Nikolai Stavrogin feels responsible for this murder he did nothing to prevent. The same scenario of murder by proxy, with all the ambiguities and uncertainties associated with it, is to be found in *The Brothers Karamazov*, in the context of the relation between Ivan and Smerdyakov.

Nikolai Stavrogin calls on Kirillov to ask him to act as a witness at the duel he cannot avoid with the son of the man he had led by the nose, who has been sending him insulting letters. Then Stavrogin goes to see Shatov, to warn him of Pyotr Trofimovich's plan to kill him.[53]

Divining the other

Meeting Nikolai Stavrogin was a life-changing event for Kirillov and Shatov. I would like to draw attention to a characteristic the two encounters have in common – a characteristic I find crucial.

Kirillov states that "Man is unhappy because he doesn't know he's happy". And he adds: "It's only that. That's all, that's all. If anyone finds out he'll become happy at once, that minute. The daughter-in-law will die; but the baby will [live]. It's all good".

Trying to understand, Stavrogin asks: "And if anyone dies of hunger, and if anyone insults and outrages the little girl, is that good?"

Kirillov answers: "Yes! And if anyone blows his brains out [on account of] the baby, that's good too. And if anyone doesn't, that's good too. It's all good, all [of it]". And he concludes: "They're bad because they don't know they're good. When they find out, they won't outrage a little girl. They'll find out they're good and they'll all become good, every one of them".[54]

This passage raises a crucial question: why does Kirillov choose the example of the little girl from the random list his visitor presented? Why does he come back to it to make his demonstration? We know that no one is aware of Stavrogin's obsession with his crime, which he will reveal for the first time to Tikhon. We can only presume that Kirillov perceived a tone of voice or some other sign showing the subjective significance of this example for his friend. Let us remember that this conversation deals with two extreme situations: a duel planned for the following day – thus, the possibility of a murder – and Kirillov's plan to kill himself, a possibility Stavrogin too has often considered. It is clear that this conversation touches upon subjects which bring it into the sphere of originary processes.[55] If we add to this the fact that the two protagonists want to explore this sphere, we bring together some of the elements found in psychoanalytic treatment, where the real of transference makes it possible to divine, and thereby to name, a scene previously excluded from the psychic world.

Divination is also straightaway at the centre of the conversation with Shatov. He divined that Nikolai would come to see him; he also divined that the latter had married Marya Timofeevna. And Stavrogin guessed that Shatov had intuited this. Then, Shatov divined that Stavrogin married Marya out of guilt:

> "Then I guessed [divined] right and you too guessed [divined] right," Nikolay Vsyevolodovitch went on in a tranquil voice. "You are right. Marya Timofyevna [...] is my lawful wife, married to me four and a half years ago in Petersburg".

> Shatov, utterly astounded, listened in silence. "I guessed, but did not believe it".[56]

Shatov is in a frenzy, he is shouting. His agitation and anguish spring from a thought he has just had: that if Nikolai's marriage to Marya is a punishment, Stavrogin must have committed a crime. What frightens Shatov is not something he simply imagines; he knows Stavrogin well enough to be convinced that the latter is capable of the worst: "Shatov hid his face in his hands, turned away, but suddenly clutched Stavrogin by the shoulders. 'Do you know why, anyway,' *he shouted*, 'why you did all this, and why you are resolved on such a punishment now!'".[57]

Stavrogin acknowledges the astuteness of his friend's remark: "Your question is *clever and malignant*, but I mean to surprise you too; I fancy I do know why I got married then, and why I am resolved on such a punishment now, as you express it".[58]

Stavrogin was to confirm this in his confession to Father Tikhon: he married to punish himself for causing the little girl's suicide, for having killed her. But Shatov guesses something essential, that I will come back to later:

> "You married from a *passion for martyrdom*, from a craving for remorse, through moral sensuality. It was a laceration of the nerves. [...] Defiance of common sense was too tempting. Stavrogin and a wretched, half-witted, crippled beggar! When you bit the governor's ear did you feel sensual pleasure? Did you? You idle, loafing, little snob?"
>
> "You're a psychologist," said Stavrogin, turning paler and paler.[59]

Tikhon intuits Stavrogin's pride. Shatov, who loves Stavrogin, intuits things at a deeper level. Under the pride, he detects the pathological sensuality of a man who is bored, who makes commitments as an amateur, because he has nothing better to do.[60]

Shatov loves Stavrogin; he is probably the only human being who ever loved him. He says as much: "Drop your tone, and speak like a human being. Speak, if only once in your life, with the voice of a man. I say it not for my sake but for yours".[61] And all at once, Shatov divined again: "Do you suppose I don't see from your face that some new menacing idea is dominating you?"[62] He is worried because he loves Nikolai. He tells him:

> "Stavrogin, why am I condemned to believe in you through all eternity? Could I speak like this to anyone else? I have modesty, but I am not ashamed of my nakedness because it's Stavrogin I am speaking to. I was not afraid of caricaturing a grand idea by handling it because Stavrogin was listening to me. [...] Shan't I kiss your footprints when you've gone? I can't tear you out of my heart, Nikolay Stavrogin!"
>
> "I'm sorry I can't feel affection for you, Shatov," Stavrogin replied coldly.
>
> "I know you can't, and I know you are not lying".[63]

Stavrogin doesn't love, he cannot feel affection. *In fact, the only thing he is attached to is his own suffering.* The hate he nurtures for himself fosters this suffering. I spoke earlier of the need we all have to be ill, sometimes very ill. But when one falls in love with one's own suffering, a complication arises: it becomes very difficult to let the suffering go, to leave it behind. To leave one's suffering is very difficult because, when all is said and done, it is the only thing the subject really has. This suffering is his tie to the world, it is what allows him to feel real. These considerations are essential when working with psychotics. The moment of greatest risk in the therapy of a psychotic comes when he starts to like life. Sometimes it is precisely at that point that such a patient commits suicide – to avoid leaving the precious possession that suffering is for him. To prevent such traumatic events, young therapists who see their clinical work as a heroic adventure should reflect on these paradoxes. Such reflection may lessen their desire to cure all patients at any cost.

Since Shatov knows and loves Stavrogin, his judgment is very valuable. Before leaving, he tells Stavrogin: "You're an atheist because you're [an aristocrat], a snob of the snobs".[64] An aristocrat is a man who is bored. Stavrogin is bored, unlike Shatov and Kirillov who – like Raskolnikov – are passionate.

Stavrogin's boredom is that of a man without a place. Having no place, he can't take the risk of loving. Neither can he be moved by art. Stavrogin is a man in whom intelligence sterilises everything.

But his boredom does not make him a man born of an idea, like the Underground Man. In *Demons*, it is Pyotr Stepanovich Verkhovensky who is born of an idea. In a letter to his editor, Dostoevsky says of Pyotr:

> my Peter Verkhovensky may not at all resemble Nechaev, but it seems to me that my aroused mind has created by imagination the person, the type, that really corresponds to the crime. To be sure, there is some value in depicting such a man, but he alone would not have enticed me. In my opinion, these pitiful freaks are not worthy of literature. *To my own surprise, this figure half turns out with me to be a comic figure.* [65]

Before they take leave of each other, Shatov tells Stavrogin to go and see the monk Tikhon. Thus, at the level of the plot, the meeting with Tikhon is the continuation and deepening of the conversation with Shatov.

But let us return to the question of divining or divination in the psychoanalytic process, based on these examples. It is important to point out that the meeting between Stavrogin and Shatov, like the meeting with Kirillov, is an extreme situation where the narcissism of each protagonist is severely tested, and where originary processes predominate. We have already seen this with Stavrogin. As for Shatov, he did not find it unthinkable that Stavrogin might come to kill him after the punch in the face he gave him at Varvara Petrovna's home – he had even bought a revolver to defend himself. He says he has been delirious, and that perhaps he still is.

Based on these examples, three conditions are necessary for divination to take place:

- narcissistic fragility that makes the encounter with the real more brutal (when I say narcissistic fragility, I mean to emphasize that the usual ego defence mechanisms are dormant). This narcissistic fragility leads to:
    - dominance of the primary and originary processes;
    - an extreme psychic state.

But these conditions do not suffice to bring about events. Think of a delusional subject who calls out to you on the street. If you respond solely in a primary and violent manner, the situation can escalate all the way to murder. What allowed the brutally frank exchanges between Stavrogin and Shatov not to degenerate into violence was no doubt mutual respect, but – above all – their shared desire to think. Thanks to this shared *desire to think*, no feeling of uncanniness was felt by either subject when his most intimate subjective stance was surmised; the desire to think gives the divination the status of a *nomination*, instead of an intrusion by the other.

I commented, in our discussion of *The Idiot*, that because the prince is not burdened by ego-support needs, he has a great capacity to identify with what others feel, and an impressive ability to *guess* the feelings of his interlocutor and name them.

Asceticism

Where is all this leading us? Doubtless to the psychoanalyst's manner of functioning. The analyst is asked to be completely receptive to the total presence of the other. Can we identify some of the conditions favourable to this attitude in an analyst?

Reflecting on *Notes from Underground*, I told myself that this novella outlines the conditions necessary for this type of thinking to exist: as I have said, all true thinking must stem from a place beyond self-esteem. I also pointed out that it is not possible to think and to protect oneself from the consequences of one's thinking. One does not formulate a thought in order to be loved or admired; an idea is presented to be shared with others, to be submitted to their judgment, to be spread around the world. In addition, an absence of self-esteem allows one to discern with precision the most subtle variations of sensibility in oneself and in others. This hypothesis of an absence of self-esteem leads to the idea of asceticism.

At times, the patient places himself between me and my thought, or slips between himself and the rest of his thought. One of the ways in which Freud defined transference was by saying that it takes the place of an association, that it is a false association. Analytic practice focusing on the treatment of trauma can make us forget this clinical observation, which is both useful and productive. The fact is that even psychotics associate. They can associate as long as their speech is rooted in a zone of the body felt and recognised for what it is.

To come back to the psychoanalyst's asceticism: we know that it has not been reached as long as the analyst places himself between himself and his patient.

Of course, I am happy when a patient expresses his or her gratitude for the work we are doing together. This indicates that introjection has taken place, or is in the process of occurring. I am happy for this person as long as these are signs of expansion or transformation in his inner world. But as far as I am concerned, I do not expect thanks from my patients. I do not hope for praise or narcissistic rewards. I am expected to do a certain work for which they pay me. It would be absurd for me to expect them to confirm that I practise my profession suitably, or to express their gratitude for what I do.

There are patients one loves as a father would love his child. I have patients I admire for the extraordinary courage with which they live their lives. I know that they love me as well, and I understand the crucial importance I have in their lives. But for me, this importance and this love are intimately linked with the work we accomplish together; when they continue to come to see me, it is not to bill and coo, but to work with me.

When an analyst does not yet have the asceticism required by this profession, he complicates things for his patients considerably. Accepting narcissistic rewards from one's patients, being open to receiving them, confines the patient to the transference, when he should make use of transference to take himself to a different place in his life or in his sensitivity. Transference is a powerful transformative tool, but it always produces a certain degree of alienation. When what is involved is idealisation of the analyst, the situation is manageable. This is so because we know that persecution will soon follow, and this expectation of seeing a reversal of the situation creates a tension, a dynamic, impels us to understand what is taking place, to find possible interpretations; it makes us dream and play with possibilities. This situation allows us to imagine what might come of the possible manifestations of transference, to dream of what the patient might become.

Things are completely different when the psychoanalyst's narcissism plays a role in the therapeutic process. This narcissism becomes an unconscious worry for the patient, who will try to respond to what he divines, or what he has perceived as the analyst's psychic expectations regarding him.

In these situations, the type of narcissism that emerges is that of the hysteric who always slips in between the other and his thoughts, between the other and his psychic investments.

As an illustration – you are reflecting out loud on a book, or on an important event you just experienced, and something you say prompts an association of ideas on the part of your interlocutor; he begins to speak passionately about the wood cabinet he just bought, using this as an opportunity to teach you the characteristics of every possible type of wood, as well as the details of tree farming. Just when you've given up and start to show interest in the felling of maple trees, he says: "But what were you saying about the book you are reading?"

Freud spoke of hysterical loquacity covering over great anxiety that originates in enormous primary fragility. This fragility is rooted in the deficiencies of the symbolic relationship with the mother. The hysteric places his words, in the form of questions, plans, experiences, between this fragility and his internal world, and later between this fragility and the world. Even thinking – genuine thinking – can be used to fill this space. Hysterical narcissism sets up a frantic rhythm of manic stuffing of the psyche, to prevent the dreaded possibility of fragility taking over the whole psyche. When a patient is trapped in the tangled web of this devouring necessity, things become complicated for both him and the analyst. Therefore, I advise young psychoanalysts to be very careful in situations where patients compliment them and their talents as therapists.

It is from the starting point of this asceticism required to exercise the profession of psychoanalyst that I would like to discuss thinking which divines the real. The "real", as I understand it here, consists of unconscious identifications and counter-identifications which clearly create a link at the time of the encounter, and serve as the foundation of the relationship between the subjects: for example, between Stavrogin and Kirillov, Stavrogin and Shatov, Stavrogin and Pyotr Stepanovich. The real consists of a combination of desires and defences, investments and counter-investments – a complex combination on which to build a reality in which it can feel good to live. Thus, to divine the real means to uncover off-stage elements previously excluded and make them accessible to thought, so as to widen the field of possibilities in one's life.

Let us start at the beginning – interpretation is not directed at the ego. Interpretation aims at a change in the subject's psychic position. This transformation means that what was unknown or inaccessible until then becomes thinkable. Interpretation, which allows thinking to hold sway over matters previously out of its reach, changes the relation to the unknown, which can itself become an object of desire. But the transformation of the unknown into the thinkable can produce pain, because this shift radically changes the place of the subject: in his relation to himself, to the world, to his past, to events in the present, to his view of the future. Thus, to desire the unknown involves accepting a certain displeasure inseparable from this quest, a displeasure softened by the promise of an accomplishment – that of widening the field of possibilities, of having greater control over one's psychic life.

This paradox is inherent to psychoanalysis: the less weight the analyst places on the sphere of transference of his ego, the better he can be fully present to the other.

But when an interpretation divines the real, this accurate guess is rooted in a point of trauma in the analyst's past; to be more precise, in the fact that he has survived a trauma. This, of course, influences the way he expresses his thoughts, and places him in a sphere beyond risk – beyond all risk, including that of death. From this position, he can bear responsibility for the effects on the other of revealing the truth in the exchanges between them. At times, the effects of this truth are violent. The fact that he vouches for the process constitutes a promise that creates a bond, and an expectation of what is yet to follow: the meaning and the history.

When the analyst engages with the other and sets aside the interests of his own ego, he accepts at a deep level the affective scandal of his presence at this encounter. From that point on, he will be able to formulate his thoughts from a place ruled by the joy of having survived his own death.

It is from this place that, unbeknownst to him, an unconscious can begin to be built. This construction presupposes that ties could be created and recognised. *Nikolai Stavrogin cannot find a dwelling place for the enormity of his madness because he refuses to create ties.*

We encounter this refusal to create bonds in the treatment of subjects who suffered great deprivation or trauma, or were exposed to cruelty in their earliest environment. These traumas, deprivations or cruel acts have prevented them from identifying with a place in the other – because this place did not exist. The impossibility of identifying with a place in the other, which is the first identification, the one that allows a subject to be constituted, prevents the closing of the psychic space. Those I have called *children of dinosaurs* reject all significant ties because, were this to happen, such an event would be associated with the promise of an unprecedented relationship that would make it possible to have *a point of view* about one's own history. Experiencing a relationship where violence does not occur allows the psychic space to close. But this inevitably involves the hypothesis of letting go of reassuring suffering, to which the subject had clung to avoid falling into the void.[66]

This is why Nikolai Stavrogin refuses Shatov's love, Liza's love, Dunya's love. From the dreadful place of his madness – therefore, from nowhere – he challenges the world to give him, despite his refusal, an unconscious.

We shall now see how this challenge is enacted.

Crime and madness

If a transitional space had existed for Nikolai Stavrogin, it would also be filled with boredom. Nikolai has no interest in himself, no *amour propre*, no vanity. What he is interested in is truth, truth and its excess. Nikolai uses boredom as a filter between himself and the world, and he breaks it down into its elements, which he uses to his benefit: gloominess to slow down time, disgust to avoid expecting anything from others, weariness in the place of a request, indifference as an enigma to counter the other's desire, while challenging the other to love him despite the barrier of the apathy that oppresses him. As for hate, that goes back a long way. He has drawn it from his mother's violent arrogance, an arrogance he transforms into pride. His use of hatred is pure negativity, a scalpel to separate, a merciless tool that hardens the other by cruelly and directly confronting him with truths that are ordinarily unbearable. Here, we might stop to discuss in greater detail the difference between pride and *amour propre*. But for the moment let us say that *amour propre* is tied to a sense of self-worth, while pride is a form of arrogance, a hate-filled fortress that encloses the horror of the threatening void which lies in wait for the subject day and night.

Unable to experience satisfaction, Nikolai finds, in the excitement of the extreme situations he creates, an outlet for the untapped strength of his desire, a desire undifferentiated from the pack of drives to which he has voluntarily reduced himself: driving women to despair, causing the suicide of a child, humiliating the powerful with his sarcasm, being insensitive to the terrible suffering he inflicts, remaining unmoved by the pleas addressed to him, not fulfilling the promises he makes and failing to stay true to the ideas he proposes. How are we to encounter a subject who has thrown his ego away like a useless rag? This is the ultimate example of a subject constituted in the obscenity of pain and the darkness of archaic passions, the shameless example of a humanity dehumanised by life, attesting to the presence of silent, boundless animality. A criminal; better to be a criminal than a madman. It is the animal strength drawn from the proximity of madness that nurtures Nikolai's excess. With these subjects, the analyst's clinical work is not to interpret, but to construct the unconscious.

Thus, instead of speaking of regression, let us speak of a way of thinking that swallows up the real in order to represent it, a way of thinking which owes its excessive character to madness and to psychotic processes at work in the representation of the world. In the face of the immensity of madness, nothing is permanently given, and the unconscious does not exist. Faced with the excessiveness of madness – I will say it again – the unconscious has to be constructed.

When Nikolai goes to see Father Tikhon, he has no idea that he is about to meet an analyst ahead of his time. He goes in order to confess his abject crime. He would like to do this without recourse to a request, but the monk confronts him with a request of his own. Tikhon plays the role of analyst in that for him the most important thing is not what Stavrogin has to confess, even though this has great importance. But Tikhon places emphasis, and draws Nikolai's attention, to the meaning of his undertaking: the act of confessing, and the benefits he expects to gain from it. In other words, the monk interprets the transference or, to be more precise, he grafts transference between him and Stavrogin, and by so doing he endows Nikolai with an unconscious.

Tikhon guesses Nikolai's pride, just as Shatov had:

> "You married from *a passion for martyrdom*, from a craving for remorse, through moral sensuality. It was a laceration of the nerves. [...] Defiance of common sense was too tempting. Stavrogin and a wretched, half-witted, crippled beggar! When you bit the governor's ear did you feel sensual pleasure? Did you? You idle, loafing little snob?"
>
> "You're a psychologist," said Stavrogin, turning paler and paler.[67]

But let us look at the meeting with the monk from the beginning. Stavrogin is aware that the monk is expecting a secret to be revealed, and he denies that he has come for this reason. Very quickly he starts to talk about the hallucination in which he sees the devil. He speaks nonchalantly, sarcastically, but he reveals the hallucination. This shows how much he trusts his interlocutor:

> And suddenly he related, in the shortest and most abrupt manner so that certain words could hardly be understood, that he was subject, especially at

> nights, to a kind of hallucination, that he sometimes saw or felt near him a spiteful being, mocking and "rational", "in various forms and in various characters". [...] This is all nonsense, utter nonsense. It is myself in various aspects, and nothing else. But even as I use that phrase, you certainly think that I am still doubtful and am not sure that it is myself, and not really the devil. [Let us note in passing that Dostoevsky had identified the mechanism of negation!] Of course I see it; I see it as plainly as I see you [...] and sometimes I see it and I'm not sure that I see it [...] and sometimes I do not know what is real: I or it. [...] And can't you possibly believe that this is indeed the devil?

And Tikhon answers: "It's more like a disease, although".[68]

Reading *Stavrogin's Confession* reveals that the hallucination about the devil was a screen hallucination, serving to mask the murder of little Matryosha, her suicide caused by Stavrogin.

> [S]uddenly [...] I saw a tiny point. The point began suddenly to take a definite form, and all of a sudden I distinctly pictured to myself a tiny reddish spider. At once I remembered it on the leaf of the geranium, upon which, too, had poured the rays of the setting sun. [Remember: Stavrogin was looking at a small red spider while Matryosha was hanging herself. In short, Dostoevsky had also understood how the displacement of a perception can be the container of a screen memory!] It was as though something were plunged through me; I raised myself and sat on my bed. That's [exactly] how it happened then. I saw before me (Oh, not in the flesh! Would that the vision had been true!), I saw before me Matryosha, emaciated, with feverish eyes, in every point exactly as she was when she stood on the threshold of my room and, shaking her head at me, threatened me with her tiny fist. Nothing has ever been so agonizing to me! The pitiable despair of a helpless creature. [...] Nothing like that has ever happened to me. [...] But it was intolerable to me, that image of her standing on the threshold with her raised and threatening little fist, merely that vision of her then, that moment "then", that shaking of her head. It is precisely that which I cannot endure, *because since then it has come to me almost every day and I know I am a condemned man.* Not that it comes itself, but that I bring it before myself and cannot help bringing it, although I can't live with it. Oh, if I could ever see her in the flesh, even though it were an hallucination! [I want her to look at me if only one more time like then, with her big feverish eyes, look straight into my eyes]. So it will go on until I go mad.[69]

And it in fact went on until the end of Stavrogin's life: until he hung himself, like Matryosha, in an attic room.

Let us look now at the way Tikhon works with the *Confession* and with Stavrogin's intention to make it public. Let's remember the last thoughts Nikolai reports having, in his manuscript. He thought of committing another crime to rid himself of Matryosha; but he realised that this was impossible. He then admitted that he "could never love anyone", and that he was governed by passions alone. But, as I said earlier, Nikolai calls "passions" all the furious impulses to which he has deliberately reduced himself.

When Tikhon finished reading the sheets of the confession, he was *indignant*, and Stavrogin heard it in his voice. He started by questioning Nikolai's decision to punish himself by making his confession public: was this a true desire for punishment? The question *irritates* Stavrogin, who starts to explain. Dostoevsky notes that he "submitted painfully, although *unconsciously*, to the need to explain himself". Dostoevsky indicates, with great genius, that Father Tikhon is right: Stavrogin refuses to face the emotional suffering involved in his crimes.

TIKHON: But you, it seems, already *hate and despise* beforehand all those who will read what is written here, and you *challenge* them [with your defiance].

STAVROGIN: Where is the defiance?

TIKHON: You were not *ashamed* of admitting your crime; why are you *ashamed* of repentance?

STAVROGIN: Ashamed?

TIKHON: You are ashamed and afraid! [...] Let them look at me, you say; well, and you, how will you look at them? Certain passages in your statement are emphasized; you seem *to be luxuriating in your own psychology* and clutch at each detail, in order to surprise the reader by a *callousness*, a *cynicism*, that [are] not really in you. [On the other hand, ugly passions and idleness have made you *unfeeling and stupid*.]

STAVROGIN: Stupidity is not a sin.

TIKHON: It is sometimes a sin, Tikhon continued, *vehemently and unrelentingly*.

STAVROGIN: [W]e have now been talking for five minutes since you read that (he nodded at the pages) and I do not see in you any expression of *aversion or shame*. [...] You don't seem to be squeamish [and you treat me like an equal].

TIKHON: I shall not conceal anything from you: I was horrified at the great idle force that had been deliberately wasted in abomination. [...] The world is full of these horrors. But you have felt the whole depth to a degree which is extremely rare.Stavrogin doesn't understand the significance of what the monk is saying; the sense to be made of this exchange is rooted in the real meaning of the confession he has given Tikhon to read. Stavrogin thinks that the monk is trying to gain his confidence by speaking of his qualities. He says sarcastically: "Have you come to respect me after these pages?" Tikhon answers bluntly: "[T]here certainly is not, nor can there be, a greater and more terrible crime than your behaviour towards the girl".

The dialogue between Nikolai Stavrogin and Father Tikhon takes place in a context where the stakes involved are the same as those between Raskolnikov and Porfiry, in *Crime and Punishment*. When we discussed that novel, I pointed out Porfiry's relentlessness in showing Raskolnikov that his lies were useless, and convincing him that it was important to confess his crime. What the monk tries to do is show Stavrogin in what way the publication of his confession is a lie. In both cases, what is needed is to create in the other a space of solitude, an intimate intimacy, in order for an unconscious to be constructed. But this is a long process. However, Raskolnikov had an advantage Stavrogin doesn't have: he has Sonya's love. It was thanks to Porfiry that he accepted to take the enormous risk of living this experience of love, at the cost of the psychotic episode to which he was subject in the prison camp. Accepting Sonya's love, which became possible only after accepting Razumikhin's friendship, triggered in Raskolnikov the long process of psychic work that would allow him to create filters between himself and the real of the world.

There is another fundamental difference between these two lives. For Raskolnikov, crime is the fruit of a passion which is attempting to create a new frame of thought from which God is absent, and in which anguish has its place. Stavrogin's abominable crime takes place in a world without God and without passion, and is born, as Shatov says, merely of the pathological sensuality of a man who is bored, who makes commitments as an amateur, because he has nothing better to do.[70]

Father Tikhon, like Porfiry, insists on *naming affects* and, by doing this, on showing that boredom and cynicism *are defences against the fear of love, which has been replaced by fear of madness.* In this encounter, where Stavrogin's fate will be decided, a crucial point is the question of contempt, one of the faces of hate.

Because Stavrogin trusts the monk, he can set aside his pride and confess his contempt for everyone; he despises others as much as himself, perhaps infintely more. Tikhon observes that it is easier for Nikolai to hate than to accept pity. He asks: "[I]f some one [...] a stranger, a man whom you will never know [...] reading your terrible confession, forgave you, in the privacy of his heart – would you feel relieved, or would it be just the same to you?" The monk adds that if answering this question is too hard to bear for Stavrogin's pride, he should say nothing, but reflect on the question for himself. In an undertone, Stavrogin admits that he would "feel easier", and then closes himself up in his megalomaniacal pride again. Now, Tikhon decides to risk everything. When speaking of the complexity of the analytic process with psychotics, Gisela Pankow often said: "With a psychotic, one must speak of something beyond his desire". To paraphrase, I would say: "With a pervert – and Nikolai holds perversion up as a badge of honour – one must speak from a place beyond the real effects of the acts he has committed, from a place that confronts these effects".

Father Tikhon decides to do the unexpected, to present the situation in a different light. Stavrogin imagined a tragic and grandiose scene: firmly ensconced in his contemptuous pride, he would reveal to the world the infamous acts of which he is guilty, and display the atrocious murder of a little girl. And people would admire this man who could commit such atrocities, this obviously extraordinary man, superhuman, who would force them to recognise the emptiness of their lives. But Tikhon asserts that this is not what will happen, and that Stavrogin would have to face what he finds unbearable: people's laughter.

> People will pretend, deliberately, not to understand the real reasons for your confession, because they are afraid of acts of this kind; they incite terror and hatred, and people seek revenge: the world loves its dirt and doesn't want it stirred. This is why it will quickly turn the whole affair into derision, for it is through derision and mockery that people unburden themselves. [...] Your madness will seem very strange, for they will consider you a little mad, but still responsible enough so that they can laugh at you. Will you endure that? Will your heart not be filled with a hatred that will destroy you? This is what I fear.

The monk does not spare Stavrogin. He tells him he is too fragile, he is mad, and he won't be able to bear the violence of the laughter. He speaks of Stavrogin's crime as *shameful, disgraceful, past all horror.* Stavrogin is deeply shaken. He says:

> Listen [...] I want to forgive myself, and that is my object, my whole object! [...] Then only, I know, that vision [of Matryosha] will disappear. [...] Christ will [not] forgive. [...] It says in the Book: "And whosoever shall offend one of these little ones", you remember. According to the Gospel there is no greater crime.

Tikhon seizes this opportunity. He assures Stavrogin that if he is able to forgive himself – that is, to comprehend the meaning of his actions and to try to love himself – then God would forgive him too. The monk suggests that instead of publishing his confession Stavrogin should go and see a hermit and, under his guidance, go into retreat for five years, or seven years, or "as many years as you find necessary". In short, he sends him into analysis to construct an unconscious, instead of letting his impulses become the standard of truth.

Hearing this, Stavrogin takes his hat and prepares to leave. Tikhon asks him to sit down. "Tikhon looked at this pose, the pose of a man suddenly turned worldly, both agitated and half crazy". Then, Father Tikhon foresees the real: "his hands pressed together in front of him, and a painful spasm [...] over his face," he said:

> I see [...] I see, as if it stood before me," Tikhon exclaimed in a voice which penetrated the soul and with an expression of the most violent grief, "that you, poor, lost youth, have never been so near another and a still greater crime than you are at this moment. [...] No, not after the publication, but before it, a day, an hour, perhaps, before the great step, you will throw yourself on a new crime, as a way out, and you will commit it solely in order to avoid the publication of these pages". Stavrogin shuddered with anger and almost with fear. "You cursed psychologist!" – he suddenly cut him short in fury and, without looking round, left the cell.

Unfortunately, the monk had guessed right. And there would be more than one murder: that of Marya Timofeevna, his wife, then that of Liza, and finally his suicide.

Let us try to understand why Tikhon was unable to help Nikolai find in the real something that would have allowed him to leave behind his perverse defences, something that could have humanised him. Tikhon named the affects, was relentless, made no concessions about the truth. Perhaps he let his identification with Nikolai show too much, showed his desire to save him too clearly, preventing himself from finding in the young man's torment an element that could be used to lead him in another direction.[71]

The nomination of affects is the first step of a journey that leads, or can lead, to form. But Stavrogin is not interested in form. He does not want to create anything, except catastrophe. Catastrophe is not a start, it is the stage before the start. Let us remember that Raskolnikov wanted to build a new world. But he felt his passion to be too small in the face of the immensity of the real – which makes him an endearing man, struggling with his desire. Stavrogin fills the real with his impulses; no empty space must remain. Raskolnikov is so full of anguish that it drives him mad. Stavrogin dumps his anguish, and his dreams, into others. Stavrogin's madness is the absence of fear. Raskolnikov is always afraid.

I was asking myself: why was Tikhon unable to help Nikolai find in the real something that would allow him to leave behind his perverse defences, something that would humanise him. But what does "finding the real" mean, and to what "real" are we referring?

We speak of a greater, wider real than the excessiveness which drives Stavrogin. The real of beginnings, the madness of the real of beginnings. This is why to love a child – a beginning *par excellence* – is so demanding, so poignant, so absolute. And this is why loving someone unfailingly produces the infinite awe of childhood. But Stavrogin has killed a child, and because a child synthesises all beginnings, Stavrogin refuses love, does not let himself be loved by Dasha (he kills himself before receiving her answer to the letter in which he asked her to come to him, knowing that she would). Refusing love was his way of staying loyal to the horror of his crime. It is the punishment he inflicts on himself. Thus, Stavrogin is consistently strict. He is not afraid of death, but rather of the force of life. Of course, he would like to forgive himself, but only on condition that he stays a condemned man forever.

Contrary to Raskolnikov, Stavrogin deprives himself of recourse to madness, the only tool that can smash the real of the act which holds him captive. And what exactly would he have found in madness, that could be of use? He would have found the exhausting, sublime quality of the emergence of the movement that serves to gather oneself together. This never-ending process is also the one which produces works of art; but these works are not what matters. For the one who creates, what matters is not the finished work, but the process. Cézanne used to leave behind, in the fields, the paintings he had just finished. Other people picked up the works he left behind.

What could be found in this real larger than immensity, this real called madness, is the constant, silent movement of gathering together, a movement in which there is no separation between what is created and the never-changing feeling, always unique, of being there. Being there, present to the real. A non-persecutory, "good" real.

To encounter a non-persecutory real of madness requires passage through another person, who can "transition" the absolute excess of this encounter. Madness is a harassing practice of lightning bolts, of the ephemeral, of burstings. But not any lightning bolts, not just any ephemeral.

Here, the stroke of lightning is always a form wounded by pain, and always to be recreated with unfailing perseverance. Such a stroke of lightning is born of patience and slowness, woven on a background of permanent emptiness, and this emptiness is woven into the flow of the movement that patience and slowness create.

How can we bring to the side of madness – madness as Hegel defined it: *an orgy of the truth where no reveler can stay sober* (Berthold-Bond, 1995) – a psychic functioning that finds narcissistic reward in the survival of a traumatic experience to which a subject is attached, a psychic functioning where using another as a prosthesis is the symbiotic figure in a scene saturated with fullness, where any emptiness is unbearable?

Healing from trauma requires the conjunction of two movements. On the part of the patient, who was able to establish the space of analysis as transitional space, a *judgment of condemnation* (Freud) must be passed on the traumatic experience. This movement goes hand in hand with the possibility of learning new experiences, like that of analysis. On the part of the psychoanalyst, there must be a willingness to use the pictogrammes awakened in him by the transferential relation (like Tikhon seeing the real concerning Stavrogin). These pictogrammes are tools that will help him guess the place in which the subject is imprisoned, as well as the place from which the latter will be able to venture into life, transforming the energy that has been utilised to sustain deadly endurance in the subject, into sustenance for the liberated strength of his enormous desire and his dreams.[72]

Notes

1 Here again, I refer you to the chapter "True Love" in my book *Letters to a Young Psychoanalyst.*

2 Freud, S. (2012a), *Contributions to the Psychology of Love. On the universal tendency to debasement in the sphere of love* (1912). S.E. XI: 165–175. My emphasis.

3 For a discussion of this subject, see my book *De l'amour à la pensée : La psychanalyse, la création de l'enfant et D.W. Winnicott.*

4 On the subject of the relation between philosophy and reflection, see the Preamble to this book.

5 Without referring to it explicitly, Gisela Pankow alludes to Winnicott's primary environment. See Pankow, G. (1981), *L'Être-là du schizophrène*, Paris, Aubier, p. 20.

6 Pankow, G., *L'Être-là du schizophrène*, pp. 67–68, 75, 77, 78, 68. My emphasis and Pankow's.

7 See "Gisela Pankow and Her Teaching", in *Letters to a Young Psychoanalyst.*

8 To learn about Dostoevsky's life at the time, as well as about the historical, cultural, ideological and social context of the period, see Frank, J. (1995), *Dostoevsky. The Miraculous Years, 1865–1871*, Princeton University Press, Chapters 22, 23, 24 and 25.

9 Frank, J. (2012), *Dostoevsky: A Writer in His Time*, Princeton University Press, p. 602.
10 Dostoevsky, F., *Letters and Reminiscences*, Koteliansky, S. S. and Middleton Murry, J. (trans.), London: Chatto & Windus, 1923 (Letter to Maikov, October 21, 1870).
11 Dostoevsky, F. (1993), *Notes from Underground*, Pevear, R. and Volokhonsky, L. (trans.), Vintage Classics, p. 130.
12 Frank, J., *Dostoevsky: The Miraculous Years*, p. 403.
13 Ibid., pp. 402–404.
14 Frank, J., *Dostoevsky: A Writer in His Time*, p. 609.
15 Frank, J., *Dostoevsky: The Miraculous Years*, p. 422.
16 Ibid., pp. 422–423.
17 Frank, J., *Dostoevsky: A Writer in His Time*, p. 638.
18 Frank, J., *Dostoevsky: The Miraculous Years*, p. 456. My emphasis.
19 Ibid., pp. 458–59.
20 Frank, J., *Dostoevsky: A Writer in His Time*, p. 459. My emphasis.
21 Dostoevsky, F. (1936), *The Possessed (The Devils)*, Garnett, C. (trans.), New York: Random House, pp. 494–495.
22 Frank, J., *Dostoevsky: The Miraculous Years*, p. 405.
23 Dostoevsky, F., *The Possessed (The Devils)*, pp. 11–12.
24 Ibid., p. 57.
25 Ibid., p. 60.
26 Ibid., p. 66.
27 Ibid., pp. 305–307.
28 Dostoevsky, F. (1993), *Notes from Underground*, p. 130.
29 See Chapter 3.
30 Dostoevsky, F., *The Possessed* (*The Devils*), pp. 548–549.
31 Ibid., pp. 654–656.
32 Ibid., pp. 673–674.
33 Ibid., pp. 632–636.
34 Dostoevsky, F., *The Notebooks for the Possessed*, Wasiolek, E. (ed.), Terras, V. (trans.), University of Chicago Press, 1968, pp. 67–68.
35 Frank, J., *Dostoevsky: The Miraculous Years*, p. 374. My emphasis.
36 Ibid. Dostoevsky's emphasis.
37 Frank, J., *Dostoevsky: A Writer in His Time*, p. 597.
38 Frank, J., *Dostoevsky: The Miraculous Years*, p. 377.
39 Dostoevsky, F., *The Notebooks for the Possessed*, p. 67.
40 Ibid., p. 180.
41 Dostoevsky, F., *The Notebooks for the Possessed*, pp. 181 and 182.
42 Frank, J., *Dostoevsky: The Miraculous Years*, p. 411. My emphasis.
43 Ibid., p. 467.
44 Frank, J., *Dostoevsky: A Writer in His Time*, pp. 646–647.
45 Ibid., pp. 647 and 649.
46 Ibid., p. 645.
47 Ibid., p. 649.
48 Dostoevsky, F., *The Possessed (The Devils)*, p. 41.
49 Ibid., p. 37.
50 Ibid., pp. 37–38.
51 Ibid., p. 44.
52 Ibid., p. 182.
53 Ibid., p. 242.
54 Ibid., pp. 240–241.
55 For the concept of the originary, see Aulagnier, P., *The Violence of Interpretation*, Routledge, 2001.
56 Dostoevsky, F., *The Possessed (The Devils)*, p. 243.
57 Ibid., p. 248. My emphasis.
58 Ibid. My emphasis.

59 Ibid., p. 258. My emphasis.
60 Ibid.
61 Ibid., p. 249.
62 Ibid., p. 258.
63 Ibid., pp. 258–259.
64 Ibid., p. 259.
65 Frank, J., *Dostoevsky: A Writer in His Time*, pp. 605–606; my emphasis (Letter to Katkov, October 1870).
66 For the notion of "children of dinosaurs", see *De l'amour à la pensée*.
67 Dostoevsky, F., *The Possessed (The Devils)*, p. 258. My emphasis.
68 Dostoevsky, F., *Stavrogin's Confession*, Koteliansky, S.S. and Woolf, V. (trans.), Hogarth Press, 1922, pp. 28–30.
69 Ibid., pp. 65–67. My emphasis.
70 Dostoevsky, F., *The Possessed (The Devils)*, p. 258.
71 I quote Gisela Pankow: "Of course these dissociations give rise to unimaginable anguish. Therefore, we must work with this *anguish to turn it into desire*, desire directed towards a unisexual body. This is the aim of my efforts of *dynamic structuring* in psychosis". My emphasis. Gisela Pankow, *L'Être-là du schizophrène*, p. 68.
72 These pictogrammes were at work when Kirillov and Shatov intuited the real about Stavrogin. Remember that it was Piera Aulagnier who defined the semantic domain of this concept, which was given a place in the unconscious at last. The pictogramme is the *representation of affect and the affect of representation*.

6

THE BROTHERS KARAMAZOV

The Brothers Karamazov is a novel about assassins. Fyodor Pavlovitch is an assassin. Dmitri and Ivan Fyodorovitch are assassins. Smerdyakov is an assassin. Katerina Ivanovna and Grushenka are assassins. Madame Khokhlakov and her daughter Liza are assassins.

Dostoevsky has Ivan say:

> "It was he [Smerdyakov], not my brother, who killed our father. He murdered him and I led him on to do it. [...] Who doesn't desire his father's death?"
>
> "Are you in your right mind?" broke involuntarily from the President.
>
> "I think I am in my right mind. [...] In the same evil mind as all of you [...] as all these [...] ugly faces". He turned suddenly to the crowd. "My father has been murdered and they pretend they are horrified," he snarled. "They keep up the fraud with one another. Liars! They all desire the death of their fathers".[1]

It was in 1880 that Dostoevsky described what Freud would call, some years later, the Oedipus complex. The fact that the inventor of psychoanalysis, while recognising that Dostoevsky's work was brilliant, nevertheless reacted so violently to this novel, clearly shows the difference between the two thinkers. Freud identified fantasy as the agency structuring psychic functioning; Dostoevsky, who did not possess the notion of fantasy, accompanied his characters along the narrow ridge separating the inventiveness of imagination from the precipitation of the act.

When he read *The Brothers Karamazov*, Freud must have recalled the period before the discovery of fantasy, a painfully exhausting period when he took every scenario he imagined as revealing an actual aspect of his personality. The torments endured by Dostoevsky's characters, similar to those experienced by Freud during his self-analysis, attest to the importance for humanity of the discovery of the role of fantasy.

At the same time, these torments make it clear that reducing the psyche to the fantasy function alone would be far too restrictive. Excluding from the psyche its interactions with the real would mean reducing feeling to a psychology of the imagination. Of course, we can understand Freud's decision, after the momentous discovery of fantasy, to set aside the reality of trauma as he continued his research. But if Ferenczi had not been there, we would have had to wait much longer to understand psychosis.

But since Ferenczi was there, there is no excuse for the fact that certain analysts are deaf to anything not related to fantasy. Since Ferenczi formulated, with Freud's support, the metapsychology of the analyses he conducted, it is no longer possible to see the real simply as that which contains terrorising material. Freud's 1924 article *Neurosis and Psychosis* confirms this. In this text, Freud states that the "normal" is a combination of the neurotic – the acknowledgement of reality – with the psychotic – the desire to alter this reality.

Indeed, any fantasy, defined by Freud as the depiction of a desire – and therefore any desire – implies surpassing the possible and presupposes that the real can act as a support for desire in this surpassing. Love, this necessary catastrophe, always gathers its strength from a living, demanding and humanising reality.[2]

Of course, the real can be an antidote to desire, as *The Brothers Karamazov* so superbly illustrates. But what is the opposite of desire?

Freud postulated the existence of the "Nirvana principle", to which Piera Aulagnier gave a very edifying definition: the desire for the absence of desire. But such an interruption of conflict is not the opposite of conflict, it is a pause, a suspension, a stasis, a falling back – there is no change in the configuration of the elements present in the opposition between drives. Based on the "death drive" concept, boredom is the opposite of desire. Indeed, being closely akin to hate, boredom opposes desire. But, if we really think about it, we can't consider boredom an opposing force; rather, it is a reactive mechanism, a defensive device in an attack, an escape route always encumbered with the desires it seeks to avoid, and which are reinforced by its vitality and strength.

An expert

Let us consult an expert who can enlighten us: the hysterical woman. She was once an unhappy, naughty little girl who set up her headquarters at the intersection of love, madness and hate. So let us turn to Liza, the daughter of Madame Khokhlakov, herself a source of wisdom on this subject:

> "I wanted to tell you of a longing I have. I would like someone to torture me, to marry me and then torture me, deceive me and go away. I don't want to be happy!"
>
> "You are in love with disorder?"

"Yes, I want disorder. I keep wanting to set fire to the house. I keep imagining how I'll creep up and set fire to the house secretly, it must be secretly. They'll try to put it out, but it'll go on burning. And I will know and say nothing. Oh, what silliness! And how bored I am!" She waved her hand with a look of repulsion.

"It's your luxurious life," said Alyosha softly.

"Is it better then to be poor?"

"Yes, it is better."

"That's what your monk taught you. That's not true. Let me be rich and all the rest poor. I'll eat cake and drink cream and I won't give any to anyone else. [...] You are awfully cross, because I don't talk about holy things. I don't want to be holy. What will they do to one in the next world for the greatest sin? You must know all about that."

"God will censure you." Alyosha was watching her steadily.

"That's just what I would like. I would go up and they would censure me and I would burst out laughing in their faces. [...] I would like to set fire to the house, Alyosha, to our house – you still don't believe me?"

"Why? There are children twelve years old, who have a longing to set fire to something and they do set things on fire. It's a sort of disease."

"That's not true, that's not true. There may be children, but that's not what I mean."

"You take evil for good. It's a passing crisis. It's the result of your illness, perhaps."

"You do despise me! It's simply that I don't want to do good, I want to do evil, and it has nothing to do with illness."

"Why do evil?"

"So that everything will be destroyed. Oh, how nice it would be if everything were destroyed! You know, Alyosha, I sometimes think of doing a lot of harm. I would do it for a long time secretly and then suddenly everyone would find out. Everyone will stand around and point their fingers at me and I will look at them all. That would be awfully nice. Why would it be so nice, Alyosha?"

"I don't know? It's a craving to destroy something good or, as you say, to set fire to something. It happens sometimes."

"I not only say it, I'll do it."

"I believe you."

"Oh, how I love you for saying you believe me. And you are not lying. But perhaps you think I am saying all this just to annoy you?"

"No, I don't think that. [...] Though perhaps there is a desire to do that, too."

"There is a little. I never can tell lies to you," she declared with a strange fire in her eyes.

What struck Alyosha above everything was her earnestness. There was not a trace of joking in her face now, though in the old days fun and gaiety never deserted her even at her most "earnest" moments.

"There are moments when people love crime," said Alyosha thoughtfully.

"Yes, yes! People love crime. Everyone loves crime, they love it always, not at some 'moments'. You know, it's as though people have made an agreement to lie about it and have lied about it ever since. They all say that they hate evil, but secretly they all love it."

[...]

"Aren't you ashamed [to be reading nasty books]? You are destroying yourself."

"I want to destroy myself. [...] Listen, your brother is being tried now for murdering your father and everyone loves his having killed your father."

"Loves his having killed father?"

"Yes, loves it, everyone loves it! Everybody says it's so awful, but secretly they all love it. I for one love it."

"There is some truth in what you say," said Alyosha softly.

"Oh, what ideas you have!" Lise shrieked in delight. "And you a monk, too! You wouldn't believe how I respect you, Alyosha, for never telling lies. Oh, I must tell you a funny dream I had. I sometimes dream of devils. [...] there are devils all over the place, in all the corners, under the table. And they open the doors, there's a crowd of them behind the doors and they want to come and grab me. And they are just coming, just grabbing me. But I suddenly cross myself and they all draw back, though they don't go away altogether. They stand at the doors and in the corners, waiting. And suddenly I have a frightful longing to revile God aloud, and so I begin. And then they come crowding back to me, delighted, and grab me again and I cross myself again and they all draw back. It's awful fun, it takes one's breath away."

"I've had the same dream, too," said Alyosha suddenly.

"Really?" cried Lise, surprised. "Alyosha, don't laugh, it's awfully important. Can two different people have the same dream?"

"It seems they can."

[...]

"You are the only person I can talk to, you know," Lise began again. "I talk to no one but myself and you. Only you in the whole world. And to you more easily than to myself. And I am not a bit ashamed with you, not a bit. Alyosha, why am I not ashamed with you, not a bit? Alyosha, is it true that at Easter certain religious sects steal a child and kill it?"

"I don't know."

"There's a book here in which I read about the trial of a man who took a four year old child and cut off the fingers from both hands, and then crucified him on the wall, hammered nails into him and crucified him. And afterwards, when he was tried, he said that the child died quickly, within four hours. That was 'quickly'! He said the child moaned, kept on moaning and he stood admiring it. That's nice!"

"Nice?"

> "Nice. I sometimes I imagine that it was I who crucified him. He would hang there moaning and I would sit opposite him eating pineapple jam. I am awfully fond of pineapple jam. Do you like it?"
>
> Alyosha looked at her in silence. Her pale, sallow face was suddenly contorted, her eyes burned.
>
> "You know, when I read about the child, I cried all night. I kept thinking of how the little thing cried and moaned (a child of four understands, you know) and all the while the thought of pineapple jam haunted me. In the morning I wrote a letter to a certain person, begging him to come and see me. He came and I told him all about the child and the pineapple jam. *All* about it, *all*, and said that it was nice. He laughed and said it really was nice. Then he got up and went away. He was only here five minutes."
>
> [...]
>
> "That person behaved honourably," Alyosha murmured.
>
> "And did he despise me? Did he laugh at me?"
>
> "No, for perhaps he believes in pineapple jam himself. He is very ill now, Lise."
>
> "Yes, he does believe in it," said Lise, with flashing eyes.
>
> "He doesn't despise anyone," Alyosha went on. "Only he does not believe anyone. If he doesn't believe in people, of course, he does despise them."
>
> "Then he despises me, me?"
>
> "You, too."
>
> "Good. When he went out laughing, I felt that it was nice to be despised. The child with fingers cut off is nice and to be despised is nice."
>
> And she laughed in Alyosha's face, a feverish malicious laugh.
>
> "Do you know, Alyosha, do you know, I would like. [...] Alyosha save me!" she suddenly jumped up from the invalid chair, rushed to him and grabbed him with both hands. "Save me!" she almost groaned. "Is there anyone in the world I could tell what I've told you? I've told you the truth, the truth. I will kill myself, because I hate everything! I don't want to live, because I hate everything! I hate everything, everything, Alyosha, why don't you love me?" she finished in a frenzy.
>
> "But I do love you!" answered Alyosha warmly.[3]

Like all the characters in *The Brothers Karamazov*, Liza teaches us that the opposite of desire is murder.

But what is a murderer? He is someone who no longer trusts anyone. And for this reason, says Alyosha, he despises everyone. But before contempt, there is the sadness of never having been loved. This sadness is recognised prior to hatred, it is taken into the hatred, but does not dissolve in it. The subject always returns to this sadness that nothing can erase, not even envy, not even the ghastly revelry of murder, which allows the discharge of extreme instinctual excitement.

Gradually, this persistent sadness succeeds in destroying all yearning in the soul, all desire. Over time, it shrouds all feelings in mist and fills the heart with indifference and disillusionment. But before inducing insensitivity, sadness will have done away with all hope.

Ivan Fyodorovich understands well the decisive consequences of loss of all hope, of the possibility of transcendence. In his poem, The Grand Inquisitor tells Christ:

> Thou didst hope that man, following Thee, too, would cling to God and not ask for a miracle. But Thou didst not know that when man rejects miracles he rejects God too; for man seeks not so much God as the miraculous. [...] Too, too well, [men] know the value of complete submission! And until men know that, they will be unhappy. [...] Then we shall give them [...] quiet humble happiness. [...] We shall show them that they are weak, that they are only pitiful children, but that childlike happiness is the sweetest of all. They will become timid and look to us and huddle close to us in fear, as chicks to the hen. [...] Yes, we shall set them to work, but in their leisure hours we shall make their life like a child's game, with children's songs and innocent dance.[4]

Alyosha and Prince Myshkin

The Karamazov brothers suffer from this sadness of having been abandoned, as well as from the sadness of not being able to love their father, who is a perverse and cruel man. It is this archaic reservoir of sadness that forces assassins to refuse all possibility of happiness. Since they cannot satisfy their desire to be loved, they will destroy with insatiable hatred any offer of love, any possibility of a lasting relation. They prefer abject solitude to the risk of being abandoned again. This foreseeable response to any new situation, or any unexpected event, eventually turns these characters, who can be fascinating, enchanting and even bewitching, into predictable, tiresome people. Their psychic functioning, serving as compensation for narcissistic injury, is unchanging and repetitive. Always self-centred, lacking humour, unable to laugh or make others laugh, they end up boring us with their suffering and their insoluble predicaments. They clearly need a psychoanalyst, and this is why they speak to Alyosha.

Alyosha gives his interlocutor his full attention, he is there in the moment, he is completely receptive to the encounter. Remember Kirillov's answer when Stavrogin asks:

> "You've begun to believe in a future eternal life?"
>
> "No," says Kirillov, "not in a future eternal life, but in an eternal life [here]. There are moments, you reach moments, and time suddenly stands still, and it will become eternal".

I am quoting Kirillov intentionally. Alyosha is acquainted with murder, not as an external event, but as a subjective possibility that he himself accepts. For Alyosha, there is no antagonism between life and death. And even less between affects and sensations, and emotions and intelligence. Alyosha's thinking process relies on sensitivity as much as on intelligence. Alyosha believes in God and in the existence of the Devil; he imagines their relation to be a dialectical one, like that between Eros and Thanatos.

Alyosha is often compared to the Prince in *The Idiot*. I find this comparison unfounded. Contrary to Myshkin, Alyosha acknowledges morbid passions but is not fascinated by them. He takes a stand, he is not merely a sieve, like the Prince, who absorbs nothing and remains empty. For Alyosha, what matters most is desire, not love. On the other hand, Alyosha takes action, creates life, opposes hate, asserts his desire. Myshkin likes Rogozhin, the man who acts out his desire in the murder of Nastasya Fillipovna; Alyosha hates Smerdiakov. Alyosha loves the aliveness of children; Myshkin causes the children to love "a walking shadow", the figure of death. For Alyosha, evil is not lies or sex, and certainly not intelligence, but rather hate, envy and murder. Therefore, evil is concrete and active, something which can be fought with actions that are real and effective.

Indeed, Dostoevsky describes Alyosha as follows:

> he was [...] a youth of our past generation – that is, honest in nature, desiring the truth, seeking for it and believing in it, and seeking to serve it at once with all the strength of his soul; seeking for immediate action, and ready to sacrifice everything, even life itself.

This portrait resembles in some respects the very astute picture of Raskolnikov drawn by Porfiry in *Crime and Punishment*. A little earlier, Dostoevsky had observed that:

> Alyosha was [...] a well-grown, clear-eyed young man [...] radiant with health. He was [...] graceful, moderately tall, with dark brown hair, with a regular, rather long, oval-shaped face, and wide-set dark gray eyes. He was very thoughtful and very serene. [...] I believe that Alyosha was more of a realist than anyone".

In short, Alyosha can be described as a realistic Raskolnikov.[5]

I say that Alyosha can act as a psychoanalyst because, in his relationships with others, he displays certain of the qualities we need in our work. First, there is his remarkable ability to identify with the other person – an ability whose devastating roots we shall discuss shortly – and his ability to set aside his Ego, and more specifically his pride. I talked about this at the start of our study of Dostoevsky, when we made the acquaintance of the Underground Man. We encountered these two characteristics in Prince Myshkin as well, and we were able to observe how their combination is also suited to the position of the pervert, and particularly that of the assassin. But Alyosha has other qualities as well: he is uncompromising in his desire, he is fearless, objective and capable of humour. I believe that our practice sometimes associates discretion with abstinence – when the analyst sets aside his ego, in the analytic work, to assert resolutely a desire upon which otherness can be constructed for the patient.

The mothers

The first thirty pages of the novel, and Chapter 8, are dedicated to the mothers of Karamazov's four children. Dostoevsky's intention is to show that the characters' childhoods have determined how they live their lives and interact with the world. More than this, Dostoevsky depicts the childhoods of these mothers, describing their own parents; in other words, he goes back three generations in the lives of his heroes, to insist on the fact that humans construct the human, and that nature has little to do with it.

Let us start with Sofia Ivanovna, Ivan and Alyosha's mother, and Fyodor Karamazov's second wife. She was "the daughter of some obscure deacon", an orphan since early childhood. She was brought up by the widow of a General. The eternal nagging of the insufferable old woman drove the young girl to try to take her own life. Fyodor Pavlovich, who happened to be travelling in the region when the girl was sixteen, asked for her hand in marriage. After making inquiries, the widow refused. But Fyodor persisted. Sofia's remarkable beauty, and her innocence, captivated this sensuous man who had, until then, only admired a coarser kind of beauty. Enchanted and driven by his powerful desire, he eloped with her, relinquishing any dowry – no small sacrifice for such a greedy man.

As for Sofia, she saw this marriage as a means to escape from her benefactress and to start a new life with a man who would be her protector. Fyodor Pavlovich did, indeed, consider himself her saviour. Now that he had saved Sofia from the old woman, she would be in his debt forever. As soon as she was in her husband's house, the young wife had to witness the orgies he organised with "loose women".[6] This brutal conjugal treatment, combined with the fact that she "had been kept in terror from her childhood", as Dostoevsky says, caused a nervous disorder and psychic collapse. People said she was "possessed by devils", that is, she had "terrible fits of hysteria" and "even lost her reason".[7]

In Karamazov's household, Sofia Ivanovna found a protector, in the person of Grigory, the servant – although nothing could stop her husband's vulgar debauchery. But Grigory berated his master "in a manner little befitting a servant" and on one occasion even "drove all the disorderly women out of the house".[8] When Sofia died, only eight years after her marriage, it was Grigory who placed a tombstone on her grave, at his own expense.

In the middle of this nightmare, Sofia had two children, born three years apart, Ivan and Alyosha. She was only twenty-four when she died. Her two children would have had the same fate as Karamazov's firstborn, Dmitri, who was abandoned by his father and would have died if Grigory had not taken care of him. But the general's widow, their mother's benefactress, came to take the two orphans to live with her. She died shortly afterwards, but she had provided for their future and their education in her will, and had entrusted their care to responsible people who brought them up and saw to it that their capital would grow.

Alyosha suddenly and inexplicably left his studies and his life in the city to return to his father's house, see his mother's grave and enter a monastery. He was twenty years old, the same age as his mother when he was born. He had been only four when she died, but he remembered her vividly; "he remembered […] her face, her caresses, as though she stood living before [him]". Dostoevsky remarks:

> such memories may persist, as everyone knows, from an even earlier age […] but they seldom stand out through a whole lifetime like spots of light out of darkness, like a corner torn out of a huge picture which has […] disappeared.[9]

One scene particularly stood out in his mind:

> He remembered one still summer evening, an open window, the slanting rays of the setting sun […] in a corner of the room the holy image, before it a lighted lamp, and on her knees before the image his mother, sobbing hysterically with cries and moans, snatching him up in both arms, squeezing him close till it hurt, and praying for him to the Mother of God, holding him out in both arms to the image […] and suddenly a nurse runs in and snatches him from her in terror. And Alyosha remembered his mother's face at that minute. He used to say that it was frenzied but beautiful. But he rarely cared to speak of this memory to anyone.
>
> In his childhood and youth he was by no means forthcoming and he talked very little, but not from shyness or sullenness; quite the contrary […] from a sort of inner preoccupation entirely personal […]. This preoccupation was so important for him that he seemed, as it were, to forget others on account of it. […] There was something about him which made one feel at once […] that he did not care to be a judge of others. […] He seemed, indeed, to accept everything without the least condemnation, though often grieving bitterly. And this was so much so that no one could surprise or frighten him.
>
> Coming, when he was twenty, to his father's house which was a sink of debauchery, he, chaste and pure as he was, simply withdrew in silence when to look on was unbearable. He did this without the slightest sign of contempt or condemnation.[10]

Ever since he was a child, Alyosha has been loved by everyone. St. Augustine, who invented original sin – an invention greatly envied by Ivan's *Grand Inquisitor* – speculated that God created man so that there could be a beginning. Alyosha is one of those rare beings who are interested in emergence, in that which brings into being, not which already is, in the unknown. Therefore, it is not surprising that he gets on well with children, who are an eternal beginning. His father comes to feel a sincere love for him, such as he has never felt for anyone before. "Do you know," he often said, looking at Alyosha, "that you are like her, the 'crazy woman'?"[11] – as he called his second wife. It is indeed true that Alyosha keeps his mother's image alive in his own person: he has swallowed her entirely.

This is no doubt why he can be patient with Liza, a capricious and insufferable girl of about the same age his mother had been when she met her future husband.

The terrible scene where Fyodor Pavlovich, drunk and full of hate, tortures his son, pushing him to the brink of madness, ends with proof of this psychic swallowing.

> "I never thought a woman ugly in my life – that's been my rule! Can you understand that? How could you understand it? You've milk in your veins, not blood. You're not out of your shells yet! My rule has been that you can always find something interesting in every woman that you wouldn't find in any other. Only, one must know how to find it, that's the point! That's a talent! To my mind there are no ugly women. The very fact that she is a woman is half the battle. [...] But how could you understand that? Even in old maids, even in them you can find something that makes you wonder that men have been such fools as to let them grow old without noticing them. Barefooted girls or unattractive ones, you must take by surprise. Didn't you know that? You must surprise them till they're fascinated, upset, ashamed that such a gentleman should fall in love with such a little slut. It's a good thing that there always are and will be masters and slaves in the world. And so there always will be a little maid-of-all-work and her master, and you know, that's all that's needed for happiness. Wait [...] listen, Alyoshka, I always used to surprise your mother, but in a different way. I paid no attention to her at all, but all at once, when the minute came, I'd be all devotion to her, crawl on my knees, kiss her feet, and I always, always – I remember it as though it were today – reduced her to that tinkling, quiet, nervous queer little laugh. It was peculiar to her. I knew her attacks always used to begin like that. The next day she would begin shrieking hysterically. You see, that little laugh was not a sign of delight. [...] That's the great thing, to know how to take everyone. Once Belyavsky – he was a handsome fellow, and a rich and he used to come here and hang around her – suddenly gave me a slap in the face in front of her. And she who was always such a mild sheep – why, I thought she was going to knock me down. How she pounced on me! 'You're beaten, beaten!' she said. [...] 'You have been trying to sell me to him,' she said, 'how dared he strike you in my presence! Don't dare come near me again, never, never! Run at once, challenge him to a duel!' I took her to the monastery to bring her to her senses. The holy Fathers prayed her back to reason. But I swear, by God, Alyosha, I never insulted the poor crazy girl! Only once, perhaps, in the first year; then she was very fond of praying. She used to keep the feasts of Our Lady particularly and used to keep me out of her room then. I'll knock that mysticism out of her, I thought! 'Here,' I said, you see your holy ikon. Here it is. Here I take it down. You believe it's miraculous, but here, I'll spit on it and nothing will happen to me!' When she saw it, good Lord! I thought she would kill me. But she only just jumped up, wrung her hands, then suddenly hiding her face in them she began trembling all over and fell on the floor [...] fell in a heap. Alyosha, Alyosha, what's the matter?"

The old man jumped up frightened. From the time he began speaking about Alyosha's mother, a change had come over Alyosha's face. He grew crimson, his eyes glowed, his lips quivered. The old wretch had gone spluttering on, noticing nothing, till something very strange happened to Alyosha. Precisely what he was describing in the crazy woman was suddenly repeated with Alyosha. He jumped up exactly as his mother was said to have done, wrung his hands, hid his face in them, and fell back in his chair, shaking all over in an hysterical convulsion of violent, silent weeping.

[...]

"Ivan, Ivan! Water, quickly! It's like her, exactly as she used to be. His mother. Spurt some water on him from your mouth, that's what I used to do to her. He's upset about his mother. His mother," he muttered to Ivan.

"But she was my mother too. Wasn't she?" said Ivan with anger and contempt. The old man shrank before Ivan's burning eyes.

Then something very strange happened, though only for a second; it seemed to escape the old man's mind that Alyosha's mother actually was the mother of Ivan too.

"Your mother?" he muttered, not understanding. "What do you mean? What mother are you talking about? Was she? Why, damn it! Of course she was yours too! Damn it! My mind has never been so muddled before. Excuse me. Why, I was thinking Ivan. [...] He, he, he!"[12]

Ivan's childhood

Alyosha has always been grateful to all those who brought him up and looked after him. Ivan, on the other hand, does not have the generosity to acknowledge his debt to others and their kindness towards him. Because of this, he has no access to love. Some people are so frightened to recognise any gift of love, feel so threatened by the idea that what they receive from others might transform them, that they prefer to destroy all links with the vitality of actual life. Contrary to Alyosha, who reveres his mother's memory, Ivan focuses on his harsh judgment of the way his father treated his mother, a judgment on which he built his avowed hatred of Fyodor Pavlovich.

Pride is rooted in this refusal to acknowledge the love one receives, in the impossibility of expecting anything from another. The fragility hidden under this rigid armour is so extreme that the smallest oversight on the part of another is experienced as an attack, an act of persecution. The one who is proud is afraid to reveal the slightest imperfection; in other words, he fears that someone may discover he is merely human. Therefore, he never asks for anything. He always speaks about himself, his projects, his accomplishments. And even when he doesn't speak of them, he thinks about them, and nothing else interests him. Indeed, he does not remember what others tell him, unless it concerns him directly. His pride renders him the marvellous child he never was for his parents. And, like a child, he takes himself for the centre of the world, for the cause of everything that happens around him.

The reader knows nothing about Ivan's childhood, except that he showed great intelligence very early. Nothing is said about his relationship with his mother. As an adolescent, he was reserved, without being bashful; he left his benefactor's family at thirteen, to go to school, and then to university, in Moscow. During his student years, bureaucratic formalities delayed his access to the inheritance left by the general's widow, his mother's benefactress, who had taken the children in after their mother's death. To earn a living while studying, Ivan wrote little newspaper articles about street incidents, and these were soon in great demand. Once he received his inheritance, he continued to write for newspaper editors, even publishing book reviews that caused him to become known in literary circles. After graduating and just before going abroad, a strange article he published on ecclesiastic courts attracted much favourable attention in a wide circle of readers. Churchmen, secularists and atheists all considered the author as one of their own. But some people concluded that the article was nothing but a brazen farce.

Why Ivan came to live in his deplorable father's house was somewhat of a mystery. It is suggested that his arrival concerned the conflict between his brother Dmitri and Fyodor Pavlovich. But given that Ivan had very little esteem for his older brother, this is highly unlikely. This mysterious absence of a reasonable cause for Ivan's arrival becomes outright strange in light of the sordid and tragic events related to the subsequent murder of his father. And, surprisingly, the reader learns that father and son get along well, that the old man accepts Ivan's influence, listens to him at times, and even starts to behave more decently. When Ivan arrived, it had been a year since Alyosha entered the monastery.

Dmitri's mother

The first-born son's mother, Adelaida Ivanovna, although beautiful, aroused no sensual passion in Fyodor Pavlovich, despite his indiscriminate love of women. He chose her and eloped with her solely to get a dowry. As for the young girl, she had married out of defiance, and imagined him to be a bold adventurer. But she soon discovered that she felt only contempt for him, and the marriage became a living hell. The spouses fought, and Adelaida even struck her husband. She eventually ran off with a seminarian, leaving her three-year-old son behind, and died in sordid circumstances not long afterwards. Thus, Dmitri was abandoned by his mother, and the consequences of this abandonment will be clearly seen in his relationship with Grushenka, and in the difficulty he has accepting Katerina Ivanovna's love.

Little Mitya survived thanks to the family servant, Grigory, who took him into his care. His father and his mother's family forgot about him. It was a cousin of his mother who offered to bring him up, but since he was often abroad, he entrusted the child to other family members, so that Mitya changed homes four times. The cousin in question was an enlightened "European", which for Dostoevsky means someone who can't be trusted.

Dmitri did not finish high school, entered a military school, was an officer in the army, fought in a duel and was demoted to the ranks, was promoted again, led a wild life and spent a great deal of money. It was during that period that he met Katerina Ivanovna – a crucial encounter in his life. We can suppose that the lack of respect his half-brother Ivan feels for him is due to the way he behaved with this woman.

When he came of age, he received an income from his father, but by then he had accumulated considerable debt. He saw his father for the first time after he came of age, when he came to Fyodor Karamazov's town to settle the question of his estate. He had grown up believing that he had some property and would be independent when he came of age. To his astonishment, he learns from his father that he has nothing, that the total value of his property has been given to him in cash by Karamazov. Dmitri almost goes mad, suspecting a trick. This disappointment nurtured his resentment, a resentment that would lead to the catastrophe that destroyed his life.

Smerdyakov's mother

Lizaveta Smerdyashehaya was the village idiot, beaten by her father, barefoot, wearing only a hempen shift. There was something monstrous about her, but this did not stop old Karamazov from having sexual relations with her on one occasion, because "there was a certain [piquancy] about it".[13] Lizaveta became pregnant and died giving birth to the child in the garden of her dastardly seducer, where she took refuge while in labour, after climbing over a tall fence! The new born was taken in by Grigory and his wife, who had just lost their baby. Thus, Smerdyakov grows up as a servant in his father's household. Aside from a stay in Moscow where he learns to be a cook, he never leaves home. Fyodor Pavlovich trusts him, completely unaware of the hate his bastard son has for him. As for his mother, Smerdyakov calls her "The Stinker", leaving no doubt as to his feelings towards her.

The father

Karamazov is an old clown, the third one we encounter in Dostoevsky's work. The first was Marmeladov, in *Crime and Punishment*, a Shakespearean king fallen from glory, lost in a "cabaret" in the slums of St. Petersburg. The second was Stepan Trofimovich, in *Demons*, a man imbued with himself, displaying insufferable unjustified smugness, a pompous intellectual believing firmly in the stories he invents, a man whose relationship with Varvara Petrovna makes it plain that he is a fearful, sentimental and irascible infant. Earlier I used his character to construct a metapsychology of the madness of folly, a last defence against schizophrenia.

I will remind you of certain characteristics of this defence. The madness of folly goes hand in hand with the inability to name affects, and with the denial of their reality. Every affect is persecutory and must find at once a representation among the manic defences. Manic representations are empty forms marked by the urgency to reject an emerging emotion. The physical agitation accompanying this urgency testifies to the attempt to expulse all sensoriality, to silence the body and, if need be, to abandon it. The typical manifestation of this attempt is the compromise in which the desperate need to control sensoriality reduces the body to its muscle structure and to voluntary movement. Stepan Trofimovich is entrapped in the madness of folly; his affects burst in upon him and persecute him. Because all affect is an impediment, rhythm is not possible. And without rhythm, there can be no well-being, pleasure, play. And since there is no reverie either, there can be no image of a future. Time is closed in on itself. What dominates is panic, as the sole response to anguish. The foolish subject is in love with his passions: not those he feels, which are dangerous and therefore prohibited, but those he invents – and which are only founded on the unreality of his world. Foolishness is afraid of sense, because sense displaces the particular towards the universal. Therefore, sense is denied, and the denial itself is then denied. Foolishness is characterised by the determination to avoid any psychic effort, any new inscription.[14]

Those who remember *Demons* must admit that some of the behaviours displayed by Stepan Trofimovich are reproduced by Fyodor Pavlovich. But the latter, contrary to Trofimovich, is completely in control of the effect he produces on others; he plays the clown to avoid conflict and direct confrontation; he is not trying to gain affection or to please others. His aim is always to exert his power, to enjoy the hate he provokes in others. But, unlike Svidrigailov, the tragic pervert in *Crime and Punishment*, he does not deposit his hate in others; Fyodor Pavlovich is a psychopath who enchants every moment of his existence by searching for the next murder to carry out.

He is an incompetent man, corrupt and extravagant. He does not work and lives on a personal income and the profits of shady transactions. As soon as his first wife ran off, he

> introduced a regular harem into the house, and abandoned himself to orgies of drunkenness. In the intervals he used to drink all over the province, complaining tearfully to everybody of Adelaide's having left him, going into details too disgraceful for a husband to mention in regard to his own married life. What seemed to gratify him and flatter his self-love was to play the ridiculous part of the injured husband, and to parade his woes with embellishments.

"Fyodor Karamazov was all his life fond of acting, of suddenly playing an unexpected part, sometimes without any motive for doing so, and even to his own direct disadvantage".[15]

Thanks to his remarkable understanding of the unconscious, Dostoevsky always describes his characters with subtlety. He seems to fear that the reader's interpretation may be too naturalist and restrictive. This often results in paradoxical formulations, as sharp as primary processes, in which clear opposites do not exist. He makes the following observation about old Karamazov: "As a general rule, people, even the wicked, are much more naive and simple-hearted than we suppose. And we ourselves are too".[16]

This observation is particularly surprising since the character has the same name as the author: Fyodor. This is why we may interpret this enigmatic "And we ourselves are too" as a slip of the pen.

> I have mentioned already that he looked bloated. His appearance at this time bore traces of something that testified unmistakably to the life he had led. Besides the long fleshy bags under his little, always insolent, suspicious, and ironical eyes; besides the multitude of deep wrinkles in his little fat face, his Adam's apple, hung below his sharp chin like a great, fleshy goitre. It gave him a peculiar, repulsive, sensual appearance. He had besides a long rapacious mouth with full lips, between which could be seen little stumps of black decayed teeth. He slobbered every time he began to speak. [Thus, when Ivan called his father a reptile, he was not speaking metaphorically.] He liked to make fun of his own face, though, I believe, he was well satisfied with it. He often pointed to his nose, which was not very large, but very delicate and conspicuously acquiline. "A regular Roman nose," he used to say, "with my goitre I look like an ancient Roman patrician of the decadent period.' He seemed proud of it".[17]

Fyodor Pavlovich is a liar. He says so himself: "But I have been lying, lying my whole life long, every day and hour of it".[18] Lying constantly to himself, he is never ashamed and he respects no one.

> And having no respect he ceases to love. And in order to distract himself without love, he gives way to passions and coarse pleasures and sinks to bestiality in his vices – and this from continual lying to other men and to himself.[19]

There is not much more to say about old Karamazov. His scandalous and violent behaviour resurfaces again and again; he also keeps posing as a victim. But what remains most obvious is his fear of death, or his infantile fear that he will be prevented from finding some new source of pleasure, when in fact he is incapable of sustaining any desire.

When Alyosha asks his father's consent to enter the monastery, they have a very strange conversation. Among other surprising things, the old man starts to speculate about whether or not there's a ceiling in hell. He thinks there is no ceiling. This dialogue is similar to the one between Raskolnikov and Svidrigailov in *Crime and Punishment*, about eternal life, when Raskolnikov is frightened and thinks his interlocutor is mad. By contrast, Karamazov's ramblings remind us of the representation of Hell that was common in Antiquity. This reveals Dostoevsky's narrative and stylistic intention in writing this book: leading us into an infernal world, one inhabited only by shadows of the living. Karamazov says:

> Yes, yes. Only [...] shadows [...]. I know, I know. That's how a Frenchman described hell: *J'ai vu l'ombre d'un cocher, qui avec l'ombre d'une brosse frottait l'ombre d'une carrosse*. (I saw the shadow of a coachman that with the shadow of a brush polished the shadow of a coach!).[20]

All this is truly terrifying. Indeed, Fyodor Pavlovich is not a father, but merely the shadow of a father: an envious rival of his children whose existence he hates because they are young and because they remind him that he has nothing to pass down except his fear. And except for Alyosha, his sons are not sons, but only shadows of sons: having neither father nor mother to love, they are not even budding Oedipuses. They are unable to hate because they are burdened with the father's hate. *They stand before the monster unarmed, and have swallowed the monster to survive.*[21]

Notes

1 Dostoevsky, F., *The Brothers Karamazov*, Garnett, C. (trans.), New York: Signet Classics, 1962, p. 621.
2 See the chapter "True Love" in the author's *Letters to a Young Psychoanalyst*, Routledge, 2016.
3 Dostoevsky, F., *The Brothers Karamazov*, pp. 527–531.
4 Ibid., pp. 236 and 238–239.
5 Ibid., pp. 33–34.
6 Ibid., p. 23.
7 Ibid.
8 Ibid.
9 Ibid., p. 27.
10 Ibid., pp. 27–28.
11 Ibid., p. 31.
12 Ibid., pp. 132–133.
13 Ibid., p. 98.
14 See *Demons*, Part II, ch. 9.
15 Dostoevsky, F., *The Brothers Karamazov*, pp. 19 and 21.
16 Ibid., p. 19.
17 Ibid., p. 32.
18 Ibid., p. 50.
19 Ibid., p. 49.
20 Ibid., p. 33.
21 The Karamazov children have the characteristics of what I call "a Réfabert". This clinical entity, described by Philippe Réfabert (French psychoanalyst; see my book *Letters to a Young Psychoanalyst*), is a person:

- in whom there is no inscription of that which did not take place
- for whom that which took place did not occur
- who stands unarmed before the monster
- who swallows the monster to survive
- who knows everything, and nothing else at all
- who is cut off from himself, from the unimaginable catastrophe in which his soul, the other in himself, is left for dead
- whose exceptional intelligence is disconnected from his body
- in whom the Id is disconnected from the Ego, and who bears the trace of the soul-murder he has suffered
- who grew up suddenly
- in whom fear of mad, raging adults transformed the child he was into a psychiatrist
- who inhabits the land of All-or-Nothing, between incest and murder, because he is cut off from the agony he lived through as a child.

7

WOMEN IN DOSTOEVSKY'S FICTION

Structure of *The Brothers Karamazov*

Early in the novel, at the gathering in Zosima's cell at the monastery, the reader is informed of the stakes around which the novel is constructed. He understands that the conflict between Dmitri Fyodorovich and his father is not a dispute about money, but rather masculine rivalry, with Grushenka at its centre. It becomes clear that Fyodor Pavlovich will be murdered, most likely by Dmitri. The reader also learns that Ivan is in love with his brother's fiancée, Katerina Ivanovna, who hesitates between them, despite the fact that Dmitri does not hide his passion for Grushenka. The segment ends with the revelation that this absurd reunion was Ivan Fyodorovich's idea, and that he was the one who *insisted on it and arranged it.* Dostoevsky lets us now know, as if in passing, to expect this man to have no scruples.

This synthetic presentation of the plot is very modern. It is reminiscent of Hitchcock, who discloses to the spectator, from the start, information unknown to other characters in the story. We might also mention Brecht, whose aesthetics have changed our perspective on theatrical performance: Brecht granted priority to the *unfolding* of the plot over its *outcome*, which he clearly considered secondary.

By presenting from the start the central elements of the plot, Dostoevsky places the reader in a very particular subjective position: by dispensing him from experiencing the suspense related to discovering a sequence of events, he allows the reader to focus on details and be attentive to their effects – in other words, to take an active role in the reading. Lovers of mystery novels are familiar with the concentration created by this approach: one tries to detect an oddity, something strange that might provide a clue for explaining the outcome. When there is no mystery about the plot from the beginning, the reader's attention is free to focus on *how* each character relates to the situations described, how he sees them, experiences them or avoids them. In other words, these aspects of the narrative reveal each protagonist's manner of relating to life, so that from then on it is their psychic functioning that interests the reader.

The Brothers Karamazov is a story about men. The main characters are shaped first of all by their relation to their mothers, and by the relations of these mothers to their husband, Fyodor Pavlovich. Secondly, the protagonists are defined by the relations they have with each other, with their father, with the law, with desire and with thought. Three of them will also be described based on the complex ties of love and passion they have formed with two women, Grushenka and Katerina Ivanovna.

Grushenka could be said to be the younger sister of Nastasya Filippovna, in *The Idiot*. Like her older sister, Grushenka was the courtesan of a wealthy man, before becoming, thanks to her volubility and her sensuality, a woman who can drive certain men mad with desire. But she does not have Nastasya's grandeur; some vulgarity is mixed with her pain, diminishing her power; her suffering does not shed light on her reflection, and she remains imprisoned in her grievance. Her brutality hides the dreams of a little girl who still believes in Prince Charming. She leaves everything to go back to her first love, who turns out to be a despicable man; and indeed, her suitors, Dmitri and Fyodor Pavlovich, do not have the stature of Myshkin or Rogozhin, nor the complexity of Ganya, in *The Idiot*.

Nastasya Filippovna is the agent of trauma because she looks for the truth under a pile of lies – she feels affection for Rogozhin and loves Myshkin because they are sincere. She is beautiful, sensual and strives to define her thinking, which would have found its formulation if the prince had not been a pervert and an idiot. Contrary to Nastasya, Grushenka uses scandal as a pitiful, cruel weapon – she does not respect herself very much, is "fond of money, that she [lends] out at a cruel rate of interest, [and] she's a merciless cheat and swindler".[1] As for serious matters, she finds them rather boring.

Katerina Ivanovna's social origins could place her on a level with Aglaya Ivanovna, in *The Idiot*. But the fact that she accepted Dmitri's money to save her father, and probably slept with him for this money, brings her closer to Grushenka. However, she believes herself to be superior to the courtesan thanks to her origins and her passion for sacrifice.

Dostoevsky's female characters are either candidates for sacrifice or scandal makers. For them, love for a man is separated from the sexual, or is expected to repair damaged sexuality; their excessive pride is rooted in a narcissistic wound they display like a trophy, to defy the world. Dmitri says about Katerina Ivanovna: "She loves her own *virtue*, not me. [...] Because [she] wants to sacrifice her life and destiny out of gratitude".[2]

Sacrifice and murder

When sexuality breaks into the psychic space, destroying all the bonds of love which tie the subject to life, life stagnates, is impoverished, decays. Dissociated from the person and no longer serving the interests of the ego which rejects it, sexuality becomes persecutory, shameful, guilty. It no longer enriches the experience of life, but remains invasive, takes up all the spaces, saturates them: eating is the same as lovemaking, lovemaking is no different than eating. When sexuality eliminates love, it remains frozen, cut off from sensations.

In women, pregenital sexuality predominates in these situations. Auto-eroticism is a defence against sexuality experienced as invasive because its subjective nature is traumatic. Traumatic sexuality cannot nurture the sphere of the ego, so it is dissociated from the ego. When sexuality is not integrated into the ego, there is a constant risk that it can manifest itself in a manner that threatens the integrity of the psyche as a whole.

Negation and sacrifice are also manifestations of pregenitality, but masochistic euphoria is often sabotaged, and is accompanied by hatred of the other and the desire to kill. But women's sacrificing for men also has another origin.

In general, women unconsciously choose someone like their mother as their first love, a partner they will try to save from melancholia. Such a project may lead them to destroy the most crucial ties they have with living, with alive life. These love relations, which hide a mother-daughter relation in reverse – now, the partner or husband holds the place of the child, while the woman holds the place of her own mother – are, of course, hopelessly tangled. Wanting to free, at any cost, the man in her life from entrapment in a deathly snare, offers the considerable advantage of dispensing her of sexuality. But the maternal spectre haunting this relation will inevitably graft onto it the remnants of old experiences imbued with guilt, hate, remorse, discouragement, various regressions and foolishness.

The reader knows nothing about Grushenka's or Katerina Ivanovna's mother. Dostoevsky provides some biographical facts about the women in his novels, but never a real story of their childhood. For Dostoevsky, woman is an essence, governed by her nature: she can be either a saint or a whore; the only exception is Sonya, who combines these two facets. But the way in which Dostoevsky's female characters treat their men confirms what I've seen in my practice and in my life. "*I will be your chattel, I will be the carpet under your feet. I want to love you forever. I want to save you from yourself*", Katerina writes to Dmitri.[3] Her sacrifice goes hand in hand with enormous pride. Ivan makes this very clear:

> [B]elieve me, Katerina, you really love him. And the more he insults you, the more you love him – that's your "laceration". You love him just as he is. You love him for insulting you. If he reformed, you'd give him up at once and stop loving him. But you need him so as to contemplate continually your heroic fidelity and reproach him for infidelity. And it all comes from your pride. Oh, there's a great deal of humiliation and self-abasement about it, but it all comes from pride. [...] I am too young and I've loved you too much. I know that I ought not to say this, that it would be more dignified on my part simply to leave you, and it would be less offensive for you.[4]

And it is also Ivan who describes most astutely the murderous side of her personality:

> Katerina has never cared for me! She has known all the time that I cared for her – though I never said a word of my love to her – she knew, but she didn't care for me. I have never been her friend either, not for one moment.[5] [Let's remember that Katerina Ivanovna said of Ivan that he is her best friends.[6]] She is too proud to need my friendship. She kept me at her side as a means of revenge. She revenged with me and on me all the insults which she has been continually receiving from Dmitri ever since their first meeting. For that first meeting has rankled in her heart as an insult. […] She has talked to me of nothing but her love for him. […] But I am going far away, and shall never come back. […] I don't want to sit beside a "laceration". But I don't know how to speak now. I've said everything. […] Good-bye, Katerina. You can't be angry with me, because I am a hundred times more severely punished than you, if only by the fact that I shall never see you again. Good-bye!
>
> I don't want your hand. You have tortured me too deliberately for me to be able to forgive you at this moment. I will forgive you later, but now I don't want your hand.[7]

Desire and its dead ends

For men, women are, of course, a cause of suffering. In Dostoevsky's fiction, men are, naturally, a source of hope for women. Valuing the truth, women demand that men keep their word, and make a commitment to love. So far so good. In these circumstances, things can take their usual course, that is, the enamoured state can exist, with its accompanying anguish. But for Dostoevsky, sexuality is a sin. As a result, his female characters are either fascinating because they accept their sexuality – but then feel too guilty to love (like Nastasya or Grushenka); or they exclude sexuality and become madwomen or maternal figures (like Katerina Ivanovna). Indeed, Dostoevsky's women do not show any particular depth of thinking. While they personify the truth or use it to denounce men's lies or cowardice, in general they themselves do not go beyond the limits of common sense. Dostoevsky's female characters are either hysterics, hysterical madwomen or hysterical maternal figures. And since the male characters are perverse or psychopaths, psychotics or hysterics, it will obviously be very difficult for the characters to be involved in veritable love relations. Thus, there is no *true love* in Dostoevsky's fiction. But there are – remarkably well described – the impediments that it usually encounters.[8]

When sexuality is dissociated from the ego, as I was saying, there is the risk that it will manifest itself in ways that are dangerous for the integrity of the psyche. This dissociation can be the result of a traumatic sexual experience, like in the case of Katerina Ivanovna or Grushenka. Usually, this experience reinforces a deficiency in the primary maternal environment. I believe that a lack of tenderness on the part of the father present at the Oedipal stage is also a crucial factor.

In the analytic process, such a dissociation may be followed by the forms of misery familiar to hysterics. I will remind you of the ones I have seen most often, and which are, of course, connected with the relations these women entertain with the men in their lives.

As we see with Katerina Ivanovna, each man serves to make it possible to complain about the others.

There is the idealist-masochist who understands everything, accepts everything: he wants to save her, although he knows not from what. He is portrayed by Dmitri, in his relation to Grushenka, who is amused by this overgrown adolescent. With unfailing astuteness, she identifies the true nature of his sham idealisation: what he "loves" is what she could become thanks to him – and she despises him because of it. With him, she will behave in a ruthless and even cruel manner – an exercise in hatred, important for her narcissistic economy. But no matter how pathetic his idealisation is, this positive, desexualised image that another has of her is beneficial to her. This is why the role of the idealist-masochist is sometimes played by the loyal homosexual friend to whom the woman can say anything about men, women, aging which destroys the beauty of the body, and – most importantly – with whom she is free to show her nastiness, the other face of envy.

Then there is the jealous man, possessive and overly attached. Dmitri illustrates this man as well. To be heavily invested as a privileged object delights her, and very quickly stifles and exasperates her. Very soon, it becomes obvious that this heavy investment has nothing to do with her, but rather with the rejecting mother of the little boy her suitor once was (remember that as a small child Dmitri was abandoned by his mother). But it is already too late; it is not easy to get out of the mud. Feeling guilty, she plays out all the scenarios of melodrama. But she has something to gain: while she takes on the anguish of the other, her own is turned inward (we will not dwell on her identification to this man; he reproduces what have become her impossible demands on her mother, after the father present at the Oedipal stage has failed in constructing a bridge between narcissistic gratitude and genital gratitude, a bridge that could be called the ego ideal).

There is the poet, whom she will mother; the alcoholic who, after making her experience terror, will allow her to hate openly. Sometimes, there is a psychoanalyst – who can't make heads or tails of what is going on.

In another sphere of her life, there are various friends with whom she is able to maintain spontaneous relations of the type that never lasts with her lovers.

And there is the brute.

The brute

The brute is not necessarily uncouth, insensitive or primitive. His social status is probably prestigious. He is admired, or even respected, in his social circle. He can be violent, but is also very generous, cultured and amusing; he is interested in a multitude of things in the world. What makes him a brute is that he refuses, with great determination, to focus on the narcissistic complaints of the woman, on her annoying tendency to transform the smallest thing into a metaphysical problem. And this is why, of all her men, the most important one, the only one she really cares for, is the brute. These are the fantasies Katerina Ivanovna was having when she first met Dmitri. These fantasies are still at work and, as Ivan understood so well, they are present beyond her desire for self-sacrifice (here, we have another example of Dostoevsky's genius: Grushenka's fantasies are not the same as those of Katerina Ivanovna, although they focus on the same man.)

With the brute, the hysterical woman, who can complain for hours about the smallest thing, always finds herself alone, regardless of the real importance of the causes of her pain. To get along with him, she must accept him as he is, take the internal resources he has to offer, without ever being able to store her own difficulties in his internal space. She will tend to the difficulties of the brute and will defend him from the whole world. But their ideas of reciprocity differ. He acknowledges what she gives him, and he loves her, without seeing her as a nurse. As for her, it is not certain that she loves him; at times, his silence, aloofness and distance are unbearable and destructive. So, she will take lovers, many lovers. But she will always be there for her brute.

A recent psychoanalytic theory has attempted to shed light on these "mysterious" masochistic tendencies in women – previously explained by the attachment of the hysterical woman to her brute, an attachment allowing her to experience the joy of having become chiefly responsible for the repetition of the initial trauma – based on the idea that the hysteric looks for a master. Pimps and macho men have demonstrated the existential validity of this paranoid hypothesis about women very convincingly. What remains to be discovered is what women are really looking for when they look for a Master. To say that they look for a master in order to reign over him doesn't solve the problem, since once she reigns over a man, the woman must renew her search. And indeed she does, if the man becomes her subject. Loyal to her symptoms, the hysteric looks for a master, but loyal to her desire, she looks for what we have called a brute. And the reason for her attachment to him – before a true analytic encounter takes place – is that he is the place where her relation to life is best integrated, real and true. Why?

Because this man, due to his own limitations, leaves intact a truth the hysteric tries to avoid by every possible means, which is that for her the question of love can only be considered if it is *first* presented as a matter of sexuality, a question of optimal sexual pleasure, integrated with the ideals she holds dear.

The brute comes together with her in bed, in the sexual encounter. She likes being loved this way, she is never more free than when he makes love to her, when she makes love to him (she will not speak of this in an analysis for years, it's her secret). She finds that his way of loving her first in her body is what suits her best. She is certain that this way of being with her is also a promise. This promise binds her and she relies on it, despite repeated disappointments when nothing else follows. But she prefers this promise to any certainty: she knows that this incompleteness allows her to be most deeply rooted in the soil of life. She has a vague sense of this, but she won't let go of this idea, this balanced and balancing idea she fiercely defends. And if certain events complicate things even more and she defiantly turns her back on this promise, all imaginable catastrophes are possible. It is sometimes after such a catastrophe that she will come to see a psychoanalyst.

In the course of her analysis, she will have love affairs of a different nature. We will discuss three types: the out-of-nowhere intense sexual fling, the homosexual affair, and love.

The love affair

She meets him at a party at a friend's house, or at a dinner out with friends. More rarely, on the street. A few minutes after their meeting, they will be in bed together. This encounter can last a few hours or a few days. She feels elated, intensely happy. She is panicked. This must be stopped right away, no matter what it takes. It has to remain an interlude, it can't continue, it was an aberration. It's impossible to contain so much happiness. After making love, she is seized by a great, ancient sadness. She cries. Suddenly, living has become a terrible task, impossible – she doesn't know why. It is urgent to destroy this, to undo the ties, to get away and escape from this new internal existence which has caught hold of her and renders her solitude so acutely necessary, so sharply defined and solid. She must get away, not to forget, but to rest. To rest. She doesn't have the strength, living will have to wait. She must destroy this. And she works hard to do it, spares no effort, goes into a wild frenzy.

It is as if a car travelling on the highway at 200 km per hour suddenly put on its brakes on the edge of a precipice: there is no more ground, no continuity, the road continues again further on, but there is no bridge to take you to the other side. This *abrupt lack of continuity* in the life of the child, this lack of integration of two periods of the child's life can explain what we view as the indifference of the hysteric. The term "inconsistency" is more useful for giving us a clue as to what underlies this attitude.

She must destroy this. She will go to see the man. She may be intending to tell him about the fatigue she feels, the impossibility. But no, in the end she just disappears abruptly. Everything has become inconsistent. He talks to her of the night they spent together, he reminds her of her joy, of her freedom, the superlatives she used. But now there is no one there. The person he is trying to reach no longer answers. Yes, she hears him speak of this woman, but what he says has nothing to do with her. Inconsistent words, inconsistent memory. The man is suffering. She sees before her a man who is suffering. The man is angry, he accuses her. She is not indifferent to how he feels, but nothing has any importance, any consistency. She doesn't care about anything, starting with herself. The man says she is crazy. She thinks that he is probably right, but whether she thinks this or something else makes no difference.

A homosexual affair is another matter. I want to emphasise its structuring effect. An encounter of this type may allow the woman to take possession of her woman's body – something her mother did not transmit to her or prevented – a reintegration of auto-eroticism into narcissism, which could open a lasting internal space of bonding with another woman in an affectionate manner – a precondition to a woman's ability to risk recognising her love for a man.

Love and psychic conflict

Now, let us speak about love. Little by little, a slowness enters the woman's life. There is no spectacular change: a different tone of voice, slight pauses in her speech, punctuating her narration, a slowing down of her movements. Her thoughts are calm, there is awareness of the passing of time, the body is a serene presence. There is also urgency, intensity, concentration. The world is more compact, full of colours. It is hard to tell whether she knows what is happening to her. It's not important, she is too busy living it to concern herself with knowing. If the woman is of a certain age, for the first time her wrinkles, some strands of white hair, will become visible. The real beauty of her mature years will make itself apparent. Love can enter her life before or after the emergence of transference love; in the latter case, it will signal the end of the analysis. If the encounter with love occurs when the question of love is about to be examined in analysis in terms of love and disappointment related to the father, it is best that the analyst be aware that most psychoanalytic stakes have been transferred onto the scene of reality. He must then help the patient *not to have anachronistic reactions* to a new experience.

Secrecy is the key word to describe the new situation, regardless of whether or not it leads to the lovers living together. In any case, this is not the woman's first lover. The secrecy has to do with the world, with protecting the intimate experience from the outside world. As if what other people think might severely injure an exceptional manner of relating to the real whose beauty is constructed out of the most delicately woven sensitivity. The relation between this fantasy and non-integration is not of any great importance, nor should we dwell on the romantic hues of this secrecy, which shuns public places and prefers to remain in the shade. What is more important to note is the absence of any excessive sentimentality (sexuality is joyfully unrestrained), and the presence of anxiety, which underscores the unprecedented character of what is taking place.

What is new is the refusal of a self-representation that excludes the connection between physical pleasure and the pleasure of thinking. Now, this connection exists. Another novelty is the permanence of a state of well-being that draws attention to the sweet silence of the continuity of living, which was interrupted by the father present at the Oedipal stage, and by his sarcastic remarks about the games she invented as a little girl to take possession of her body, and project herself into the time when she would be the woman she was to become.

This inability of the father to feel intense tenderness for his daughter's attempts to build a bridge between the sensations of her body and the demands of appearances has grave consequences. The lack of respect for the serious nature of these childish games can, from then on, make it impossible for the pleasure associated with the enactment of representations of bodily sensations to be integrated into the totality of representations – the condition needed for this pleasure to be a pleasure for another as well. And the distance to be bridged becomes an abyss. The father's brutal behaviour has *prohibited* the connection between physical sensations and their imaginary extension into the future, preventing them from finding a way to take hold there. The inability to make this connection has also prohibited the spontaneous joy that would ensue. This dissociation, this non-integration between the living body of the little girl and fantasies about the body of the woman to come results, after adolescence, in a separation between the living body of the little girl and the subjectively experienced body of the woman. This radical dissociation between the representations of pregenital sexuality and genital sexuality, whose integration *is directly dependent on the* tenderness *of the father present at the Oedipal stage*, has blocked the constitution of a minimum of identificatory security, without which the subject cannot risk experiencing love – this experience that brings together, in such a complex and mysterious manner, the body and the psyche. The absence of this tenderness has created a gap between these two types of representations. As a result, the working through of her capacity to love must recognise in advance the effects on the woman of *the injury inflicted by the father on the child's thinking*. But this dissociation was also a means of avoiding the psychic pain associated with the betrayal associated with the injury (the betrayal is more devastating than the injury).

If integration can only be achieved at the cost of recognising disillusionment with the father, it is better to avoid love. Two enactments of indifference: rendering thinking unreal and anesthetising sensitivity, testify to the *work of disinvestment* of the representations set in motion by the advent of love. This work serves to avoid recognising the paternal offence, and to elude the unthinkable anxiety tied to the lack of a bridge between representations of pregenital and genital sexuality. The paternal offence has disturbed the representations of the little girl pertaining to love for herself, including, of course, the validity of her thoughts about this love.

In this regard, let me make an observation: in recent years, clinical interest in trauma seems to be accompanied by the relinquishing of the idea that infantile sexuality is at the foundation of psychic functioning. I cannot conceive of psychoanalytic treatment of trauma that would not draw on the pregenital to reorganise the psyche. A form of therapeutic practice that does not take into account the role of sexuality in narcissistic development cannot claim to be psychoanalysis; it would be essentially nothing more than philosophical reflection on being.

But let us return to our discussion. In an adult woman, a lack of integration between the representations of pregenital and genital sexuality is experienced concretely either as chronic dissatisfaction with everything she accomplishes, or as bursts of exuberant passion rooted in the magical thinking of childhood. There is no continuity in the transition from one affective sphere to another; this transition takes place by intermittent leaps. Dissatisfaction with one's accomplishments goes hand in hand with a sense of worthlessness: both are the result of a thought process which, lacking validation by the father, has lost the certainty of its direct link with reality, and cannot guarantee that the relation between its formulations and the reality to which they refer is reliable.

Another consequence of dissociation is the inability to decide: should she be in the world with other people and waste one's time, living a "lie" and a "pretence", or withdraw from the world, take time to be alone and safe from sexuality, to make a new start possible? The need for hiding the new love in her life arises partly as a result of this belief in the omnipotence of solitude.

While she needs to keep this important relationship secret, attacking its continuity is the temporary compromise she makes in order to deal with the anxiety that always threatens to invade the scene and destroy everything. At first, this attack will be subtle (but continuous): she will be very late for a meeting, she will cancel engagements at the last minute, she will unexpectedly go away for a few days. The telephone is an ideal way to keep communication fragmented: the conversation can be interrupted at any time, and initiated any time, even at unsuitable hours. Another considerable advantage of the telephone is that it separates the body from the word, sexuality from its practice. And for this reason, it makes it possible to speak about the body and about desire and sets in motion fantasmatic activity – recognised as such – related to sexuality. Very quickly, these telephone conversations will become actual *preliminaries*. Of course, the man in question must interpret all these attacks as postponements that are part of the game of desire.

What can we say about the men such a woman loves? Although they are as different from each other as there is variety in life, each one has three characteristics whose combination allows her, for the first time since her childhood, to rebuild a structuration process which broke down then and has remained broken since.

First, he is able to talk, without shame, about the great importance sexuality has for him, about his love for this woman's body and for the pleasure it gives him. Second, he respects, appreciates and always takes into account her thinking. But he completely rejects her sterile auto-erotic musings which cut her off from the reality of the world and from the other. The tendency to such daydreaming is another effect of the dissociation created by the lack of integration of sexuality into the ego, the lack of integration of sexuality and thinking. On a phenomenological level, this lack of integration can be said to be reflected in the inconsistency sensed in a hysteric (man or woman), interpreted as indifference, withdrawal or falseness. This musing is always present in the background. Standing between the subject and her perceptions, between the subject and her thoughts, it constantly interferes with the process of subjective appropriation of experiences as they unfold. This relative derealisation of experience always allows the woman who struggles with the hysterical prohibition of femininity to avoid feeling entirely responsible for what happens to her: *un*able to explain the whys and wherefores of her past, she often feels cheated by life and sinks into a state of indifference that can last a long time. But the man she loves categorically denies this interpretation of things and rejects just as categorically the complacency that supports it.

Although to be loved like this allows the woman to obtain vengeance for the paternal offence, she is still filled with anxiety in the face of this new happiness.

And an unconscious sense of disloyalty to the father causes her to feel guilty for being loved as a subject in a woman's body. She also finds it difficult to accept the idealisation associated with her beloved's love, as it is with any love. To defend against it, she can choose to interpret the intensity of this love as weakness on the part of her lover.

Suicide is a different matter. It is always an attempt to stop the unbearable anguish associated with a lessening of dissociation. Suicide is also an attempt to end once and for all the anguish that is part of the renewal of energy released in anticipation of greater integration. This is why suicide sometimes intervenes to put an abrupt end to a real moment of happiness. A psychic explosion caused by the sudden encounter of two kinds of representations usually kept apart by lack of integration, suicide is always a triumph of dissociation, a last attempt to keep it intact, a final loyalty to the paternal prohibition of an orgasmic experience of the ego, capable of bringing about the integration of these two kinds of representations.

Indeed, idealisation can quickly compromise well-being by introducing a fluctuation between hypomania and depression sometimes aggravated by more or less serious somatic manifestations. As time passes, this new love starts to persecute her more and more. She feels "small", "stupid", "unworthy", "pathetic". At first, we could say that all this is to be expected, since feeling unworthy is part of being in love. But this feeling, which in her case is combined with anguish and guilt, often degenerates, leading to panic. The woman says nothing about this (to "confess" her feelings to her lover would make her feel even more "worthless"). To fight off the panic, she reinforces her attacks on love.

To start with, she really makes herself "small", "stupid", "pathetic". In the analysis, she does the same thing. And if her lover does not give up and abandon her in the face of this persistent debility, if the analyst succeeds in helping her recognise the relation between her rejection of this love and the old disappointment with her father, the unconscious will adopt another strategy. She still feels persecuted, and her stupidity will take another form: talking incessantly, she will try to make everything inconsistent; her way of exposing a sequence of facts about the most minute details of her daily life resembles the thinking of subjects who turn all troubling psychic questions into physical symptoms. Her feelings of inadequacy and her need to put herself down are overwhelming; she is desperate and displays clearly the narcissistic injuries caused, in retrospect, by the paternal offence. Stupid, wounded, silent, suffering and anesthetised, she is boring, heavy. Hatred is also part of the picture. In order to preserve a minimum of narcissistic stability, she is only marginally present, she is "indifferent", unreachable. Never have the attacks on the continuity of the relationship been so obvious, so shameless. She is inconsistent, irresponsible, frivolous. Hateful and hard to take.

The lover is expected to maintain, no matter what, the intensity of their sex life as an indestructible core. He does not have to spare her his irritation or his anger, but he must show tenderness as well – in other words, keep loving her.

The abandoned lover

As for the analyst, he is expected to help her put an end to the repression of aggressivity, in order to recognise that this aggressivity is the source of the attack on her relationship with her lover, of her feelings of unworthiness and, finally, of inhibition of the thinking process. When this working through can be achieved in analysis, the woman recovers her intelligence, her joy, her desire to be appealing and seductive, without being overwhelmed by persecutory internal objects. At the same time, she can let the new love enrich her life, transform her, so that she can connect her thoughts and her feelings, show her fear of loss, and speak of her jealousy. After this work on aggressivity, psychic elaboration of her anger towards her father becomes possible. This final stage of the work puts an end to the dissociation between the thinking process and sexuality and enables her to formulate a story; this will signal the end of the analysis.

If the lover manages the situation as best he can, but the analyst has not sorted out the essential elements of an Oedipal conflict, not taking seriously enough the real narcissistic difficulties present, the violent attacks on the continuity of the relationship with the lover intensify, with dangerous consequences. The dissociation makes it impossible to resolve deadlocks and the pressure created by an intense sex life that finds no means of psychic symbolisation becomes unbearable. The violent attacks turn into spectacular scenes and even physical fights. The aim of this acting out is to put an end, even at the cost of destroying the relationship, to the excess of psychic work left undone.

Because the anxiety involved in such a situation often leads to depersonalisation, the acting out strategy is used to reestablish dissociation at once. The easiest way to do this is to bring in a second relationship, to introduce another man in the configuration. For a time, the illusion of having two spaces in which to work out the same problem serves as an outlet for psychic tension. This reprieve is short-lived, of course. Since each space brings its own set of questions, the patient will try to "integrate" them by provoking another drama: she will reveal to her lover the existence of his rival (or to her long-time partner the existence of the lover).

For her to have come to such a confusion of feelings, to have been thrown in such disarray, the psychoanalyst must have made a great many mistakes.

As for the lover, he doesn't know what to think or how to feel. This combination of hatred, suffering and inhibition weighs on him. And he finds this showdown between two men – a homosexual dramatisation of the woman's unbearable narcissistic wounds – boring and exhausting. Irritation turns to sadness; he retreats, he gives up. Ivan does the same with Katerina Ivanovna, when he has had enough of being subjected to her hatred.

> "Oh, Alyosha, if you only knew how light my heart is now! Would you believe it, I sat here eating my dinner and was nearly ordering champagne to celebrate my first hour of freedom. It's been going on nearly six months, and all at once I've thrown it off. I could never have guessed even yesterday, how easy it would be to

> put an end to it. [...] I fell in love with her [...] she worried me. I sat watching over her. [...] And all at once it's collapsed! I spoke this morning with passion, but I went away and roared with laughter. [...] Yes, it's the truth".
>
> "You seem very happy about it now," observed Alyosha, looking into Ivan's face which had suddenly grown brighter.
>
> "And yet how she attracted me! How attractive she was when I made my speech! How she attracts me awfully even now, yet how easy it is to leave her. Do you think I am boasting? [...] But how she tormented me! It certainly was [...] a 'laceration'. She knew how I loved her! She loved me and not Dmitri," Ivan insisted. "Her feeling for Dmitri was simply self-laceration. All I told her was perfectly true. But [...] it may take her fifteen or twenty years to find out that she doesn't care for Dmitri but loves me whom she torments. She may never find it out at all, in spite of her lesson today. Well, it's better this way. [...] I [am going] away for good".[9]

When the beloved deserts the field of love, he leaves behind him a psychic body in ruins, like a city that has been bombarded. And, we should point out, the psychoanalyst's ineptitude worsens the damage: narcissistic injuries become scars, and short-circuited ideals become a permanent breakdown.

She can still recover, find a link with life by using the disaster as a means of challenging the other. But because hatred holds a predominant place here, the chances for a new romantic encounter to occur – with the acceptance of difference that it requires – are very slim.

Or she can stop everything. If she chooses psychosis as a refuge from the world, we must not assert, in retrospect, that she always had a predisposition to psychosis. Here, psychosis is the result of the conjunction between the failure of a real relationship in the present and the collapse, brought about by psychoanalysis, of solid defences, exposing a secret, primitive region in which nothing can be built (without extensive preparation).

Being a place for the other

Among Dostoevsky's female characters, Sonya in *Crime and Punishment*, Marmeladov's daughter, is an exception. To describe Sonya Semyonovna, I spoke of the selfless space she became after she attained nothingness: a space that can contain, a space for passing through – depending on the need. I said that this indetermination opens onto the infinite, and that it is frightening.

To be nothing, to be a place, requires the setting aside of one's own ego. The lack of ego needs in the Sonyas of the world allows all possible identifications, allows interest in everything, is a solid foundation for projects of all kinds, and offers unquestioning hospitality to the radical difference and particularly of the other. Let us remember what Raskolnikov thought of Sonya: "He was afraid of Sonia too. Sonia stood before him as an irrevocable sentence. *He must go his way or hers.* At that moment especially he did not feel equal to seeing her".[10]

Why is Sonya's selflessness so frightening? Why does it create a distance, why is it threatening? Because to have left all vanity behind, to have abandoned all traces of ego, transforms Sonya into a space that can *contain* everything. Beware if you are told: "You can tell this person *everything*". Be careful, because this person may be able to *hear everything*. Sonya's position is not unlike that of a good primary mother and that needed by a therapist to do his work.[11]

In terms of the actual love relation between Sonya and Raskolnikov, two things are particularly noteworthy. First, Raskolnikov is the one who comes to Sonya. Elsewhere in Dostoevsky's fiction, and often in real life, women are the ones who choose their men. Second, although love for Raskolnikov is what she experiences first, when desire appears, her usual equilibrium is destroyed; love must submit to this new requirement: that it be coupled with desire.

Being purely a space for the other is not a privilege reserved for women. This could lead to a discussion about the relation between bisexuality and love – a very broad subject we will have to leave for another time. Let us remember only that Myshkin and Alyosha were recognised as such places by Nastasya Filippovna and by Grushenka; this is no doubt why two men are considered identical by some commentators. I will quote the two pertinent passages:

Nastasya Filippovna to Myshkin:

> Haven't I dreamed of you myself? […] I dreamed of you long ago, when I lived five years all alone in his country home. I used to think and dream, […] and I was always imagining someone like you, kind, good and honest, and so stupid that he would come forward all of a sudden and say, "You are not to blame, Nastasya Filippovna, and I adore you!" I used to dream like that, till I nearly went out of my mind.[12]

And Grushenka about Alyosha:

> "He is the first, the only one who has pitied me, that's what it is. Why did you not come before, you angel?" She fell on her knees before Alyosha. "I've been waiting all my life for someone like you [to] come and forgive me. I believed that […] someone would really love me, not only with a lustful love!"[13]

Alyosha, contrary to Myshkin, knows how to speak to women, is not afraid of his desire and does not refuse sexuality.

In Dostoevsky's work, Alyosha is Sonya's twin brother.

The gift of the ego

Women start with love and then integrate desire. Whether this integration will be difficult or not depends on the relationship the woman had with her mother. According to a certain psychoanalyst, sexuality is the only place from which the mother is excluded. Even if he is right, this place has to be preserved: a task that is not so easy.

Winnicott introduced the concept of the *good enough mother*; that is, not too persecutory. This definition is very interesting in many respects and has numerous ramifications. I will speak more at length about persecution, the mode in which a subject, man or woman, usually encounters the outside, the strange, the unexpected, the unknown. This persecutory quality, highlighted by Piera Aulagnier, is not taken into account very often in the reflection about new situations encountered in life and experienced as threatening by the subject. This omission is a consequence of Freud's theory on paranoia, asserting that any feeling of persecution must be seen as a projection of one's own hatred onto another person. From this point of view, the impression of a threat is always the result of a projective process, the real does not exist, and everything is explained as fantasmatic processing of the encounter with the world or with the other.

Both Winnicott and Aulagnier, following in Ferenczi's footsteps, insisted, each in his own way, on the real importance of the care given to the child, on the effects of the real encounter between the mother and the baby, the mouth-breast encounter, for structuring the psyche. If the mother did not love her daughter, if the benefits of the homosexual relation mother-daughter did not come to be represented by the subject, the relation between the daughter now a woman and a man who loves her can become unbearable, persecutory, through loyalty to a mother incapable of loving. Clinical experience demonstrates this: in these circumstances sexuality can be a manic defence against the recognition of the maternal deficiency, and love can become either an idealised relation, or a relation focused on repairing the woman's beloved, an endless work of repair which repeats the work the child carried out with an irreparable mother.

What I want to emphasise above all is that a man's love for a woman not loved by her mother is a love that persecutes her so terribly that, out of loyalty to her mother, the woman may destroy all ties with this man. Interestingly, in these circumstances persecution is not the result of projected hatred; it is, rather, an attempt to protect the representation of an internalised mother whose endless repairing requires enormous psychic energy. To accept the man's love would mean disinvesting the impossible-to-accomplish psychic work, which nevertheless organises in large measure the subject's functioning. For this reason, such a disinvestment would require rearranging the entire identificatory configuration, in which the father's place is no doubt ambiguous.

I have often stressed the importance of the father in the organisation of the hysterical obstacles of femininity; I did so especially to highlight his role in Oedipal concerns. Speaking now of loyalty to failed/imagined maternal love, I am stressing the immense difficulty a woman who carries this burden can encounter in attempting to accept love and desire. And we ask ourselves: how can these difficulties be treated in clinical practice?

In my book *De l'amour à la pensée* (From Love to Thought), I described in detail various forms of transference as they relate to the father present at the Oedipal stage. I will now examine this question from another perspective, since the mother/daughter relation is not something directly accessible to a man. This doesn't mean that it's easier for a woman to deal with this matter; in fact, I think it's much more complicated, and the ready insistence of most women on the ease of it only confirms this.

But since I referred to clinical practice, let us start at the beginning; let's look at the first necessary condition: the greeting. Of course, the term is a metonymy. But some people take it literally, telling themselves: "Greeting the patient well is important". But what is the difference between greeting the other in a therapeutic setting and the greeting one is given in a shoe store, an hotel, an airplane or a travel agency, by a person trained to greet the public? Of course, we do not display the phoney smile or any feigned kindness – negative definitions – but how can we give a positive and metapsychological definition of this thing called greeting? Yet, as you will see, it's as easy as being under a beautiful, starry sky, or on a Mediterranean beach: the required minimal condition is to make the gift of an ego, an ego that contains, delimits, carries. But if there is no ego to meet the one who arrives, it is not possible to undertake therapy with the subject. The ego that the analyst offers is a place and, as I have been saying for some time, *the first identification is to a place.* There must be an ego that can take care of the ego of the person who arrives, because, obviously, the ego precedes the subject. Read, or reread, Winnicott. In France, after Lacan's specular concept of the ego, with its anticipation of the total image of the body, which condemns the child to alienation, the ego has become the "yucky poo" of psychoanalytic theory. Even Aulagnier, loyal to her teacher, tries to eliminate the ego by replacing it with her "I". Applying Lacan's theory has often resulted in clinical difficulties with serious and dangerous consequences for patients and analysands. Removing the illusion/disillusion dialectic from psychic functioning violates the very core of desire. But reading Lacan's text on the mirror stage reveals much greater complexity and subtlety. While the child contemplates his image, which gives form in advance to a wholeness not yet felt in the body – a phenomenon at the origin of alienation, according to Lacan – the mother is talking to the child, and this has an effect on what will follow from the baby's experience of meeting his reflection in the mirror. In other words, Lacan speaks of a simultaneous emergence of the image and the identification of the subject, a simultaneity abandoned later in his theorisation. After having discussed this question in *De l'Amour à la pensée*, I came back to it in *Letters to a Young Psychoanalyst*, to say that Loup Verlet considers this simultaneity, recognised and later abandoned by Lacan, as an example of the founding paradox of a change in the frame for thought. According to Verlet, the illustration *par excellence* of such a change is the revolution brought about by Newton, which Verlet considers identical to the work of psychoanalysis. Nothing less![14]

Thus, when you speak of this and some well-informed person will ask – fortunately there are those who are informed – if I have become an advocate of the strong ego theory, you can say that I have always thought that the ego has to be reinforced. But, let us specify, this must be done at the start of the analytic process, not at the end; reinforcing the *ego* is a prerequisite for conducting clinical work with the *subject*, for doing analysis. And I have always said that a difference must be made between the therapeutic process and analysis. And for those who don't know it yet, let us point out that it was with this question of the strong and weak ego, a question raised by American analysts, that the great and unruly upheaval started, and that Lacan initiated the major reexamination that allowed us to recognise that Freud's conceptual apparatus was very clear and rigorous, freed from psychological overtones and separated from philosophy. We must not confuse this brilliant re-examination with the imposture that Lacanian filiation has become.

You can also remind anyone who asks you that I am indebted to Winnicott, who does not consider the origin of the ego to be specular but believes the originary mirror to be the mother's face. You can add that it is based on this concept that the ego is seen as anterior to the subject – a reminder of the obvious fact that the mother is there before the baby and that, without maternal care, there is no baby – and that this preexistence of the ego is what allowed me to propose the concept of a "tension principle".[15] This concept explains the interconnection between life drive and death drive, which renders the inadequate notion of *primary masochism* unnecessary. The *tension principle* sheds light on an experience that would not be possible if the mother's ego was not there to contain and carry the infant's space, filtering the stimuli and the drives so as to render them not frightening, and by doing so, to nurture and strengthen the baby's sense of existing in reality. Finally, you can explain that although I think the offer of the ego must be made from the start, this does not imply that the analyst has a strong ego, but only that he makes it available, and that this offer is inevitably fragile, fortunately fragile, like human life itself.

Women and their mothers

Once the analyst's ego is made available, what is the next thing to do?

Mother and daughter. Two women. What do women talk about among themselves? Some say that there are no mother/daughter relations, or woman-to-woman relations, but only mother/mother relations. And what do mothers talk about among themselves? They say that all men are children who are afraid of women's desire. Of course, this is the deathly aspect of mothers, but it exists; for a man, who was once a son, this experiencing of the deathly aspect of mothers may have been direct and massive and is therefore easier to recognise and to name. Things are more difficult for a woman because this relationship between two women where one holds the place of mother is also a promise of the feminine, a feminine at the crossroads between love and death. A feminine feeding itself on the murder of men.

Barbey d'Aurevilly wrote a short story called *The Story Without a Name*, which illustrates the horror of isolation in a world of mothers, of imprisonment in mother/daughter incest. Let us be clear: all incest goes back to the mother; a father who rapes his daughter holds the place of incestuous mother. In the story, Madame

Ferjol wants her daughter Lasthenie to become a woman, without encountering the world, or any man. To accomplish this, Lasthenie must make love in her sleep, while she is insensitive and unconscious; after this, she gives birth to a dead child.

"*You are mortal, you must always think two things at once*",[16] Leslie Kaplan wrote, drawing her inspiration from Heraclitus, in *Toute ma vie j'ai été une femme* (I Have Been a Woman My Whole Life). First observation: to say that one must always think two things at once is proof that a woman can always reject the temptation of the same, a morbid offering made by the archaic mother. And the first association that comes to mind is to think of one's life and one's death at the same time, to avoid sameness. Indeed, Kaplan goes on to say: "We live, we die, every moment". And we are reminded of Hegel's assertion that "*the life of the Spirit* [...] *endures* [*death*] *and maintains itself in it*".

But Leslie Kaplan has her reasons for asserting that *she has been a woman her whole life*. You might not know that "Leslie" in English is a neutral name, like Dominique or Claude in French. But in French, Leslie is perceived at once as a feminine name; for people of my generation, this is probably to some extent thanks to Leslie Caron, an actress who must have made life easier for Leslie, the young American living in Paris.

In other words, if one's name is Leslie in America, or Claude or Dominique in France, *one always thinks two things at once*: one thinks that despite having a woman's body, one can be thought to be a man; or, on the contrary, despite having a man's body, one can be thought to be a woman. In short, this ambiguity of names brings us to the question of bisexuality, a central theme of Freudian theory which, as you may know, was the cause of serious conflict between Freud and Fliess, when the latter reminded his friend that it was he, Fliess, who invented the concept.[17]

At this moment in time, when psychoanalysis is fiercely attacked and discredited, if we want to maintain that our practice is something other than a nebulous, esoteric practice, we must show that our work is based on clearly defined, distinct conceptual tools, and that those who do not work with these concepts, acquired after lengthy theoretical and clinical experience, are engaging in a practice other than psychoanalysis. To refer to our use of the conceptual apparatus, developed patiently over more than a century, is not only a way of acknowledging our debt to those who have constructed and shaped the field of our practice, but also a way to confirm the validity, vitality and pertinence of a practice that stands the test of ever-renewed inquiry, always new because it testifies each time to a distinctive encounter with the real of desire, anguish, pain and deathly predicaments. Any other attitude would be rooted in belief in the all-powerfulness of thought and would therefore remain in the infinite swampy sphere of mothers, that is, under the reign of Thanatos.

Let me open a parenthesis here to say that Lacan, who believed and said that ideas belong to everyone, and who did not hesitate to gather those useful to him from any source, ended up complaining that others are using his ideas without quoting him.[18] It's proof that those who think ideas belong to everyone are above all those who use other people's ideas. Are men more likely than women to commit such an indiscretion? A self-satisfied psychologist may say that this could be so because men do not give birth. This assertion is not to be dismissed out of hand: there is always some truth in every darn foolishness, just as there is a little reality in delusion.

Why am I insisting on this question? Because I just had an unpleasant experience. After I wrote this text, I started to reread the texts that came to my mind while I was preparing my own. This is what I usually do: I write first, then I look at the bibliography and reread the texts that I feel will clarify my discussion. Thus, I read Barbey d'Aurevilly's short story again, and I took up François Perrier's seminar *L'Amour*. An association of ideas induced me to look up "L'Amatride", the 26 January 1971 seminar. I remembered that it was after reading this seminar that I looked for the novella "The Story Without a Name", recommended by a writer friend. This was forty years ago. I was very proud, I must say, to have formulated the idea that through morbid loyalty to impossible maternal love a woman experiences the love of a man as persecutory. In fact, I am still very proud to have pointed out that this feeling of persecution is not at all projective in nature. And then I read the first two paragraphs of Perrier's text:

> I shall start with an "aphorism": "There is no woman for whom love, the hope of finding love, the right to love, the assumption of love, does not refer back to the mother and to the 'incestuous' relationship mother-daughter-mother".
>
> What makes being loved, or responding to a man's love impossible or unbearable for certain women is related to this question.[19]

Cryptomnesia notwithstanding, I can't deny the blow to my pride. Perrier's text continues: "Speaking of the clinical setting now, let us attempt to examine the hypothesis of the "inability to be a hysteric", particularly for a woman".[20] In short, read this text, read the whole seminar; Perrier's writing is mad, brilliant, it is good for the mind and the body. In conclusion, I will quote the conclusion of "L'Amatride":

> Recently someone told me the story I am about to relate. It was a patient whose elderly mother, almost blind by then, used to say: "My son, I no longer see well, but even if I don't, do I still have beautiful eyes?" And he would answer: "Yes, you still have beautiful eyes." And she would say: "That reminds me of something." This old lady told her son: "When my mother was dying, I was at her bedside and I told her: "Mother, you have such beautiful eyes." And my mother answered: "How strange that you should say that, it's what I told my mother when I buried her."
>
> [...]
>
> For a possibility of sublimation in the feminine sense of the word to come into existence, for imagining the capacity of a woman to refer to herself, to her femininity, to the female in her being, to the real of her body, to the desire of the man and to love and pleasure at the same time, what was needed

was not only words, but perhaps traditions, or counter-traditions, or dramas, or wars, or people killed – but in any case, what was needed was three generations of women, *three generations of a gaze*. The beautiful appears to serve as the last bastion against death, and as a transfiguration that obscures the non-representable of the Lacanian small "a". Woman is a source of beauty for man, but what is poorly understood is that woman is a source of beauty for herself, although sometimes this involves anguish. If, in the gaze she gives her image in the mirror in order to gain confidence, to identify with another woman, to make herself beautiful or make herself lovable or desirable, she does not have in reserve, as it were, two other gazes inside her own eyes to support her in the face of the impossible question of desire and pleasure, *she takes refuge in the certainty that it is unbearable to be loved. From then on, a man's love is an aggression that causes her to run away, to hate passionately or to need to betray.*[21]

The bedrock of bisexuality

Freud saw bisexuality as the bedrock of what cannot be analysed: the acceptance of the feminine in men and penis envy in women. But despite the frequent presence of these two figures of the difficulty encountered by patients in their attempts to free themselves of the repetition which holds them captive, preventing them from changing, we must remember that these resistances to analysis are defences. But defences against what?

Freud's answer is only partial. Although in the man's case Freud recognises the narcissistic difficulty going back to the relationship with the father, in the woman's case he sees this obstacle as seemingly unavoidable: an outcome of hereditarily acquired resistances, a biological given[22] – despite having also written that for a woman the end of analysis coincides with identification with her father.

As for me, I suggest that we consider the stakes related to the question of penis envy as the sign of a deficiency or a perversion in the relation to the mother who provided care to the infant, and therefore as a sequel of the lack of inscription of primary homosexuality.

The clinical management of this problem aims at making it possible for the woman to gain access to the masculine, which requires her to assume her phallic position. Remember that according to Freud the libido is always masculine, that is, on the side of the masculine. To bring a woman towards the *phallic position* means to recognise her right to think, to desire, to choose, to decide and to act. Of course, this may refer back to the relation with the father. But the inscription of the masculine, the ability to assume the libido, do not depend solely on the father; this is, first of all, a matter of detaching oneself from the deathly maternal element. Some psychoanalysts think that this kind of clinical work can lead to the "hysterisation" of all conflict, which is foolishness, since hysteria in women is the classic manifestation of the impasses of penis envy. The danger that can, in fact, exist is the creation of a paranoid position: the energy made available by disinvestment of the morbid representation of the relation to the mother can be placed momentarily in the service of the ideal ego. The experience, in the transference, of the freedom to desire and the recognition of one's right to think, is accompanied, thanks to separation from the paralysing maternal, by increased intensity of all pleasure, which can sometimes trigger great anxiety. The framework of paranoid certainties tries to contain both excessive pleasure and excessive anxiety.

Freud admits that in women also aspiring to virility is in accord with the ego *at a certain period*, in the phallic phase, before development leading to femininity".[23] But the theory did not seem to concern itself very much with this *passage*, which relies on the masculine nature of the libido, preferring to place emphasis on the erogenous transactions between clitoris and vagina. While we wait for women psychoanalysts to discuss these questions in greater detail, I would like to observe only that clinical practice and experience refute the distinction that defines the clitoris as an "active" erogenous organ, while describing the vagina as a "passive" erogenous organ.

I suggest that what is important here is to point out that insufficient attention given to the stage in which a woman comes to live her libido and integrates it as an element of masculine nature will result in neglecting the devastating effects produced when this aspiration to virility is inhibited, instead of being integrated into the subject's psychic functioning. This inhibition will constitute an impediment to desire, and lead to neurotic imbecility and to social figures of the ideal ego being used to avoid the psychic work necessary for self-realisation.

Again, it is up to women psychoanalysts to show that maternity is not limited to the displacement of penis envy through children, and to show how the experience of pregnancy and childbirth parallels great accomplishments of the mind, but extends beyond this limit, given its consequences in the sphere of the real.

Notes

1 Dostoevsky, F., *The Brothers Karamazov*, p. 116.
2 Ibid., pp. 114 and 115. Dostoevsky's emphasis.
3 Ibid., p. 114.
4 Ibid., p. 180.
5 Ibid.
6 Ibid., p. 176.
7 Ibid., p. 180.
8 See the chapter "True Love", in *Letters to a Young Psychoanalyst*.
9 Dostoevsky, F., "The Brothers Karamazov", pp. 214–215.
10 Dostoevsky, F., *Crime and Punishment*, p. 389.
11 The reader can refer to the section, *The Sonya Solution* above.
12 Dostoevsky, F., *The Idiot*, pp. 159–160.
13 Dostoevsky, F., *The Brothers Karamazov*, pp. 328–329.
14 De Macedo, H., *Letters to a Young Psychoanalyst*, Letter 28.
15 "Le concept de Masochisme primaire et le Principe de Tension", in *Epistolettre*, no. 43 (publication of the Fédération des Ateliers de Psychoanalyse), March 2015.
16 Kaplan, L., *Toute ma vie j'ai été une femme*, p. 81.
17 In his book *La Pensée et le féminin*, a work of reference on this question, Wladimir Granoff provides facts making it possible to shed a different light on this "controversy". He reminds the reader that the question of bisexuality is central to the research

conducted and published by the young Sigmund Freud, on the sexual behaviour of fish, while he worked in Ernst von Brücke's laboratory. See the chapter "Le modèle de la dissection" in Granoff's book.

18 See Lacan's Preface to Anika Lemaire's book *Jacques Lacan*, Brussels: Pierre Mardaga, 1977.

19 Perrier, F., "L'Amatride", in seminar *L'Amour,* in *La Chaussée d'Antin II*, Collection 10–18, Paris: Christian Bourgeois, 1978, p. 195.

20 Ibid., p. 202.

21 Ibid., p. 208. Perrier's emphasis, then mine.

22 Oddly, in the key text on this question, Freud speaks of a biological given only when referring to the refusal of the feminine in men, in their relations with other men. See *Analysis Terminable and Interminable* (1937), S.E., 23, pp. 216–253, London: Hogarth.

23 Freud, S., *Analysis Terminable and Interminable*, p. 251.

8
THE GRAND INQUISITOR

The quest-for-happiness society

In our society, where we engage in the quest for happiness, we are unhappy. Every day, all the time. We have reasons for being unhappy: they have to do with work, or with being out of work; with raising children, or with not having children. With our health, with our vacations. Every day, we have reasons for dissatisfaction, reasons to be unhappy, malcontent.[1]

These literary observations, which show Kaplan's understanding of the injunction to be happy and of the absurdity of claiming the contrary, were soon followed by Pierre Dardot and Christian Laval's work of reference *The New Way of the World*. These authors point out that what is unbearable for those in power in our refusal to accept the happiness they press on us is that this happiness goes hand in hand with the perspective advocated by the neoliberal market. In this perspective, unhappiness is simply very poor management of our health and pleasure capital. Unhappiness results from rejecting the only valid criterion in the modern world, one that depends on adapting to a highly variable definition of happiness, itself dependent on market fluctuations.[2] The difficulties created by this great adaptability to economic requirements can be lessened, or eliminated altogether, by the drugs supplied by pharmaceutical companies, absolutely essential for the successful conduct of behavioural therapies. Let us remember that the World Health Organisation defines mental health as the ability of a subject to cope with adversity.[3]

We have to admit that capitalist actors have made considerable political efforts, over the past several decades, in order to change drastically the elements to be considered, based on Margaret Thatcher's vision for the future, as formulated in the 1980s: "Economics are the method; the object is to change the soul".[4]

Changing the frame of thought and the soul are central themes in Ivan Karamazov's poem about the encounter between Christ and *The Grand Inquisitor*. The latter has the son of God arrested, right after witnessing the miraculous resurrection of a little girl. Christ had decided to visit his children "in Spain, in Seville, in the most horrible time of the Inquisition, when fires were lighted every day to the glory of God, and 'in the splendid act of faith the wicked heretics were burnt'".[5]

The frame of thought

The Grand Inquisitor, "an old man, almost ninety [...] with a withered face and sunken eyes, in which there is still a gleam of light", accuses Christ of having been deaf, in the desert, to the words of "the spirit of self-destruction and non-existence", on the pretext that this warning was a temptation. Christ pretended not to hear "the dread Spirit" warn him that men care more about their needs than about their desires:

> But Thou wouldst not deprive man of freedom [...] thinking what is that freedom worth, if obedience is bought with bread? [...] Thou wouldst to go into the world [...] with some promise of freedom which men in their simplicity and their natural unruliness cannot even understand. [...] "Thou wast warned,'" he says to Him. "Thou hast had no lack of warnings, but Thou didst not listen to those warnings. Thou didst reject the only way by which men might be made happy".

The Grand Inquisitor admits that Christ was right to insist that beyond sustenance, man needs a reason to live:

> In that Thou wast right. For the secret of man's being is not only to live but to have something to live for. [...] Didst Thou forget that man prefers peace, and even death, to freedom of choice in the knowledge of good and evil? [...] Thousands and tens of thousands shall follow Thee, [but] what is to become of the millions and tens of thousands of millions of creatures who will not have the strength to forgo the earthly bread for the sake of the heavenly? Or dost Thou care only for [...] the great and strong, while the millions, numerous as the sands of the sea, who are weak but love Thee, must exist only for the sake of the great and the strong? [...] Canst Thou have simply come to the elect and for the elect?

The Grand Inquisitor proclaims the truth of our own conclusion: "It's long [...] since we have been on *his* side and not on Thine", and the fact that, as the Devil admonished Christ, there is need for an organised power – *for universal union* – to bring *peace to mankind*. "We have taken the sword of Caesar, and in taking it, of course, have rejected Thee and followed *him*. [...] Thou are proud of Thine elect, but Thou hast only the elect, while we give rest to all."

Thou didst hope that man, following Thee, would cling to God and not ask for a miracle. But Thou didst not know that when man rejects miracles he rejects God too; for man seeks not so much God as the miraculous. [...] Too, too well, [men] know the value of complete submission! And until men know that, they will be unhappy. [...] But Thou didst think too highly of men therein, for they are slaves, of course [...] man is weaker and baser by nature than Thou hast believed him! Can he, can he do what Thou as didst? By showing him so much respect, Thou didst [...] cease to feel for him, for Thou didst ask far too much from him – Thou who hast loved him more than Thyself! Respecting him less, Thou wouldst have asked less of him. That would have been more like love, for his burden would have been lighter. He is weak and vile.

We have corrected Thy work and have founded it upon *miracle, mystery* and *authority*. And men rejoiced that they were again led like sheep, and that the terrible gift that had brought them such suffering, was, at last, lifted from their hearts. Were we right teaching them this? Speak! Did we not love mankind, so meekly acknowledging their feebleness, lovingly lightening their burden, and permitting their weak nature even sin with our sanction?

Then we shall give them [...] quiet humble happiness. [...] We shall show them that they are weak, that they are only pitiful children, but that childlike happiness is the sweetest of all. They will become timid and look to us and huddle close to us in fear, as chicks to the hen. [...] Yes, we shall set them to work, but in their leisure hours we shall make their life like a child's game, with children's songs and innocent dance.

But we shall tell them that we are Thy servants and rule them in Thy name. We shall deceive them again, for we will not let Thee come to us again. That deception will be our suffering, for we shall be forced to lie.

And all will be happy, all the millions of creatures except the hundred thousand who rule over them [...] *we who guard the mystery*. [...] There will be thousands of millions of happy ones and a hundred thousand sufferers who have taken upon themselves the curse of the knowledge of good and evil. Peacefully they will die, peacefully in Thy name, and beyond the grave they will find nothing but death. *But we shall keep the secret*, and for their happiness we shall allure them with the reward of heaven and eternity [...] and [we] accept lying and deception, and lead men consciously to death and destruction [deceiving] them all the way so that they may not notice where they are being led, that the poor blind creatures may at least on the way think themselves happy.[6]

Raskolnikov's theories

Christ and the Grand Inquisitor walk in the footsteps of Roskolnikov; their exchange reformulates his theories. Roskolnikov has preceded us all in the adventure we now pursue without God, with only our anguish and desire; in his time, this required a radical change of the frame of thought established by religion.

For Christ, both God and desire exist. He knows that desire cannot be sustained without the anguish that accompanies it. But he offers a possibility to ignore it, thanks to the gift of a life after death.

Supposing that all men are able to choose desire over pleasure means believing in a community of extraordinary men, as Raskolnikov defines it. Christ's uni-dimensional perspective does not take into account the great psychic difficulty of the task. It leaves the social aspect aside, counting on spontaneous organisation of the human community. Raskolnikov's nightmare in prison illustrates the abominable consequences of such a supposition.[7] Today, certain political projects choose a similar theoretical position, which uses ready-made formulas to resume the complexity of the political and organisational consequences of the current emergence of insurrectional resistance movements in Brazil, Greece, Spain, Tunisia, Egypt, in Teheran, in Ukraine, in England and in the United States.

The other possibility, posited by the Grand Inquisitor, is to form a group of extraordinary men entrusted with the secret that there is no life after death. This group sacrifices itself to lessen the suffering of the "feeble slaves" who make up the flock of sheep, as Raskolnikov says. In order to achieve his aims, the Grand Inquisitor introduces a hierarchy: he establishes the power of the Church, transforms desire and thinking into sins, and demands obedience and submission.

Margaret Thatcher and her cronies used the same strategy. Her plan to change the soul, that is, the frame of thought, was built day after day on a foundation supported by all cultural and political actors. Contrary to the Grand Inquisitor's plan, desire was not forbidden: it simply did not exist. It was replaced by performance, based on objectives set in view of meeting corporate requirements established according to variable market conditions. The subject has disappeared; the reign of the individual has been restored. And let us not confuse the individual with particularity. Feeble or not, all those belonging to the anonymous mass of slaves are members of a new species: that of the self-entrepreneur.[8] The suffering of the masses no longer counts, transcendence is over. We are all summoned to be cannibals who must survive in the fierce world of competition. There is no more room for friendship or a minimum of respect, sensuality is banished, ousted by drives and instincts – we are animals and proud of it. The world invented for us by Thatcher and her associates is a cruel world. Power is in the hands of the financial establishment, which will survive and prosper by adopting hate and murder as national strategies. Remember Margaret Thatcher's steadfast support of Auguste Pinochet, one of the greatest criminals of the twentieth century: responsible for torture, kidnapping, the murder of political opponents and their children, author of Operation Condor – an alliance between Chile, Uruguay, Argentina and Brazil, involving the elimination of political activists by having them dropped, alive and tied up, from airplanes into the ocean. She was also successful in preventing Pinochet's extradition from England to Spain, where he would have been tried for atrocities perpetrated against Spanish citizens.

In their book, Pierre Dardot and Christian Laval also describe in detail this changing of the *frame of thought*: how neoliberalism replaced liberalism; they describe the crisis of liberal capitalism and the birth of neoliberalism in a strong State acting as the guardian of private law, and the birth of the new rationality.

We believe we are living in a liberal democracy where the idea of public law is respected by the government and serves as a reference standard for the citizens of the State. This reference creates the collective understanding that public law determines and delimits, in the society, a space where many types of practices are carried out: political, social, cultural. This understanding produces symbols. But Dardot and Laval show that this fictional understanding has lost its ability to generate symbols. Public law has lost its content, and social practice has been privatised. This means that the State has become a corporation, and the citizen an entrepreneur. The rule of law, which established rules and prohibitions, has been replaced by the norm, whose role is to shape behaviour; this norm is presented as natural. The definitions of the normal and the abnormal replace those of "legal" and "illegal", considered the province of the law. This change is effected in the name of medical knowledge. But the medical norm has become the social norm, which is based on a new social rationality that destroys all collective organisation. Choice is still possible, but within the range of possibilities set out in advance by the firm. The firm can be a factory, a hospital, a government ministry. The hierarchical structure of possibilities reflects the norm established based on the best economic performance at a given moment. In short, there is no vacuum, the entire space is filled to saturation, in view of achieving a functioning that will not produce sense, but only "enterprise", in other words, more of the same. There is no thought since there is nothing external; there is only management of the enterprise. This privatisation of everything is not accepted by all those who are subjected to it, myself for one. The universal does not exist either. My way of thinking in terms of "partial totalisation" – Sartre's term – is out of date. Politicians are no longer required to set out practices, or to arrange for the temporary coherence of these practices. Normative reasoning focuses only on the fragmented fields of activity it has created. There is no longer a plan, only objectives. I will no longer die, but simply disappear. I have no history, just a function and a career. I have no future, only evaluations. I don't have to be real, I just have to follow the norm.

The major change consists in a new control through competition, in rapid growth of financial capitalism, in corporate governance and State governance. From now on, society will be modelled on the corporation, culture will be corporate culture, and the new subjectivity, if this term still has some meaning, will be self-enterprise. Performance will surely lead to asceticism and guilt, ethical considerations and anguish will be replaced – I guarantee it – by management of the soul, modelled on corporate management. *The production of the neoliberal subject*, authoritarian kingdom of consensual clichés, is the one put forth and advocated every day by the media, in talk shows, reality shows, etc: *the market of the individual and of the loss of experience*, as Serge Daney called it in 1992.[9] Of course, this ordinary perversion will produce collateral effects, losses, damages; it's unavoidable, there is always a price to pay: disintegration of the personality, demoralisation, desymbolisation. But not to worry: the concept of *mental health* shall be redefined.

In his book *Mental Health*, Mathieu Bellahsen traces the concept of "mental health" from its origin in post-war progressive schools of thought, to today's neoliberal reorganisation of psychiatry.[10] The progression begins with a statement by the philosopher Georges Canguilhem: "Health is the luxury of being able to fall ill and recover", and leads all the way to our current definition of mental health: "*the ability to adapt to a situation one cannot change*".[11]

Today, health is a *right*. And not claiming this right is considered a sign of dysfunction. This positive definition of health is an invocation to *happiness*. Bellahsen invented the term "mentalhealthism" to speak of the paradox constituting one of the ideological elements of the neoliberal conceptual framework. This term also illustrates the mixture of sentimentality and mediocrity so well-thought-of and widely used in several sectors of the new culture, where naturalism reigns and where new actors at a loss for ideas try to convince us that their inability to create metaphors will allow us to describe more clearly the times in which we live, and our contemporary way of being artists. The fact is that they have convinced many people that we are unable to produce a conception of the world, and are condemned to admit our limitations.

Since, as everyone knows, there is no such thing as the unconscious, what is needed is an industrial procedure for the treatment of psychic suffering: classification, management, standardisation. Governments have stopped doing political work, so there are no health policies; we submit instead to the demands of "science", promoted by "experts" on the corporate world – hospitals are corporations – and on the latest research conducted by pharmaceutical companies. When a patient – even suffering from schizophrenia – cannot be treated with a drug, he is not a patient but an *ab-normal* individual. What can be done with him?

Of course, he can appear on a television show, or write a book telling his own story, or create an "installation" for a museum. It's all very good, because it's entertaining. When we see an *ab-normal* person on television, we are glad to be normal. So *ab-normality* has a good side, it can be useful for a little while. Of course, it can't be shown on the screen over and over – and that's a problem for those who are *ab-normal* – because seeing it all the time is not at all amusing. A bit of it is fine, just for fun, as long as there is variety, a smidgen of *ab-normality*, a fragment of tragedy, a dab of monstruosity, but no more than that. Of course, the question remains of how to treat the *ab-normal* person afterwards: after the television program, or the tour of the play, or the publication of the book and the interviews to the press; it's a real problem, like the disposal of nuclear waste, but we will soon find a solution – maybe only temporary – but something in any case.

In short, today we have an overview of the development of the idea of happiness, and this development raises certain questions: after the destruction of the old order, of the family, of our old conventions, the assertion of individual rights takes place within the framework of the neoliberal capitalist society. On the pretext of asserting one's (false) individuality, we are led to develop forms of thinking that are not at all singular in nature, but which, on the contrary, follow new conventions and create new clichés. We see the emergence of more or less overt forms of authoritarianism, dictatorship and "soft" totalitarianism.

In our new World Republic, is happiness a right? Is it a conquest, a project, a promise? Is it individual or collective? Limited? Ever-expanding? Risk-related? Related to boredom? Is it a lie? Is it denial? Is it an illusion? Or is this the right question to ask at all?

This reflection seeks to find answers to the urgent question of how to live together and develop a perspective different from that of our modern-day societies, how to formulate a new concept of collectivity and make use of innovative new practices which already exist.

Happiness during the French Revolution

In March 1794, Saint-Just declared that "happiness is a new idea in Europe". This statement established a relation between happiness and the revolutionary spirit of the liberation movement: liberation from the duties and obligations related to the old feudal order and its privileges. It proclaimed that happiness and freedom, just like happiness and equality, go together.

This proclamation had been preceded by the American Declaration of Independence (1776), which stated that all men are endowed with "unalienable rights" which include "life, liberty and the pursuit of happiness".

Saint-Just's statement is found in the Law of Ventôse (March 1794), which decrees that the property of opponents of the Revolution be confiscated and redistributed to the needy: "Let us teach Europe that we do not intend there to be one unhappy man or one oppressor on French soil. Let this example bear fruit throughout the world. Happiness is a new idea in Europe."

Saint-Just also discusses the "law of self-preservation".

> It (government) is less to make a people happy than to prevent it from being unhappy. Do not oppress, that's all. Everyone will know well [how] to find happiness. A people, among which would be established the prejudice that it owes its happiness to those who govern, does not retain it for long.[12]

So, it is not a matter of defining happiness as such. At the time of the French Revolution happiness was related to victory over poverty and oppression, to the defeat of internal and external enemies; it was indistinguishable from the fervour and enthusiasm of revolutionary action.[13]

Happiness and psychoanalysis

The focus of psychoanalysis is not happiness, but the living. But it is worthwhile to ask what psychoanalysis can say about happiness, and about its own links with political matters.

We must start by saying that there once was a time when, in a certain place, psychoanalysis was promising happiness, on condition that the subject adapt to the norms of his society. It was in the United States in the 1950s. This inanity was denounced, and made room for a practice based on Freud's definition of mental health: the ability to love *and* to work; being sane enough to recognise reality, *and* crazy enough to do whatever it takes to change it.

The first part of the Freudian definition is the foundation of psychoanalytic theory: man is a sexual being and man thinks – and continuous psychic work is required for these two aspects to function in harmony.

The second part of Freud's definition of mental health reaffirms the continuity he observed between normal mental functioning and psychopathology; dysfunctions and excesses seen in the latter shed light on the resources of the former and widen the field of its possibilities. In this context, the excessive is that which allows a subject to believe in the all-powerful nature of his desire, an illusion essential to any love relationship or to passionate investment in a work project.

The tension produced by the constant effort to bring together these two distinct aspects of our human nature produces conflict. And conflict produces anxiety, the twin of desire.

These characteristics of psychic functioning presuppose the existence of the unconscious, constituted by the integration of three elements Freud recognised: rituals honouring the dead (freeing ourselves of the enormous burden of the tradition of past generations, which "weighs like a nightmare on the brain of the living" (as Marx said), meaning burying the dead so that they stop coming back as ghosts, separating the living from what is deadly), the prohibition of murder and the prohibition of incest.

If a human community is not founded on these three elements, its humanity is missing and at the centre of its life there will be hate and the enjoyment of murder. This perpetuates endlessly the repetition of the same monotonous, deadly scenario.

The "new way of the world" and the positive definition of mental health offer the diabolically seductive promise of ridding us once and for all of anxiety and hate. How can we decline such an offer?

This is the theme of Dardot, Laval and Bellahsen's discussion. The excerpts from Dostoevsky quoted above reveal the attitude on which such a project is founded: total contempt for the people. This contempt springs from a triple denial: that of desire, anxiety and hate, the three elements that compose our humanity.

But what does psychoanalysis offer, instead of this perversion which proposes to replace the tension of desire with the management of the pleasures authorised by those in power? (Let us note that, essentially, such a substitution is no different from Bolshevism or the post-war revolutionary movements modelled on the Russian or Chinese revolution).

Knowing that any desire to widen the field of possibilities is usually associated with displeasure caused by tension, psychoanalysis supposes that when an analysis is over, this tension will be accepted, and even welcomed, by the subject. Interest in displeasure shifts to transforming the relation to the real world. Tension is recognised as essential for this process. The anxiety that always accompanies desire loses its heaviness and becomes a means to maintain desire and fulfil it. The certainty of death loses its shadow, and nurtures psychic vitality and strength, like a wild beast looking for its prey, when this prey is life itself, with all its richness, its demands, its transience. Of course, the satisfaction of desire is a form of happiness. But there are no guarantees and happiness is not a state. It is a process, endless and always in progress, like revolution.

But when hate, destruction and murder fill the entire psychic space, before this process can unfold, an unconscious has to be constructed, so as to intertwine hate and destruction with desire, in order to place them in the service of life.

In other words, when a political theory does not ignore the existence of the unconscious, as neoliberalism does, when it overlooks the conflicts involved and the anxiety they produce, how can it take into account in its particular propositions these fundamental aspects of our humanity? And what tools will it recommend to deal with hate, which will inevitably show its ugly face after the euphoria of insurrection?

In an interview Sartre granted me and three Brazilian friends on 12 July 1978,[14] he reminded us that "the masses have no memory" and that "cultural agents" are always needed to transmit history.

While in *The New Way of the World* Dardot and Laval describe the *frame of thought* neoliberal capitalism imposes on us, in their most recent essay, "The Common: An Essay on the 21st-Century Revolution",[15] they try to identify the conditions allowing the creation of a *new* frame of thought.

I will reproduce briefly what I wrote earlier about this concept developed by Loup Verlet:[16] establishing a new frame of thought is a frightening experience for the person who undertakes this task. It is frightening to travel along the path leading from the moment when the subject begins to abandon a conceptual framework to the moment when a new frame of reference is created. To describe this journey, Loup Verlet invokes the concepts of crossing over and paradox. When a subject takes the risk of going beyond the limits imposed by a conceptual paradigm, and ventures towards the unthinkable which doing so involves, he enters a paradoxical situation. Because this crossing involves "the more or less radical suspension of the epistemological premises [on which his frame of thought is built], [he]*seeks grounding in that which (does) not yet (exist)*". But this venturing, involved in any creative thinking, is a dangerous psychic state, a borderline state. In such a state, the subject draws his energy from the excess of his desire. He needs considerable energy for everything he is in the process of creating: a new frame of thought for a new subject. In any case, in this uncertain period of transition, the danger of sinking into madness is ever-present.

What I find interesting in Dardot and Laval's writing is their way of paying attention to this crossing, which is a transition. Speaking of the possibility of a revolution, which is a change in the conceptual framework, they refer to Cornelius Castoriadis, a political thinker who takes the unconscious into account. They admit being endebted to this reflection and they find, in institutional psychotherapy, the theoretical tools needed to elucidate their concept of a "founding practice". They ask what political theories can be elaborated based on the new forms of political combat and social experimentation currently seen in different parts of the world. From this perspective, they attempt to understand these recent insurrectional initiatives, in order to formulate theoretical and practical political proposals.

As for my search for ways to deal with hate once the revolutionary elation is over, the problem I find with Cornelius Castoriadis is that he bases his thinking on the hypothesis that the unconscious is always already constituted. Indeed, Castoriadis was married to Piera Aulagnier, the only psychoanalyst who formulated a metapsychology of psychosis, and he himself worked as a psychoanalyst. In short, his view of the unconscious is based on clinical experience. But he did not treat psychotic patients.[17]

The construction of the unconscious

Working with psychotic patients requires constant reformulation of the conditions allowing the members of this therapeutic community, which is, in fact, a countercultural community, to *construct* the unconscious.[18] Why is this community a counter-culture? Because its members have in common the fact that they are unable to live in ordinary society, which demands that they adapt to its rules and customs, and which rejects those who refuse the reality it sets forth. The psychiatric practice based on this perspective was initiated (in France) during the Second World War in a Saint-Alban hospital whose director, François Tosquelles, was a Catalan refugee from Spain, at the time of the Civil War. The objective was to create a new type of organisation, that I call *a society of care*, flexible and dynamic enough to be open to the unexpected, so that what is being *instituted* can always bring into question existing practice. This society of care has its own rules of functioning, despite the great diversity of its forms. This allows sudden, sometimes dazzling, phenomena to occur in the midst of daily routine. Generating these constant passages, crossings and changes in quality implies an uninterrupted process of constructing the unconscious, based on Freud's well-known triad – ritual honouring of the dead, the prohibition of murder and the prohibition of incest – which will be safeguarded by the laws of the society of care. To do so, the *institutions* of this society, thanks to their flexibility, must be able to create and/or promote what Freud considers the process which brings the unconscious into being: primary repression. Thanks to primary repression, the energy associated with the pleasure taken in committing murder and incest places itself in the service of desire and life. Of course, this displacement is not possible without the enormous effort of psychical working out and accompaniment of subjects caught in the whirlwind of actions which discharge affects mixed with emotions. In some cases, this work lasts a whole life through. In other words, if in a society of care what is being instituted takes priority over what already exists, to create an opening for the unexpected, the unknown, the dazzling discovery and the perpetual beginning of life, these phenomena must be, at the same time, *agencies of repression*, so that hate does not contaminate all interactions and the social life of the members, and each subject's persecutory anxiety remains, as much as possible, within tolerable limits. This concurs with the definition given by Jean Oury, Tosquelles' disciple, who considers psychosis to have a double root: the social and the psychical. What follows is a summary presentation of the principles of institutional psychotherapy.

After the war, at the centre of this movement, the most extraordinary psychiatric experiment of all time was conducted by Jean Oury, founder and director of the *La Borde Clinic.*

Jean Oury is a poet. He understood very early that he was not gifted for living. He says so quite clearly in the magnificent book of conversations with Marie Depussé, *À quelle heure passe le train?* With the unfailing tactfulness of love, she points out his unshakable fate, making it possible for him to say exquisite things about his early understanding of this impasse. Perhaps this is what defines artists, gifted people, geniuses: the recognition of one's own limits at an early age. Or an early decision about what constitutes one's limits. Deciding is not the same as recognising, but they can have similar effects. In Oury's case, since he was not gifted for life, he entrusted that task to Félix Guattari. He told Félix that he did not have time, that he was very busy at La Borde, and that it was Félix who had to go out into the world, and then come back and tell him about it. This is how Oury tells the story to Marie Depussé. For me, this makes the relation between the two men very clear.

Of course, Montaigne and La Boétie come to mind (Depussé mentions them). But I think above all of Alyosha, who is told by the *starets* to go into the world – the *starets* is the very special Russian monk we discussed earlier. But in this case, it takes two people to make one Alyosha: Jean and Félix, one inside and one outside. And it's even more complicated when one has known poverty, like Jean Oury, who came from a poor family. One knows the hard and cruel face of the world. So, one does not mix the living with the deadly. Having known poverty can act as prevention against imposture, making one intolerant to insistence on appearances, to the overly comfortable, and making it possible to recognise quickly the gifts life makes, and to appreciate the superfluous. Depussé says of Oury: "He is a gentleman with the impertinence of the slums".[19] It was Oury himself who referred to *The Brothers Karamazov* and to Alyosha; he was very familiar with the book.

Oury liked Kierkegaard. Tosquelles' admiration for the philosopher no doubt inspired this interest. In his doctoral thesis on Nerval, the Catalan had said of Kierkegaard that "his philosophical work and his life are so intertwined that it is not possible to understand one without the other".[20] Making one's life coincide with one's desire expresses the Sartrean ideal, which Oury and Guattari knew very well, and which made them give precedence to the *subject*, rather than the *structure*. Treating psychosis requires a *decision*, a Sartrean concept, a decision which favours the precarious, making anxiety the epicentre of the being, the place which gives it its consistency and nurtures its desire.

A rereading of Sartre's *Search for Method* makes clear the extent to which Oury and Guattari are inspired by him. In Oury's case, Sartre's proposition to consider Kierkegaard the philosopher who maintained, contrary to Hegel, that knowledge cannot contain the real, and that the scandal of subjectivity must be taken into account, supports his search for detail which interprets and/or modifies the functioning of the collective or the group. Detail, group and the collective are ideas Sartre emphasises in his critique of Marxist theory, which is neither opposed or loyal to Marx. Sartre's uncompromising judgment and his ferocious attack of the Marxist intellectuals of his time reaffirms the teachings transmitted by Tosquelles, who was drawing on his political experience in the POUM party (the Workers' Marxist Unification Party in Spain). The POUM, a Spanish revolutionary organisation, Marxist and anti-Stalinist, was founded in 1935 and was declared illegal in 1937. It participated actively in the Spanish Civil War against General Franco. Violently repressed by both Franco supporters and Stalinists, the POUM survived in Spain and in exile, particularly in France, and continued its fight against the Franco dictatorship. The organisation had a Trotskyist orientation and brought together two factions resulting from the split of the Spanish Communist Party.

Sartre's critique, which condemns what he sees as intellectual imposture and, at the same time, designates Marxism as a requirement if reflection is to be dialectical, provided Oury with the design for a method, a *praxis* that he constantly perfected and supported. Like Tosquelles, Sartre was a thinker who hated and denounced intellectualism, who rejected simplistic classifications, who taught loyalty to the boundless complexity of relations between men all over the world, who always took care to give preference to movement rather than totalisation, to what emerges rather than what is established, to change rather than certainty, to the search for transformative answers rather than strict conclusions, to risk-taking rather than cautious progression, to deeds rather than ideas, with the understanding that each of these pairs is to be seen as a set of dialectical tensions in which the prioritised option does not minimise the importance, power and field of application of the second option.[21]

Tosquelles, Oury and Guattari were all interested in the unconscious aspect of politics:

> Madmen [come] from a world that speaks and performs its act without a net in the circus of the unconscious. I see no other way of approaching them and reinstating in them a state of "living with others" than to enter the circus and play with them in the same conditions of danger.[22]

Identifying the unconscious aspect of politics and constructing the unconscious in a "society of care" is the same thing. Tosquelles proposes a method:

> How to help them feel better? [...] To create a setting, establish byroads, that is, speak of anything at all, taking care not to let anything slip past you, so that

> the work is effective. We can say that the method is like individual analysis: not intrusive.[23]

I feel it is essential to point out that all these questions, and all this work of structuring have only one objective: to facilitate verbal exchange, spoken expression, within the "society of care". The continuous focus on the therapeutic aspect of institutional events goes hand in hand with the constant requirement to construct the unconscious, to make the life of the community livable. This is in line with the clinical concerns indicated by Tosquelles:

> The dialectics of transference have to be considered, and the physician has at his disposal his countertransference and his science. I have given priority to counter-transference over science because this is often the weak point that causes the work to fail. I therefore ask myself whether [recourse to] structural analysis is not an attempt to avoid this sometimes burdensome analysis of transference and countertransference.
>
> I agree that such an analysis is necessary. [...] The same thing can be said of the analysis of the social interactions taking place around the patient. But we know that these analyses [...] are expressions of the patient's and the doctor's resistance to undertake the analysis of these relations as introjected objects, and not as subjects of discourse or reflection.[24]

We could refer to Lévi-Strauss, but Lévi-Strauss did not have to treat anyone.[25]

History of the construction of the unconscious

Are there historical examples of this requirement to construct an unconscious? The Mothers of the Plaza de Mayo, in Argentina, an event I described in the Preamble of this book: these women who for years, every Thursday, demanded the return of their children, who had been killed or had disappeared, and through their action demanded that the murder be acknowledged, that its prohibition be instituted. In the meantime, their action expressed hatred for the murderous regime.[26] Of course, this demand is, first of all, an act of resistance, a condemnation of crime as a mode of government. Such a demand was not heard in France concerning the Vichy regime or the murders associated with colonisation. In my view, the lack of such a demand plays a role in the existence of the *Front National*, and in the current plans for creating a neo-Nazi party, proposed by Dieudonné and Alain Soral.

The experiment of the Social Psychoanalysis Clinic founded in a Rio de Janeiro favela by Helio Pellegrino in Brazil, also described in the Preamble, illustrates the construction of an unconscious, a construction associated with the creation of a new conceptual framework for a large population excluded from representation by poverty. The project concerned constructing the unconscious of a subject and a citizen in that Brazilian population. Since most psychoanalysts who founded the Clinic were physicians, the experiment started with treatment of all sorts of illnesses existing in the community: from rickets in children due to poor nutrition, to various infections, as well as treatment of the physical and psychological effects of alcohol and drug addiction. This management of physical health, combined with patient teaching of the basic rules of hygiene, and work to build sewage facilities and provide drinking water and electricity – all these things changed the inhabitants' image of themselves as people condemned to perpetual sickness and contagion. These measures acted as an *agent of repression* of hate turned against oneself. In addition, from the beginning, to treat emotional health, the psychoanalysts worked with the healers in the favela.[27]

This collaboration also acted as an *agent of repression*: respected and recognised by the psychoanalysts as custodians of an ancestral therapeutic practice, and as teachers and guardians of one of the community's cultures of reference, the healers were able to set aside (to some extent) their belief in their supernatural powers, a belief generating all kinds of superstitions. This is how, little by little, that which had been attributed solely to destiny and occult powers, and therefore uncontrollable, can come to be recognised as universal human anguish felt by everyone in the face of desire and death, an anxiety which is always specific and rooted in the unique history of a particular subject.[28]

When a murderous power has been destroyed, thanks to a revolution or an insurrection, an institution is put in place, which functions as an agent of repression. In the name of what I call the *principle of the people*, which represses the lack of structure characterising the throng, this institution is charged with dealing with the hate associated with the establishment of a new power after the destruction of the old regime. This management of hate is no doubt inseparable from the creation of a new frame of thought. Dante was expressing a similar opinion when he said: "Let us be pitiless so the people will not be". Of course, this has to be accompanied, as it was in the *Social Psychoanalysis Clinic* experience, by symbol-generating mediations – a term used by Françoise Dolto – making it possible for hate and destructiveness to be interwoven with desire, and be placed in the service of life, facilitating the creation of initiatives intended to produce the repression needed to institute the prohibition of murder, the prohibition of incest, and rituals for the dead. Let us remember that these three fundamental principles make it possible to establish the anxiety/desire dialectic, with the whole range of configurations created by this dialectic.

The enormous and endless work of changing the frame of thought, made necessary by the recognition that God does not exist, is ever-present in Dostoevsky's writing. In *Demons*, Dostoevsky has Kirillov say:

> I have no higher idea than disbelief in God. I have all the history of mankind on my side. Man has done nothing but invent God so as to go on living and not kill himself; that's the whole of universal history up till now.[29]

Becoming aware that God does not exist means, for man: "to recognise at the same instant that one is God oneself. [...] If you recognise it you are sovereign, and then you won't kill yourself but will live in the greatest glory".[30]

This perspective is reminiscent of Spinoza's *Ethics*. Spinoza is the forerunner in this domain; for him, the fact that God and nature are indistinguishable is a source of joy. Contrary to the philosopher, Dostoevsky, like Freud, thinks that a world without God brings man face to face with the tragic character of his anguish and desire. Man is unhappy because he is afraid to assume his desire. Kirillov calls this desire self-will, which is "the attribute of my divinity. [...] Self-will! That is all, by which I can show in the main point my insubordination and my new fearsome freedom. For it is very fearsome".[31]

A world without God is a world where desire reigns supreme, but this desire is sometimes fearsome, and can lead to murder or madness. It can also lead to a pure "idea", an ideology created to fill the space left empty by God, that soothes men's anguish and serves to justify in their eyes all sorts of atrocities, like those set forth by Pyotr Stepanovich in *Demons* and by the Grand Inquisitor in *The Brothers Karamazov*.

Freud proposed a *strategy of existence* based on the prohibition of murder, the prohibition of incest, and the place given to the dead. In this framework, it is possible to recognise that desire in a world without God is tragic, and to see that its association with hate is possible, without excluding the joy that accompanies it, the joy celebrated by Spinoza.[32]

Complexities, complexities! What is there to do?

Continue on!

Notes

1 Kaplan, L. (2006), *Toute ma vie j'ai été une femme* (All My Life I have Been a Woman), play.
2 Dardot, P. and Laval, C. (2014), *The New Way of the World*, Verso.
3 See Bellahsen, M. (2014), *La Santé mentale. Vers un Bonheur sous contrôle* (Mental Health: Towards a Happiness under Control), La Fabrique Éditions.
4 In *The Sunday Times*, 1 May 1981.
5 Dostoevsky, F., *The Brothers Karamazov*, p. 229.
6 Ibid., pp. 230–241. My emphasis.
7 Dardot, P. and Laval, C., *The New Way of the World*, Chapter 13.
8 Ibid.
9 Daney, S., article in *Libération*, 20 January 1992.
10 Bellahsen, M., *La Santé mentale*.
11 Ibid.
12 Saint-Just, *Republican Institutions* (1793–1794), Fragment 3.
13 Here, I am referring to a day of reflection organized by Leslie Kaplan in November 2014, on the play *La République du Bonheur*, by Martin Crimp, directed by Di Fonzo Bo, M. and Vigier, É.
14 MEDIAPART, http://www.mediapart.fr/journal/culture-idees/150713entretien-inedit-avec-jean-paul-sartre-12-l-amitie-est-un-outil-politique
15 Dardot, P. and Laval, C. (2019), *The Common: An Essay on the 21st-Century Revolution*, Bloomsbury Academic.
16 See above, ch. *Crime and Punishment*, "Raskolnikov", concept of an unprecedented practice.
17 For a discussion of Piera Aulagnier's groundbreaking work, see my book *Letters to a Young Psychoanalyst*, the chapter titled "Freud, Michel Neyraut, Piera Aulagnier".

18 We have already alluded several times to the concept of construction of the unconscious, or its foreshadowing. See, particularly, the chapters herein titled "The Sonia Solution", "Prince Myshkin", "Stavrogin" and the discussion on Ivan Karamazov.
19 Oury, J. and Depussé, M. (2003), *À quelle heure passe le train?* Conversations sur la folie, Paris: Calmann-Lévy, p. 15.
20 Quoted by Apprill, O., *Une avant-garde psychiatrique, le moment GTPSI (1960–1966)*, Eppel, 2014, p. 99.
21 Sartre, J.-P. (1968), *Search for Method*, Vintage.
22 Tosquelles, F., "Discussion critique de la thèse de Claude Poncin", *Essai d'analyse structurale appliqué à la pratique institutionnelle*, Association Culturelle du personnel de Saint-Alban, 1995.
23 Ibid.
24 Tosquelles, F., "Discussion critique de la thèse de Claude Poncin", op. cit., quoted by Apprill, O., in *Une avant-garde psychiatrique, le moment GTPSI*, op., cit. I will note in passing that Tosquelles' use of the concept of introjection shows his interest in the work of Ferenczi.
25 GTPSI archives, quoted by Appril, O. in *Une avant-garde psychiatrique, le moment GTPSI.*
26 See Preamble above.
27 *Pai e Mae de Santo*, Father and Mother of the Saint, that is, earthly ministers of the gods of Nago mythology: the divinities the Blacks of Africa brought with them when they came to Brazil as slaves.
28 We could say that these *agents of repression* result from the action of the "projective super-ego" described by Freud in his 1927 text *Humor*. I have already discussed at length this late correction made by Freud, so that the super-ego ceases to be considered simply a "severe master". I indicated the disastrous clinical consequences that could have been avoided if this correction had been made earlier. See *The Celestina Superego and the Dulcinea Superego*, in *Letters to a Young Psychoanalyst.*
29 Dostoevsky, F. (1936), *The Possessed*, Garnett, C. (trans.), New York: Random House, p. 628.
30 Ibid., p. 629.
31 Ibid.
32 Regarding the connection between Freud and Spinoza, see *Freud and Spinoza* in *Letters to a Young Psychoanalyst.*

REFERENCES

Apprill, O. (2014), *Une avant-garde psychiatrique, le moment GTPSI (1960–1966)*, Eppel.

Aristotle (1981), *The Politics*, Sinclair, T.A. (trans.), Penguin Classics.

Aulagnier, P. (2001), *The Violence of Interpretation*, Sheridan, A. (trans.), Routledge.

Bakhtine, M. (1984), *Problems of Doestoesvky's Poetics*, University of Minnesota Press.

Bellahsen, M. (2014), *La Santé mentale. Vers un Bonheur sous contrôle* (Mental Health: Towards a Happiness under Control), La Fabrique Éditions.

Berthold-Bond, D. (1995), *Hegel's Theory of Madness*, State University of New York Press.

Bleuler, E. (1950), *Dementia praecox or the group of schizophrenias*, Oxford, England: International Universities Press.

Crimp, M. (2014), *Dans la République du Bonheur* (In the Republic of Happiness) (play), directed by Di Fonzo Bo, M. and Vigier, É.,

Dardot, P. and Laval, C. (2014), *The New Way of the World*, Elliott, G. (trans.), Verso.

Dardot, P. and Laval, C. (2019), *The Common: An Essay on the 21st-Century Revolution*, Bloomsbury Academic.

De Macedo, H.O. (ed.) (1988), *Le Psychanalyste sous la terreur*, Paris: Matrice-Rocinante.

De Macedo, H.O. (1994), *De l'amour à la pensée*, Paris: L'Harmattan.

De Macedo, H.O. (2016), *Letters to a Young Psychoanalyst*, Routledge.

De Saint-Just, L.A. (2003), "Fragments sur les institutions républicaines", in *L'Esprit de la révolution*, Éditions10/18.

Dostoevsky, F. (1915), "Akulka's Husband", in *The House of the Dead*, Garnett, C. (trans.), London: Heinemann.

Dostoevsky, F. (1915), *The House of the Dead*, Garnett, C. (trans.), London: Heinemann.

Dostoevsky, F. (1922), *Stavrogin's Confession*, Koteliansky, S.S. and Woolf, V. (trans.), Hogarth Press.

Dostoevsky, F. (1923), *Letters and Reminiscences*, Koteliansky, S. S. and Middleton Murry, J. (trans.), London: Chatto & Windus.

Dostoevsky, F. (1936), *The Possessed (The Devils)*, Garnett, C. (trans.), New York: Random House.

Dostoevsky, F. (1945), *The Double* in *The Short Novels of Dostoevsky*, Garnett, C. (trans.), New York: Dial Press.

Dostoevsky, F. (1960), *Notes from Underground*, Garnett, C. (trans.), Dell Publishing.

Dostoevsky, F. (1962), *The Brothers Karamazov*, Garnett, C. (trans.), New York: Signet Classics.

Dostoevsky, F. (1968), *The Notebooks for the Possessed*, Wasiolek, E. (ed.), Terras, V. (trans.), University of Chicago Press.

Dostoevsky, F. (1993), *Notes from Underground*, Pevear, R. and Volokhonsky, L. (trans.), Vintage Classics.

Dostoevsky, F. (1996), *The Idiot*, Garnett, C. (trans.), Wordsworth Classics.

Dostoevsky, F. (1997), *Winter Notes on Summer Impressions*, Patterson, D. (trans.), Northern University Press.

Dostoevky, F. (2000), *Crime and Punishment*, Garnett, C. (trans.), Wordsworth Classics.

Dostoevsky, F. (2004), *The Double: Two Versions*, Translated with an Introduction by Evelyn Harden, New York: Ardis Publishers.

Dostoyevsky, F. (2016), *The Dream of a Ridiculous Man*, Garnett, C. (trans.), CreateSpace Independent Publishing Platform.

Ferenczi, S. (1949), "Confusion of the Tongues Between the Adults and the Child", *The International Journal of Psychoanalysis*, 30: 225–230.

Frank, J. (1995), *Dostoevsky. The Miraculous Years, 1865–1871*, Princeton University Press.

Frank, J. (2003), *Dostoevsky: The Mantle of the Prophet, 1871–1881*, Princeton University Press.

Frank, J. (2012), *Dostoevsky: A Writer in His Time*, Princeton University Press.

Freud, S. (1900). *The Interpretation of Dreams,* S.E. IV & S.E. V, London: The Hogarth Press.

Freud, S. (1911), *Formulations Regarding the Two Principles in Mental Functioning,* S.E., 12: 218–226. London: Hogarth.

Freud, S. (1912a), *Contributions to the Psychology of Love. On the universal tendency to debasement in the sphere of love,* S.E. XI: 165–175.

Freud, S. (1912b), "The Dynamics of the Transference", *in Papers on Technique and Other Works*, S.E., 12: 97–108.

Freud, S. (1920), *Beyond the Pleasure Principle*, S.E. XVIII, London: The Hogarth Press.

Freud, S. (1924), *Neurosis and Psychosis*, S.E., 19, London: Hogarth.

Freud, S. (1937), *Analysis Terminable and Interminable*, S.E., 23: 216–253, London: Hogarth.

Gauchet, M. (1999), *The Disenchantment of the World*, Burge, O. (trans.), Princeton University Press.

Granoff, W. (1976), *La Pensée et le féminin*, Éditions de minuit.

Green, A. (1980), Preface, in Dostoevsky, F. *Le Double*, Gallimard.

Kaplan, L. (2003), "L'Expérience du meurtre", in *Les Outils*, Paris: POL.

Kaplan, L. (2006), *Toute ma vie j'ai été une femme* (All My Life I have Been a Woman), play.

Kaplan, L. (2008), *Toute ma vie j'ai été une femme*, Paris: POL.

Lacan, J. (1977), Preface, in Lemaire, A., *Jacques Lacan*, Brussels: Pierre Mardaga.

Mann, T. (1996), *The Magic Mountain,* Woods, J. E. (Trans.), Vintage.

Masson, J.M. (Ed.) (1985), *The Complete Letters of Sigmund Freud to Wilhelm Fliess, 1887 –1904.* Cambridge: Harvard University Press.

Oury, J. and Depussé, M. (2003), *À quelle heure passe le train? Conversations sur la folie*, Paris: Calmann-Lévy.

Pankow, G. (1981), *L'Être-là du schizophrène*, Paris, Aubier.

Perrier, F. (1978), "L'Amatride", in seminar *L'Amour*, in *La Chaussée d'Antin II*, Collection 10–18, Paris: Christian Bourgeois.

Perrier, F. (2008), *Structure hystérique et dialogue analytique*, Paris: Albin Michel.

Sartre, J.-P. (1968), *Search for Method*, Vintage.

Slonim, M. (1950), *The Epic of Russian Literature from Its Origins through Tolstoy*, Oxford University Press.

Sylwan, B. and Réfabert, P. (2010), "Fliess et Freud, un transfert psychotique", in *Freud, Fliess, Ferenczi. Des phantômes qui hantent la psychanalyse* (The Ghosts of Psychoanalysis), Paris: Hermann.

Turgenev, I. (2008), *Fathers and Sons*, Oxford Paperback.

Tosquelles, F. (1995), "Discussion critique de la thèse de Claude Poncin", *Essai d'analyse structurale appliqué à la pratique institutionnelle*, Association Culturelle du personnel de Saint-Alban.

Verlet, L. (1993), *La Malle de Newton*, Paris: Gallimard, coll. "Bibliothèque des Sciences humaines".

Vidal-Naquet, P. (1990), Preface to *Tragédies de Sophocle*, Gallimard.

Winnicott, D.W. (2005), "Dreaming, Fantasizing and Living", in *Playing and Reality*, Routledge Classics.

Yovel, Y. (1992), *Spinoza and Other Heretics*, Princeton, NJ: Princeton University Press.

INDEX

Note: Page numbers in italics refer to those in notes/references.

Kolibri 360 GmbH
Ferdinand-Jühlke-Straße 7
99095 Erfurt, Deutschland
produktsicherheit@kolibri360.de